Child Health and Nutrition from Conception to Age Two

Shoba Suri
Editor

Child Health and Nutrition from Conception to Age Two

Policies and Practices in Public Health

Springer

Editor
Shoba Suri
Senior Fellow-Health Initiative
Observer Research Foundation
New Delhi, Delhi, India

ISBN 978-981-95-7867-2 ISBN 978-981-95-7868-9 (eBook)
https://doi.org/10.1007/978-981-95-7868-9

This Springer imprint is published by the registered company Springer Nature Singapore Pte Ltd.
The registered company address is: 152 Beach Road, #21-01/04 Gateway East, Singapore 189721, Singapore

Foreword

The first 1,000 days of human life—from conception to a child's second birthday—represent a critical window of opportunity that lays the foundation for lifelong health, nutrition, and well-being. This period is not only pivotal for individual development but also holds profound implications for the future of societies, influencing economic resilience, social stability, and public health outcomes. Recognizing the urgency and the utmost significance of this transformative phase, this volume, *Child Health and Nutrition from Conception to Age Two—Policies and Practices in Public Health* presents a comprehensive exploration of the policies, practices, challenges and interventions necessary to optimize health and nutrition outcomes during this crucial period.

By bringing together the expertise of leading researchers, practitioners, and policymakers, it provides an integrated understanding of the multifaceted aspects of child development. The volume combines cutting-edge scientific research, evidence-based practices, and insightful real-world case studies to offer actionable strategies for improving outcomes during the first 1,000 days. It is designed to serve a diverse audience, including policymakers, healthcare professionals, researchers, and caregivers, empowering them to guide informed decisions to transform the trajectory of a child's lifelong health.

The unparalleled growth and development in the first 1,000 days, characterized by rapid neural and physical changes, set the stage for future potential. Adequate maternal nutrition, responsive caregiving, and a nurturing environment during pregnancy and early childhood are essential to ensure optimal outcomes. Conversely, the consequences of neglecting this period can be severe, leading to developmental delays, stunting, and heightened vulnerability to chronic diseases in adulthood. This book underscores the importance of public health interventions, policies, and community-driven efforts in addressing these challenges, emphasizing that early investment in child health yields lifelong dividends.

As we navigate the complexities of public health in a rapidly changing world, it is imperative to acknowledge the interconnectedness of maternal and child health, nutrition, and social determinants. This book serves as both a call to action and a resource for innovation, offering insights that are adaptable across diverse cultural and healthcare contexts. It aspires to catalyze dialogue, inspire collaboration, and drive transformative change in child health and nutrition practices worldwide.

In conclusion, the contributors to this volume share a unified vision: a future where every child is afforded the opportunity for a healthy start to life. As you engage with the knowledge and perspectives presented in these pages, I urge you to reflect on their implications, and to join us in our collective commitment to advancing the health and well-being of children from conception to age two. Together, let us shape a world where every child thrives.

New Delhi, India

Prof. Vinod Paul
Former Member, NITI Aayog

Preface

In the journey of life, the first 1,000 days—from conception to age 2—represent a critically formative period. During this time, the foundations for lifelong health, nutrition, and well-being are established. Understanding this pivotal phase is not just an academic pursuit; it is a pressing global imperative that affects the future of individuals and societies alike. It is with this understanding that we present "Child Health and Nutrition from Conception to Age Two—Policies and Practices in Public Health," an edited volume designed to illuminate the complexities and opportunities surrounding child health and nutrition.

This collection brings together a diverse group of experts, each contributing their unique perspectives and insights into the multifaceted issues that confront health and nutrition during early childhood. The scope of this volume is both broad and deep, addressing critical topics such as maternal health and nutrition, the intricacies of fetal development, and the unique challenges faced during infancy. By weaving together scientific research, case studies, and practical strategies, we aim to provide a comprehensive and accessible resource for a wide range of stakeholders, including policymakers, healthcare practitioners, researchers, parents, and caregivers.

Moreover, this volume champions an evidence-based approach, synthesizing the latest findings and best practices to ground our discussions in scientifically supported methodologies. The importance of public health policies in shaping child health and nutrition cannot be overstated; therefore, we critically evaluate existing interventions while offering recommendations to address gaps and enhance strategies aimed at safeguarding the well-being of our youngest citizens.

As global health challenges continue to evolve, so too must our responses. This book is designed to be a resource for action, providing insights that are not only relevant within localized contexts but also adaptable across diverse cultures and health systems. We aspire to catalyze dialogue and inspire innovation in programs and policies aimed at addressing the fundamental health and nutrition needs of children worldwide.

Our journey begins with an exploration of the vital role of maternal nutrition and health, which sets the stage for optimal fetal development, preventing complications at birth and mitigating future health risks. As the spotlight shifts to the postnatal period, we delve into the challenges infants face as they transition from the womb into the world. Each chapter contributes to a larger narrative, aiming not only to spotlight existing problems but also to elevate successful programs and policies that have shown promise in improving child health outcomes globally. In closing, the contributors to this volume share a collective vision: a future where every child is afforded the opportunity for a healthy start to life. The knowledge contained within these pages is meant to empower individuals and communities alike, ensuring that we all play our part in shaping a healthier future for the next generation. We invite you to engage with this work, to reflect on its implications, and to join us in our commitment to the health and well-being of children from conception to age 2.

The volume is divided into five sections as follows: Section 1 on Prenatal Development explores the 1000-day period beginning from pregnancy. Adequate nutrition, healthcare, and a healthy lifestyle during pregnancy are crucial for the baby's growth and development. Good prenatal care ensures the baby receives essential nutrients, minimizes complications, and establishes a foundation for a healthy life.

Section 2. Critical Interventions to Promote Child Nutrition explores the first 2 years of a child's life as a period of rapid growth and development. During this time, the brain develops at an astonishing rate, and critical neural connections are formed. Adequate nutrition, responsive caregiving, stimulation, and a nurturing environment are crucial for optimal brain development and the establishment of cognitive, motor, and socio-emotional skills.

Section 3. Child Nutrition and Development delves into the experiences and conditions a child encounters during the 1000-day period, which can have long-lasting effects on their health and well-being throughout their life. Malnutrition, infections, inadequate healthcare, and lack of stimulation during this critical period can increase the risk of developmental delays, growth stunting, compromised immune function, and even chronic diseases later in life.

Section 4. Intervention and Support recognizes the significance of the 1000-day period, interventions and programs that have been developed to improve child health and development during this crucial time. These interventions often focus on improving maternal health, promoting exclusive breastfeeding, providing adequate nutrition, ensuring access to healthcare, and promoting responsive caregiving practices.

Section 5. Strengthening Health System in 1000-day period highlights the vital importance of comprehensive health and nutrition services, which are foundational for lifelong wellbeing. Employing data-driven approaches will further enhance policy-making and service improvement, while collaboration across sectors such as health, nutrition, and education will support better child development.

By prioritizing the health, nutrition, and overall well-being of children during the 1000-day period, we can set them on a path towards a healthier and more prosperous future. "The first 1000 days of a child's life are not just a window of opportunity; they are the blueprint for a lifetime of health and well-being."

New Delhi, India Shoba Suri

Introduction

This book is about the critical window of opportunity in a child's life, which begins with the conception till the age of 2. The term "first 1000 days" encompasses the period from conception until a child's second birthday. This time is significant for the advancement and maturation of the offspring and the impact on their future health. Numerous factors impact this time frame such as maternal health, breast-feeding, introducing solid foods, and socioeconomic factors. Nutritional treatments may inflict permanent impacts on biological and metabolic growth, resulting in later changes in body function due to adaptations. Children and adults alike may experience non-communicable diseases such as diabetes, cardiovascular and chronic respiratory diseases, cancers, and neurodegenerative disorders during their lifetime including obesity and impaired growth.

The development of the human brain in the first 1,000 days is critical for life-long health, cognition, and emotional well-being. Rapid neural development occurs during this period, including forming key brain structures, synaptic connections, and myelination. In utero, the brain develops foundational structures, while postnatal growth focuses on connectivity, sensory processing, and cognitive abilities. Proper nutrition, responsive caregiving, and stimulation are vital during this time to support optimal brain development. Adverse factors like malnutrition, stress, or neglect can have long-term effects, emphasizing the importance of interventions to promote a nurturing environment during this sensitive period. Improving nutrition in the first 1,000 days of life as the optimal, and in their view, the only, point of intervention at which the intergenerational cycle of malnutrition can be broken.

Emerging research in epigenetics highlights how the interaction between genetics, and the in-utero environment can influence long-term health. While genetic inheritance provides the blueprint, environmental factors such as nutrition can affect gene expression, potentially shaping future health outcomes. Insufficient intake of calories, proteins, fatty acids, or essential micronutrients during pregnancy can impede these developmental processes, negatively impacting the baby's neurodevelopment. Several key nutrients play vital roles during this time. Zinc is essential for developing the autonomic nervous system, hippocampus, and cerebellum. Iron is necessary for myelination, influencing brain processing speed. Long-chain polyunsaturated fatty acids in breast milk, fish oil, and egg yolks are vital for brain and eye development. Since the mother's diet is the sole source of nutrition for the baby, any deficiencies in calories, proteins, or essential nutrients can lead to developmental delays, birth defects, and cognitive difficulties. For instance, folate is critical for early brain and spinal cord development. Insufficient folic acid before and during early pregnancy can result in neural tube defects such as anencephaly or spina bifida, which can cause severe disabilities or even death.

The infant stage, spanning from birth to a child's first birthday, is a critical period for forming eating habits and food preferences that often persist throughout life. For mothers, who can breastfeed, breast milk stands out as a unique "superfood," providing unmatched nutritional and immune benefits. Research underscores the crucial role of breastfeeding in supporting infant health and development. Breast milk not only aids in brain development but also protects against infections and diseases. It reduces the risk of Sudden Infant Death Syndrome (SIDS), respiratory infections, and necrotizing enterocolitis, particularly in premature infants.

Infancy provides a unique opportunity to foster healthy food preferences. A mother's diet can influence an infant's taste preferences even before birth, and breastfed infants are exposed to various flavors through breast milk, helping them develop a preference for healthier foods. A well-balanced diet should include proteins, fruits, vegetables, whole grains, unsweetened dairy products, and minimally processed foods to ensure proper growth during the toddler years.

Experts generally agree that early childhood is an ideal time to establish healthy eating patterns. Young children need a balanced diet consisting of protein-rich foods, fruits, vegetables, whole grains, and unsweetened dairy products. It is equally important to limit intake of saturated fats, sugars, and sodium to promote healthy growth and maintain a healthy weight. The consequences of poor nutrition and unhealthy eating habits during early childhood can have long-lasting effects. Rapid weight gain during the first 2 years of life is linked to an increased risk of obesity and other health issues later in life. Research indicates that children who are overweight or obese early on are more likely to continue these challenges into adulthood. Additionally, inadequate nutrition in early childhood can lead to health problems that are passed down to future generations, as undernourished children are more likely to have undernourished offspring.

Stunting, which affects approximately 22% of children under five worldwide, results from prolonged undernutrition and has significant long-term consequences on health, development, and productivity. It often starts during pregnancy due to poor maternal nutrition, including deficiencies in energy, protein, and micronutrients such as iron, zinc, and folic acid. A meta-analysis found that maternal anemia and malnutrition substantially increase the risk of intrauterine growth restriction (IUGR) and low birth weight (LBW), both of which are precursors to stunting. After birth, insufficient breastfeeding, delayed introduction of complementary foods, and lack of dietary diversity further worsen the child's growth. Study reported that exclusive breastfeeding for the first 6 months, coupled with the timely introduction of nutrient-rich complementary foods, can reduce the risk of stunting by up to 19%.

Healthcare interventions such as vaccination and deworming help reduce the infection burden contributing to stunting. Furthermore, investing in clean water, sanitation, and hygiene (WASH) initiatives is crucial to preventing environmental enteropathy and improving overall child nutrition. Stunting in the first 1,000 days is a multifaceted issue with far-reaching consequences for physical growth, health, and economic productivity. Research shows that both nutrition-specific and nutrition-sensitive interventions, particularly in low-resource settings, are essential to addressing the root causes of stunting and breaking the cycle of intergenerational malnutrition.

Epigenetic modifications in gene expression occur through mechanisms such as DNA methylation, histone modifications, and gene silencing by non-coding microRNAs. These changes to the epigenetic landscape, shaped by both internal and external factors, can have immediate and long-lasting effects on gene activity. Various environmental stressors have been shown to induce epigenetic alterations that are linked to several diseases. These stressors include tobacco-related diseases, the effects of air pollution on immune function and inflammation, and exposure to endocrine-disrupting chemicals. Research on how environmental stressors influence the epigenome provides valuable insights into the mechanisms connecting these stressors to disease development. This study area is significant for understanding how environmental factors and nutrition during the first 1,000 days of life can influence long-term health outcomes.

Feeding practices have a significant impact on the development of gut microbiota. Breast milk, which contains over 200 complex non-digestible oligosaccharides, provides a food source for beneficial microorganisms. These oligosaccharides resist digestion in the small intestine and pass into the large intestine, where they encourage the growth of specific beneficial bacteria. To replicate this effect, many infant formulas are now supplemented with oligosaccharides like fructo- and galacto-oligosaccharides, aiming to promote healthy gut microbiota from an early age.

Nutrition and feeding during the first 1,000 days of life play a crucial role in determining the risk and progression of respiratory diseases, with mechanisms such as epigenetic modifications contributing significantly. The development of microbiota also has an impact, as it can influence immune responses, inflammation, and allergies, which in turn affect the susceptibility to various respiratory conditions. A 2015 study demonstrated that poor maternal nutrition, particularly a high-fat diet before and during pregnancy, leads to placental inflammation and insufficiency, which can hinder fetal growth and impair lung development. This, in turn, increases the likelihood of respiratory distress syndrome at birth and chronic lung diseases later in life.

On the other hand, maternal diets rich in vegetables and fruits during pregnancy are associated with a lower risk of allergic respiratory diseases, such as asthma and allergic rhinitis, compared to diets high in processed foods and oils. The Mediterranean diet, which emphasizes the intake of fruits, vegetables, olive oil, fish, and fiber, is a protective dietary pattern for mothers. It potentially normalizes gut microbiota and reduces the risk of allergic diseases. Supplementation with Omega-3 fatty acids from fish, along with essential micronutrients like vitamins D and E and zinc during pregnancy, has also been linked to a reduced risk of conditions such as asthma, allergic rhinitis, and atopic dermatitis in children.

Breastfeeding offers both short- and long-term protection against respiratory infections due to its rich content of secretory IgA antibodies, anti-inflammatory cytokines, and other protective factors. Studies show that exclusive breastfeeding for the first four months reduces the risk of respiratory-related hospitalizations in infants and significantly lowers the incidence and mortality of lower respiratory infections.

Micronutrients play a pivotal role in respiratory health. Antioxidants such as vitamins C and E, selenium, and carotene help reduce oxidative stress, delay the onset of asthma, and improve related outcomes. Zinc and iron support immune function by inhibiting viral replication and enhancing T-cell activity, respectively; deficiencies in these nutrients can weaken immune defenses. Vitamins D and A have specific roles in preventing respiratory diseases, including modulating immune responses and improving lung function. While most vitamins have protective effects, some studies have linked high doses of folic acid after the first trimester to an increased risk of asthma. Early interventions and adherence to a balanced, nutrient-rich diet—such as the Mediterranean diet—can provide significant health benefits for both mothers and their children.

Children who receive proper care and nutrition during the first 1,000 days are better prepared to resist chronic diseases such as diabetes, obesity, and cardiovascular conditions in later life. Research studies have highlighted how early nutrition impacts the developmental origins of health and disease. Good nutrition during this critical period reduces the risks of non-communicable diseases, leading to better health outcomes in adulthood. A systematic review underscores that interventions in the first 1,000 days result in a 20–40% reduction in stunting and significantly lower risks of chronic diseases in adulthood. It emphasizes a holistic, multi-sectoral approach to address the complex drivers of malnutrition, focusing on maternal and child health, nutrition, and environmental factors.

Optimal maternal nutrition is critical for fetal development. Adequate energy, protein, vitamins, and minerals during pregnancy reduce the risk of low birth weight (LBW) and other complications. Iron and folic acid supplementation, for instance, are proven to reduce maternal anemia and improve birth outcomes. Evidence shows that iron-folic acid supplementation during pregnancy significantly reduces LBW by 29%, contributing to healthier infants. Antenatal care ensures that expectant mothers receive essential medical check-ups, advice on nutrition, and access to interventions such as vaccinations and parasite control. These measures help to prevent complications and support healthy fetal growth. Exclusive breastfeeding for the first six months of life is a cornerstone of the first 1,000-day framework. Breast milk provides essential nutrients and antibodies, promoting healthy growth and reducing the risk of infections. Complementary feeding should begin at 6 months, with nutrient-dense foods introduced alongside breast milk. A varied diet is crucial for continued growth and development, helping to prevent stunting and micronutrient deficiencies. Complementary feeding programs have been shown to reduce stunting when nutrient-rich foods are included.

Preventing and treating illnesses, including diarrhea and respiratory infections, are essential for safeguarding nutritional status. Early childhood vaccinations and deworming programs help protect children from infectious diseases that can undermine nutrition. Access to clean water, sanitation, and hygiene (WASH) is vital for preventing environmental enteropathy, which impairs nutrient absorption and contributes to stunting. Evidence from studies shows that improved sanitation significantly reduces stunting and other nutrition-related health problems.

Micronutrient deficiencies, such as lack of vitamin A, zinc, and iron, are prevalent during the first 1,000 days and can have long-term consequences. Targeted interventions, such as vitamin A supplementation and zinc fortification, can reduce mortality and improve growth.

Conclusion: The first 1,000 days of a child's life provide a crucial opportunity to lay the foundation for long-term health and well-being. It is widely recognized that many of society's most pressing challenges stem from the quality of nutrition and care provided to children during this critical period. The nutrition children receive in these early years influences a wide range of outcomes, from their risk of developing chronic illnesses to their academic achievements, with negative consequences creating a significant societal burden. Ensuring optimal nutrition for young children is a collective responsibility, requiring action from healthcare providers, educators, community leaders, and policymakers. Improving children's nutrition during the first 1,000 days requires collaboration between policymakers, healthcare professionals, community organizations, and families. When children are supported in reaching their full developmental potential, society benefits. A comprehensive approach is needed to enhance child nutrition from conception to age 2, which includes policies that support breastfeeding, maternal nutrition, access to health services, and education on proper infant feeding. Public health strategies must be tailored to specific regional and cultural contexts to ensure their success.

Shoba Suri

Contents

Contributors

Ananya Awasthi Anuvaad Solutions, New Delhi, India

Manjula Bahuguna Society for Nutrition, Education and Health Action (SNEHA), Mumbai, India

Kruti Dalal ARMMAN, Mumbai, India

Rupal Dalal Centre for Technology Alternatives in Rural Areas, IIT Bombay, Mumbai, India

Sushmita Das Society for Nutrition, Education and Health Action (SNEHA), Mumbai, India

Hema Divakar Past President, Federation of Obstetric and Gynecological Societies of India (FOGSI), Mumbai, India

Habib Hasan Farooqui Public Health Foundation of India, New Delhi, India

Sebanti Ghosh Public Health (MNCAH) and Nutrition Expert, Delhi, India

Aparna Hegde ARMMAN, Mumbai, India

Tejal Barai Jaitly ARMMAN, Mumbai, India

Anuja Jayaraman ARMMAN, Mumbai, India

William Joe Institute of Economic Growth, Delhi, India

Shweta Khandelwal Social and Economic Empowerment, IPE Global Limited, New Delhi, India

Praveen Kumar Lady Hardinge Medical College and Associated Kalawati Saran Children's Hospital, New Delhi, India

Saroj Kumar Institute of Economic Growth, Delhi, India

Hrishikesh Pai Visiting Professor, D Y Patil University, Navi Mumbai, India

Ishika Pahuja Institute of Economic Growth, Delhi, India

Seema Puri Institute of Home Economics, Department of Food and Nutrition, University of Delhi, Delhi, India

Priya Rampal Oxford Policy Management India Pvt Ltd, Delhi, India

Subhasree Ray Section Head - Wellness at TVS Motor Company, Hosur, Tamil Nadu, India

Neha Sanwalka Hirabai Cowasji Jehangir Medical Research Institute, Jehangir Hospital, Pune, India

Anshu Sharma Institute of Home Economics, Department of Food and Nutrition, University of Delhi, Delhi, India

Aamir Siddiqui Social and Economic Empowerment, IPE Global Limited, New Delhi, India

Rajesh Kumar Sinha Jaipuria Institute of Management, Jaipur, India

Jennifer Spencer Society for Nutrition, Education and Health Action (SNEHA), Mumbai, India

Bhuvaneswari Sunil ARMMAN, Mumbai, India

Shoba Suri Observer Research Foundation, New Delhi, India

Sheila Vir Public Health Nutrition and Development Centre (PHNDC), New Delhi, India

Sanjay Zodpey Public Health Foundation of India, New Delhi, India

Part I
Prenatal Development

Chapter 1
An Overview of Prenatal Development and Its Significance

Hema Divakar and Hrishikesh Pai

Introduction

The prenatal period, derived from the Greek word *peri* (around) and the Latin word *nasci* (to be born), refers to the time surrounding birth. In developed countries, with expert neonatal care, this period spans from 22 completed weeks of gestation (typically around 154 days) to 7 completed days after birth, when the birth weight is usually 500 g. However, in many developing countries, the prenatal period is completed at 40 weeks of conception or when the birth weight exceeds 1000 g [1].

Each year, there are over 213 million pregnancies globally [1], resulting in approximately 300,000 maternal mortalities, 2 million stillbirths, and 2.4 million newborns death [2]. Approximately 190 million or 89% of these pregnancies take place in low-resource environments where they are often poorly managed [3]. In low- and middle-income countries (LMICs), the prevalence of insufficient antenatal care (ANC) after registration is about 22.25%. Inadequate ANC is most observed in South and Central Europe and Caribbean nations with a recorded rate of 29.83%. Conversely, the lowest rate is found in Central and Western Asia and Oceania at 13.72% 000[4].

The lack of ANC increases the threat of adverse birth effects. Approximately 60% of preterm deliveries follow annually in sub-Saharan Africa and South Asia [5]. India alone accounts for 12% of the world's preterm births, resulting in over 750,000 neonatal deaths each year [6]. In 2019, approximately 77.6% of pregnant women in the United States received first-trimester prenatal care, a critical period for early detection and intervention. The report of the Centers for Disease Control and

H. Divakar (✉)
Past President, Federation of Obstetric and Gynecological Societies of India (FOGSI), Mumbai, India
e-mail: drhemadivakar@gmail.com

H. Pai
Visiting Professor, D Y Patil University, Navi Mumbai, India

S. Suri (ed.), *Child Health and Nutrition from Conception to Age Two*,
https://doi.org/10.1007/978-981-95-7868-9_1

Prevention (CDC) suggested that 3% of babies in the United States are born with major structural birth defects.

From 2000 to 2019, the under-five death rate due to birth defects decreased from 3.4 per 1,000 live births to 2.9. Despite this decline, the increase in under-five deaths attributed to birth defects increased from 4.6 to 7.6% over a certain period. This change varied notably depending on the level of national income [7]. In 2019, the under-five mortality rate due to birth defects was lower in high-income countries compared to LMICs, being 1.3 versus 3.0 per 1,000 live births, respectively. Factors contributing to these outcomes include infectious diseases, harmful medications, environmental exposures, maternal health, and genetic predispositions [8].

Given the critical importance of prenatal development, this chapter aims to delineate the significant stages in prenatal development, examine the factors influencing it, and analyze the impact of inadequate prenatal care. Furthermore, it seeks to evaluate current policies and propose new directions to improve these outcomes.

Overview of Prenatal Development and Its Significance

The Germinal Stage

The germinal stage (pre-embryonic period) spans the first 2 weeks post-conception, (able no 1). The zygote undergoes rapid mitotic division (cleavage), forming a morula by day 3. Continued division converts the morula into a blastocyst, comprising an inner cell mass (future embryo) and a trophoblast (part of the placenta). By days 6–10, the blastocyst implants into the uterine lining, initiating the embryonic stage and forming critical structures like the placenta and amniotic sac. Evidence indicates that approximately 60% of naturally conceived pregnancies do not successfully implant (Fig. 1.1) [9].

The Embryonic Stage

The embryonic stage begins upon zygote implantation into the uterine wall, spanning week's 3–8 post-conception. During this period, vasculogenesis initiates as mesodermal cells differentiate into hemangioblasts, forming blood islands that produce angioblasts, which coalesce into primitive blood vessels. Angiogenesis later expands this network, extending into the placenta to establish maternal-fetal circulation for oxygen, nutrient, and waste exchange. By week 3 (day 22), the neural tube forms, developing into the brain and spinal cord, while growth follows cephalocaudal and proximodistal patterns (Table 1.1) (Fig. 1.1) [10]. By week 4, head formation and heartbeat begin, with gill- and tail-like structures gradually regressing. Organogenesis progresses rapidly: the neural tube closes by week 4, limb buds appear by week

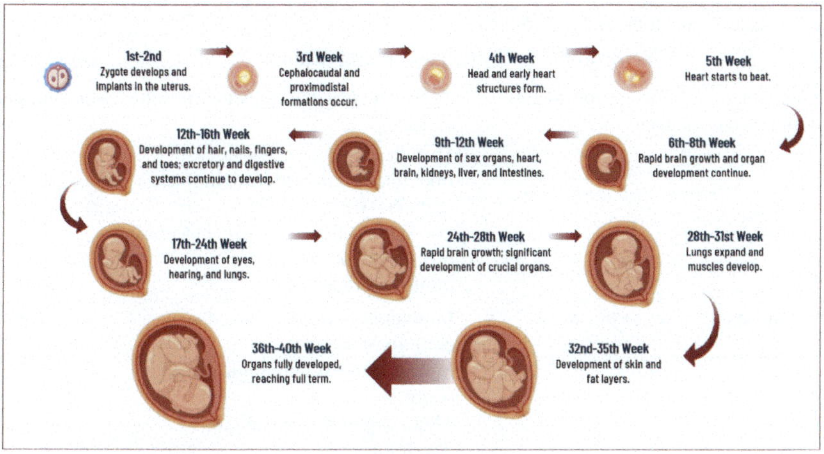

Fig. 1.1 Stages of prenatal development

6, and major organs emerge by week 8, though immature. By the end of this stage, the embryo measures ~1 inch (4 g), responds to touch, and moves. Approximately 20% of embryos fail due to genetic abnormalities or teratogens (e.g., alcohol), often unnoticed by the mother. Proper regulation of these processes is critical for viable development (Table 1.1) (Fig. 1.1) [10].

The Fetal Stage

By the 9th week, the embryo transitions to the fetal stage, reaching kidney bean size. Between 9 and 12 weeks, it adopts a more human-like form as the "tail" recedes and genital differentiation begins. By the 12th week, major organs—heart, brain, kidneys, liver, intestines, and external genitalia—develop, with the fetus measuring ~3 inches and weighing ~28 g. From 12 to 16 weeks, hairs, nails, and teeth form, while digestive and excretory systems mature. By the 14th week, limbs elongate, facial features refine, and fingernails and toenails emerge, further refining human morphological features [10]. By week 16, the fetus measures the size of avocado and undergoes rapid nervous system development (Table 1.1) (Fig. 1.1) [11].

Between weeks 17 and 24, light sensitivity emerges, auditory development begins, and respiratory growth continues. At 20 weeks, reflexes like sucking and hiccupping appear, alongside sleep-wake cycles. From 16 to 28 weeks, the brain nearly doubles in size, with most neurons formed by 24 weeks, though still primitive, while glial cells develop further. By this stage, the fetus weighs up to 635 g, responds to sound, and can feel pain. Viability outside the uterus occurs between 22 and 26 weeks, as critical organs (lungs, heart, stomach, intestines) mature. From the 7th (28th–31st week) to the 9th month (32nd–35th week), muscle strength and lung capacity

Table 1.1 Stages of prenatal development

Stage	Time period	Key events and features	Size/weight
Germinal stage (pre-embryonic)	Conception to 2nd week	– Zygote undergoes cleavage (mitotic division) – Morula (day 3) → Blastocyst – Implantation into uterine lining (days 6–10) – Formation of trophoblast (placenta precursor) and inner cell mass (embryo precursor)	Microscopic
Embryonic stage	3rd to 8th week	– Implantation marks start of embryonic stage – Vasculogenesis and angiogenesis begin – Major organ systems begin developing – Cephalocaudal and proximodistal development patterns	1 inch/4 g
	22 days	– Neural tube (Brain and spinal cord) form	0.1 inch/ <1 g
	4–5 weeks	– Heart begins to beat	0.2–0.3 inch/ 1 g
	6–7 weeks	– Limb buds and facial features form	0.5 inch/1.5 g
Fetal stage	9–12 weeks	– Tail regresses; resembles human form – Genitalia begins to differentiate – Major organs (heart, brain, liver, kidneys) formed – External genitalia visible	3 inches/28 g
	12–16 weeks	– Hair, nails, teeth develop – Face becomes more defined – Fingernails and toenails form – Movements such as thumb-sucking begin – Quickening may be felt by mother	4.5 inches/ 100 g
	17–24 weeks	– Eyes respond to light – Auditory system matures – Reflexes (sucking, swallowing, hiccupping) emerge – Brain growth accelerates – Most neurons in place by 24 weeks	Up to ~635 g
	25–28 weeks	– Continued brain and lung development – Weight and length increase – Fat accumulates under the skin	1000 g

(continued)

Table 1.1 (continued)

Stage	Time period	Key events and features	Size/weight
	29–35 weeks	– Muscles strengthen – Lungs mature – Fat increases for thermal regulation	2.26 kg ~7 inches
	36–40 weeks (full term)	– Final maturation of organs – Ready for birth – Responsive to stimuli, movements well-coordinated	~2.72 kg ~18.5 inches

increase, with weight reaching approximately 2.26 kg and a length of about 7 inches; fat accumulation in the 8th month aids insulation. By the 9th month (36 weeks), the fetus nears delivery at ~2.72 kg and ~18.5 inches. From 37 to 40 weeks, all organ systems are fully developed for survival post-birth (Table 1.1) (Fig. 1.1) [12].

Factors Affecting Prenatal Development

Prenatal development is a complex process influenced by a variety of factors that can significantly impact the health and well-being of the developing fetus. The following factors—genetic inheritance, maternal health and nutrition, environmental exposures (such as toxins and pollutants), lifestyle choices like substance use and stress levels, socio-economic status, and access to healthcare—play crucial roles in ensuring a healthy pregnancy.

Environmental Factors

Environmental factors play a crucial role in prenatal development, as they can significantly influence a baby's growth and health. Factors such as maternal health and nutrition, the intrauterine environment, and exposure to teratogens (e.g., alcohol, drugs, or pollution) can affect fetal development.

Maternal Physical Health

It is reported that 10–30% of pregnant women worldwide are classified as obese [13]. In obesity, adipose tissue causes an increase in inflammatory cytokines like IL-6 and IL-10 and adipokines, creating a chronic inflammatory environment that can impair placental utility and nutrient transference to the fetus (Fig. 1.2). This can result into intrauterine growth restriction (IUGR), altered fetal metabolic programming, as well as an augmented threat of metabolic disorders, cardiovascular disorders (CVD), and neurodevelopmental abnormalities in the offspring later in life. An investigation by An et al. revealed that having a BMI exceeding 28 kg/m^2 was associated with 16% of miscarriage risk. Similarly, Haque et al. observed an 8% augmented risk of miscarriage with overweight and 26% of elevated risk with obesity [14].

According to the global health statistics, type 2 diabetes mellitus (T2DM) is also a significant concern especially among women, with around 8% of adult females affected globally [15]. According to the studies, it is reported that maternal hyperglycemia leads to macrosomia (large birth weight) and augmented adiposity, potentially leading to birth complications such as shoulder dystocia by 15–45%. Wu et al. observed the link of gestational diabetes mellitus (GDM) with congenital anomalies ($P < 0.001$) birth defects like cleft lip and palate, clubfoot, heart defects, neural tube defects, and down syndrome [16]. Another study revealed that during GDM, approximately 40% of fetuses exhibit congenital malformations across numerous organ systems, such as gastrointestinal, genitourinary, cardiovascular, and neurological systems such as anencephaly, holoprosencephaly, and syntelencephaly (Fig. 1.2) [17].

Nutrition

The nutrients a mother consumes play a key part in shaping the progress of organs, brain, immune system strength, and overall growth of the fetus. Insufficient or unbalanced nutrition leads to a variety of complications, like low birth weight (LBW), preterm birth, and potential long-term cognitive and developmental issues. Inadequate nutrition can likewise upsurge the threat of stillbirth, small birth weight, poor growth, and delays in child development (Fig. 1.2) [18]. According to the United Nations International Children's Emergency Fund (UNICEF), over 20 million newborns worldwide are affected by LBW each year. The primary mechanism through which nutrition affects prenatal development is by influencing DNA methylation patterns in the fetus via the maternal diet, thereby altering gene expression and potentially predisposing the child to certain health conditions later in life (Fig. 1.2) [21].

Nutrients such as folate found in leafy greens, legumes, and fortified cereals are essential for neural tube formation and the prevention of neural tube defects like spina bifida. The suggested daily dose of folate during pregnancy is 600 μg, and its deficiency can lead to health issues, including megaloblastic anemia, regarded as abnormally large and immature red blood cells. Omega-3 fatty acids are also crucial for supporting healthy cell membranes, reducing inflammation, and aiding brain function. Pregnant women should aim to consume up to 284 mg of Omega-3 fatty acids daily, as a deficiency can affect brain and visual development. Adequate nutrition, including vitamins C and D from fruits, vegetables, and sunlight, is vital for fetal immune system development. The Recommended Dietary Allowance for vitamin C is approximately 85 mg per day, necessary for collagen synthesis, iron absorption, and immune function, while vitamin D requirements range from 600 to

800 IU per day, supporting calcium absorption, bone health, and immunity. Additionally, vitamin D reduces the risk of maternal bacterial vaginosis and associated preterm birth [19].

Micronutrients (MNs) such as iron (120 mg/day), zinc (15–45 mg/day), and iodine (250 mg/day) are essential for placental function, oxygen transport, and thyroid hormone production. MNs deficiencies can lead to neurodevelopmental impairments: iron deficiency may cause cognitive deficits, learning difficulties, and behavioral problems; zinc deficiency can impair synaptic plasticity, affecting learning and memory; and iodine deficiency can result in congenital hypothyroidism, leading to irreversible brain damage and intellectual disabilities (ID), if not promptly addressed. Studies suggest that 25% of first conceptions are associated with MN insufficiencies, including zinc, iron, vitamins C and D, envisaging long morbidity and mortality for both the mother and the infant [20]. In Sub-Saharan Africa (SSA), the occurrence rates for pre-term delivery (PTD), small gestational age (SGA), LBW, stillbirth, neonatal, and maternal mortality are 12, 16.5, 13, 28.7, 27.7%, and 546 per 100,000 live births, respectively. Additionally, a systematic analysis revealed that the overall burden of neural tube defects (NTDs) due to malnutrition is 1.67 per 1000 live births [23]. Multi-micronutrient (MMN) supplementation in expectant mothers offers a promising approach, potentially plummeting the incidence of stillbirths by 9–11% [21].

Intrauterine Environment

The intrauterine environment, also known as the prenatal environment, is the environment within the uterus where a fetus develops during pregnancy. This environment plays a crucial role in shaping the health and development of the fetus. Amniotic fluid that engulfs the fetus serves as a protective cushion enabling movement and promoting musculoskeletal development. The placenta, an organ unique to pregnancy, facilitates nutrient transfer and oxygen from the mother to the fetus while eliminating waste products. Additionally, hormones such as progesterone, human chorionic gonadotropin (hCG), estrogen, and thyroid-stimulating hormone (TSH) are integral to regulating pregnancy and supporting fetal development (Fig. 1.2) [22]. However, research indicates that disturbances in these factors affect approximately 1.5 million fetuses globally [23]. Studies have also shown that disruptions in intrauterine conditions, such as hormonal imbalances or irregularities in amniotic fluid can be associated with reduced placental perfusion due to elevated blood pressure and vascular constriction, resulting in a significant deficit ($P < 0.01$) in fetal growth. According to the WHO, TSH deficiency can lead to maternal iodine deficiency, which may cause severe neurological impairment and mental retardation in children, affecting about 46.2% of such cases [24]. Additionally, fetus exposed to hyperglycemia in utero is at high risk to develop insulin intolerance in about 4.7% in their childhood [25].

Exposure to Teratogens

Teratogens include various factors such as maternal medical conditions, environmental toxins, and substances like alcohol and drugs. These agents have the potential to cause abnormalities in the developing embryo and impairments in neurodevelopment (Fig. 1.2) [25].

Alcohol

The leading and extensively acknowledged illustration of teratogens affecting fetal growth is fetal alcohol syndrome (FAS), known for causing birth defects and neurodevelopmental disabilities. Ethanol, the main component of alcohol, affects stem cell differentiation through its impact on RNA, leading to epigenetic changes, and oxidative damage. These effects can alter differentiation balance, favoring one lineage over another (e.g., mesodermal over neural), contributing to developmental abnormalities. The precise mechanisms involve complex interactions between RNA damage, epigenetic modifications, and gene expression regulation, ultimately influencing the fate of stem cells. It is estimated that FAS or fetal alcohol spectrum disorders (FASDs) affect at least 1% of live births [25].

Research has indicated that FAS significantly increases the risk of stillbirth by 40–80% among women who consume any amount of alcohol during pregnancy. Similarly, among pregnant women who consume more than seven drinks in a week, the comparative peril of PTD was found to be 3.26 (OR: 0.80–13.24) compared to those who abstain from alcohol [26]. Additionally, another study highlighted that the infants exposed solely to prenatal alcohol consumption, particularly instances of binge drinking, showed delayed visual neurodevelopment during the first 6 months after birth ($P < 0.001$) [27].

Smoking

Globally, more than 50% (approximately 52.9%) of women smoke during pregnancy, which significantly upsurges the threat of birth defects, including LBW in one out of every five babies born to smokers. Exposure to cigarette smoke during pregnancy can introduce harmful substances like nicotine and carbon monoxide to the fetus. These compounds can diminish oxygen levels and hinder the delivery of essential nutrients, potentially causing developmental complications, LBW, and an elevated hazard of preterm labor. Moreover, these toxins can impair fetal brain development and function [28]. Infants exposed to cigarette smoke, either directly or indirectly, have a threefold increased risk of Sudden Infant Death Syndrome (SIDS), and these infants often have weaker lungs, making them more susceptible to various health issues. Studies conducted in Italy ($n = 220{,}927$), Spain ($n = 382{,}340$), and Boston ($n = 206{,}244$) have reported varying occurrence of orofacial clefts in infants exposed to maternal smoking [36]. Additionally, heavy smoking throughout gestation is allied to an OR of 1.35 for PTD (birth before 37 weeks) [29]. Prospective analyses have also shown that maternal smoking increases the risk of placental abruption by 20.4% and is also associated with a higher risk of placenta previa, indicating an increased likelihood of placentation abnormalities [30].

Substance or Drug Use

Illegal drugs such as cocaine and opioids are substances that significantly impact the body and can cause severe health complications, particularly when consumed during pregnancy. Approximately 5% of expectant mothers are believed to use one or more addictive substances during pregnancy [31]. Cocaine exposure affects cortical thickness, induces hyperconnectivity between thalamus and frontal regions, and alters efficient connectivity in areas like medial frontal lobe, amygdala, supplementary motor area, and insula, impairing information processing, sensory-motor integration, and cognitive functions, potentially contributing to syndromes including autism spectrum disorder (ASD) and attention deficit/hyperactivity disorder (ADHD) [36]. Studies have confirmed that drug use is correlated with 70–90% of decreases in birthweight [40]. According to a meta-analysis, heroin use by pregnant women increases the relative risk of delivering LBW infants by 4.61% compared to non-drug-using mothers. It is also associated with a higher frequency of prematurity and SGA infants. Furthermore, maternal methadone use significantly raises the odds (RR 1.81) of LBW, respiratory illness, third-trimester hemorrhage, preeclampsia, and death [40].

Socioeconomic and Psychological Factors

Maternal well-being and fetal health are significantly impacted by socioeconomic and psychological factors. Women from lower socioeconomic backgrounds may face challenges such as limited access to healthcare, and heightened stress, all of which can negatively affect pregnancy outcomes. These factors can increase the risk of complications such as preterm birth, low birth weight, and developmental delays.

Inadequate Prenatal Screening

Prenatal check-ups are crucial for the well-being of both mother and baby with each trimester focusing on specific areas (Fig. 1.2). In the first trimester, check-ups confirm pregnancy, assess maternal health, and identify risks through physical exams, blood tests, and ultrasounds. The second trimester involves frequent visits to monitor fetal growth, anatomy, and screen for conditions like Down syndrome, along with checking blood pressure, urine protein for preeclampsia, and glucose tolerance for gestational diabetes. In the third trimester, the focus shifts to childbirth preparation, tracking fetal movements, fundal height, and baby's position, and managing complications like gestational hypertension or diabetes. Psychological support is also vital throughout pregnancy. A global survey shows prenatal depression prevalence ranging from 15 to 65%, with an average of 17%. Addressing anxiety, depression, and stress improves maternal mental health and pregnancy outcomes. Regular counseling sessions help in providing emotional support, managing concerns, and preparing women for postpartum, fostering secure, and empowered parents [32].

According to the CDC report, the percentages of prenatal care in higher income countries (HICs) increased to 91.7% for white mothers, 85.2% for Hispanic mothers, and 84.1% for black mothers. However, among LMICs, only 11.3% pregnant women received prenatal care, where 49.9% reported a lack of antenatal screening [33]. According to a review, a lack of serum analytes, including alpha-fetoprotein, HCG, unconjugated estriol, inhibin A, and pregnancy-associated plasma protein A (PAPP-A) during 20 weeks of gestation, could increase the risk of Down syndrome in the fetus by 60% [34]. Another study reported that improper screening of coda (the proportion of cell-free DNA in the mother's blood that originates from the placenta) can lead to false positive results, resulting in the termination of 7% of pregnancies. Similarly, a meta-analysis revealed that cell-free DNA screening failures increase the risk of trisomy in pregnancy by 5.4%. Trisomy is a genetic condition where a fetus has 47 copies of a chromosome, instead of the usual 46. It can lead to premature pregnancy or miscarriage (Fig. 1.2) [35].

Maternal Stress and Depression

Maternal stress and depression during pregnancy are significant concerns due to their potential impacts on both the mother and the growing fetus. These conditions can lead to a variety of severe consequences, like PTD, LBW, and developmental issues in the child. Maternal stress can result from various factors, such as financial instability, relationship problems, lack of social support, and concerns about the pregnancy itself. The prevalence of maternal stress and depression in LMICs is estimated to be 29.2% antenatal and 24.4% postnatally. Prenatal maternal stress has a significant effect on infant brain development (Fig. 1.2). This process is driven by the secretion of stress hormones like cortisol, which can pass through the placental barrier and impact the development of the fetus directly [35]. Elevated cortisol levels in the fetus can disrupt normal neurodevelopment, leading to microstructural changes in the neonatal amygdala and reduced hippocampal volumes in infants, with gene moderations further influencing these associations. This can result in long-term consequences like cognitive deficits, behavioral regulation difficulties, and augmented defenselessness to mental health disorders later in life [36].

Additionally, maternal stress has been observed to impact the development of fetal central nervous system, contributing to 35% of fetal activity as well as influencing changes in the heart rate and body movement. Furthermore, research indicates that pregnant women experiencing stress face a higher risk of preterm birth, with rates reported as high as 54%. Moreover, heightened anxiety levels during gestation have been associated with improper development of the fetal left amygdala, potentially leading to emotional symptoms, behavioral issues, difficulties in peer relationships, and overall challenges in early childhood ($P = 0.002$) [36].

Genetic Factors

Genetic features play a crucial role in fetal growth impacting different facets of fetal growth and development (Fig. 1.2). Approximately 16% of women worldwide are affected by these factors. Gene polymorphisms, a variation in DNA sequences that occur in at least 1% of the population during prenatal development resulting from mutations or recombination during meiosis. These mutations can be induced by environmental factors such as radiation, chemicals, or maternal health conditions, leading to the development of polymorphisms [37].

The studies have indicated that gene polymorphism in the 1298A > C gene methylenetetrahydrofolate reductase (MTHFR) gene ($P < 0.05$), and MTHFR C677T gene ($P \leq 0.001$) increases the risk for NTDs during fetal development due to decreased conversion of homocysteine to methionine [38]. On the other hand, a study conducted in Brazil found that human bone morphogenetic protein 4 gene (BMP4) rs17563 polymorphism during embryonic stage in pregnancy causes non-syndromic cleft lip (NSCL) or is devoid of cleft palate in children (OR = 0.70) [39].

Gene variants or mutations occur due to a variety of factors, including errors during DNA replication, environmental influences like radiation or chemicals, and inherited mutations from parents. It is different from gene polymorphism a specific type of genetic variation where two or more alleles exist at a locus within a population, often with each variant occurring at a frequency of at least 1% [52]. These variants can impact prenatal development by altering the normal process of cell division, differentiation, and organ formation, potentially leading to congenital anomalies or developmental disorders. The prevalence of gene variants impacting birth outcomes such as neurodevelopmental disorders, congenital anomalies, and genetic syndromes become apparent or diagnosable as the child grows and develops that can be diagnosed during adolescence is reported to be 40.5% [40]. A study conducted in Nigeria identified a sickle cell trait prevalence of one in four individuals with significant associations noted between this trait and prenatal issues such as IUGR attributed to genetic variations in the hemoglobin subunit beta (HBB) gene (variation in HBB gene can lead to sickle cell anemia, which impairs the blood's oxygen-carrying capacity, potentially causing fetal hypoxia and developmental complications) ($P < 0.001$). In Brazil, the prevalence of sickle cell trait varies from 1.1 to 9.8%, while sickle cell disease affects 0.8–60 per 100,000 live births (Fig. 1.2) [42].

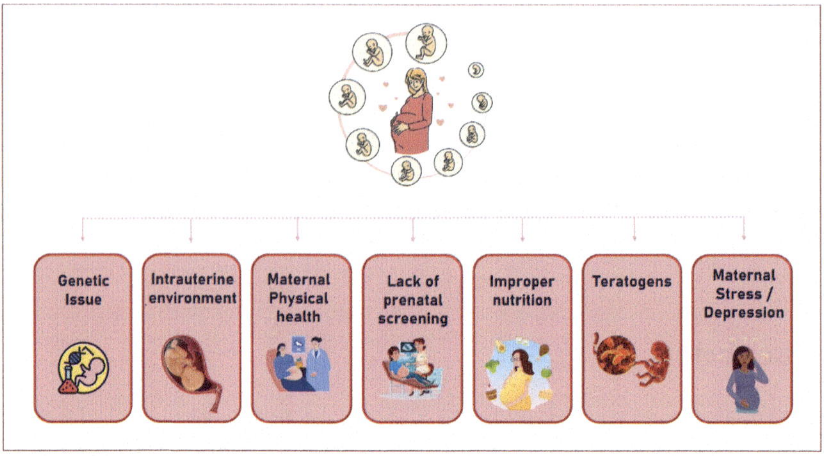

Fig. 1.2 Factors affecting prenatal development

Impacts of Inadequate Prenatal Development

Inadequate prenatal development can lead to adverse outcomes such as LBW, preterm birth, and developmental delays, all of which significantly increase the risk of health complications in early life. These conditions may contribute to long-term cognitive, emotional, and physical challenges, affecting a child's academic performance, social integration, and overall quality of life. The potential consequences of insufficient prenatal development include.

Brain Development

Insufficient prenatal development can have profound effect on cognitive and emotional growth, and lifelong impairments (Fig. 1.3). A study conducted in Swedish found that iron deficiency (anemia) during gestation is related with a 4.9% incidence of ASD, a 9.3% incidence of ADHD, and a 3.1% incidence of intellectual disability (ID) in children. Similarly, exposure to antidepressants such as selective serotonin reuptake inhibitors (SSRIs) during prenatal period is linked to a 38% increased risk of ADHD. Hypertensive disorders during pregnancy (HDP) that complicate 5–10% of gestations are also allied with an augmented risk of ASD and ADHD in infants globally [41].

Depression experienced by mothers during pregnancy has been related to negative developmental effects in their children. A study discovered that by 24 months, newborns whose mothers suffered from prenatal depression showed lower cognitive abilities and language difficulties ($P < 0.93$). Additionally, Donald et al. reported a

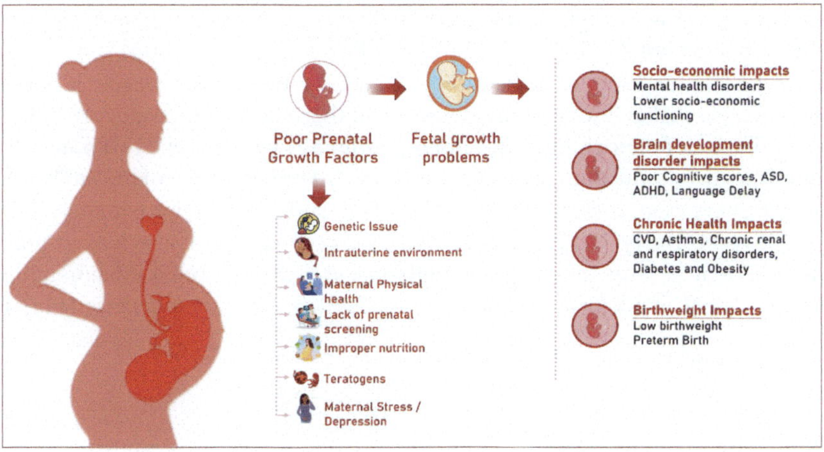

Fig. 1.3 Impacts of poor prenatal development

noteworthy connotation between antenatal stress and negative cognitive abnormalities in boys ($P < 0.05$), as well as expressive language delays in the overall cohort ($P < 0.05$) and specifically in girls ($P < 0.05$) [42].

Birth Weight Impacts

Inadequate prenatal development, chronic stress, and anxiety during pregnancy, with prevalence ranging between 1 and 26% in LMICs, can lead to unhealthy coping behaviors such as poor diet or inadequate prenatal care, further influencing birth weight outcomes (Fig. 1.3). Maternal depressive indications have been more frequently allied to LBW than with pre-term birth. A meta-analysis of 20 studies on HDP revealed that the upsurge in depressive symptoms was interrelated to 1.4–2.9 times higher risk of LBW in LMICs and an average 1.2 times greater risk in the United States [43]. The worldwide prevalence of LBW stands at 14.6%, with a range between 12.4 and 17.1%. This translates to roughly 25 million infants born with LBW each year. Notably, 95% of these cases are identified in LMICs with South Asia contributing nearly 52% of the worldwide occurrence [44].

Chronic Health Conditions

A prenatal growth restriction significantly enhances the risk of metabolic syndromes such as future obesity by 29% through a process known as "fetal programming." Moreover, children who go through accelerated growth due to GDM are at a high risk of becoming overweight in adulthood ($P < 0.001$). Similarly, poor fetal growth and LBW weight notably elevate diabetes risk later in life ($P < 0.0001$) with 90% of adults in LMICs developing diabetes post-GDM during prenatal stages. It is found through a research that low vitamin D levels in mothers during pregnancy are linked to a greater danger of their children developing asthma, wheezing, and respiratory tract infections with a significance level of $P < 0.01$ [45]. The deficiency of iron and protein during pregnancy can increase the risk of CVD in children by approximately 17.4% and 1.1%, respectively. Protein restriction during pregnancy can also lead to smaller nephron size in 30% of infants, potentially causing chronic renal inflammation in adulthood due to inadequate amino acid availability for nephrogenesis (Fig. 1.3) [48].

Socioeconomic Impact

Improper prenatal development is linked to neurodevelopmental disorders and cognitive impairments, affecting educational attainment and employability, leading to reduced income and increased reliance on social welfare systems (Fig. 1.3). These combined effects create a cycle of poverty, restricting access to healthcare and further education, thereby impeding social mobility and overall quality of life. Research indicates that newborns exposed to maternal stress both during the antenatal and postnatal periods often experience insecure emotional problems and poor social skills ($P < 0.05$) [46]. Another systematic analysis revealed that maternal depression is associated with several outcomes in adolescents: oppositional defiant disorder or conduct disorder in 59%, ADHD in 52%, aggression in 28%, non-aggressive rule-breaking behavior in 7%, and externalizing behavior in 85%. Similarly, SGA infants are linked to a higher frequency of mood disorders in adulthood (OR: 1.26) and lower socioeconomic functioning (OR: 1.77) [47].

Policies, Programs, and Public Health Initiatives on Child Health Outcomes: Challenges and Statistical Data

Policies, programs, and public health initiatives have been specifically designed to enhance child health outcomes, encompassing comprehensive care, immunization, and nutritional support programs. Although these efforts have significantly benefited pregnant women in LMICs, they continue to face persistent challenges, including disparities in access, resource limitations, and logistical barriers.

Comprehensive Care Programs

The continuum of care (CoC) framework 2006–2012 for maternal, neonatal, and child health ensures comprehensive and continuous care for adolescence through pregnancy, childbirth, postnatal care, and childhood. Effective implementation of CoC initiatives is found to substantially reduce the mother, neonatal, and child mortality rate by 40–44% [48]. Additionally, the global under-five mortality rate has declined from 75 demises per 1,000 live childbirths in 2000 to 38 deaths per 1,000 live births in 2019 by the framework of CoC. Between 2000 and 2017, the global maternal mortality ratio (MMR) reduced by nearly 38%, averaging a 2.9% annual decline. Despite this progress, an average annual reduction of 6.4% is required to meet the sustainable development goal (SDG) target of 3.1, which aims to lower the MMR to fewer than 70 demises per 100,000 live deliveries [49]. However, disparities in completing the CoC persist globally. For instance, 60% of women in Cambodia completed the CoC during the 2010 Cambodia Demographic and Health Survey (CDHS), but this figure dropped drastically to 5% by the end of 2010. Tanzania reported a mere 10% adherence to the recommended CoC, encompassing four ANC visits, skilled delivery attendance, and postnatal follow-up. Ghana demonstrated disparities with 86.1% of women accessing ANC but only 25.4% receiving timely postnatal care, and just 8% completing the full CoC. In Cambodia, 90% of women receive ANC with 71% continuing with skilled birth attendance and only 60% completing the entire service spectrum. In Pakistan, the CoC rose from 15% in 2006 to 27% in 2012, indicating the progress but still leaving substantial room for improvement. Nepal reported that only 27% of women utilize maternal and neonatal health services, which are crucial for plummeting morbidity and mortality rates, and refining overall maternal and neonatal health [50]. Shortage of medical facilities, out-of-pocket expenses, insufficient knowledge about pandemics, and dietary deficiencies hinder adequate ANC [51].

Immunization Programs

Maternal immunization is a highly effective strategy for preventing infections in both the mothers and their newborns. Vaccinating pregnant women induces pathogen-specific antibodies that can protect infants during their vulnerable early months. A significant achievement in global health is the substantial decrease in neonatal tetanus cases worldwide. This success is largely due to the World Health Organization's (WHO) Maternal and Neonatal Tetanus Elimination (MNTE) Program, which focuses on lowering the incidence of MNT to a phase where it no longer poses a risk to public well-being. This is achieved by ensuring that maternal tetanus vaccination status is reviewed during ANC and administering the tetanus vaccine as needed. This initiative, which includes widespread tetanus toxoid vaccination for pregnant women, improved prenatal hygiene, and female's immunization of childbearing age, led to a significant drop in neonatal tetanus deaths—from 14 to 5%—over two decades (1990–2010) in participating countries [52]. From 1999 to 2016, over 150 million women received at least two dosages of these vaccines by MNTE program and additional campaigns. By March 2018, 45 out of 59 countries had accomplished eradication status, well-defined as fewer than 1 case per 1,000 live births annually, leading to a 96% decrease in neonatal deaths caused by tetanus since the late 1980s [53]. Gavi, the Vaccine Alliance, is a global health corporation that brings together public and private sectors to expand access to vaccines in LMICs and manage over half of all donor health assistance. The majority of funding for global immunization efforts has facilitated the vaccination of over 822 million youngsters since 2000, preventing more than 14 million deaths [54].

The combined efforts of Advisory Committee on Immunization Practices (ACIP), the American College of Obstetricians and Gynecologists, the American Academy of Family Physicians, the American Academy of Pediatrics, and the National Vaccine Advisory Committee have resulted in higher vaccination rates during gestation in the United States. For instance, influenza vaccine coverage among pregnant women increased from about 15% in 2008 to almost 45–50% during 2013–2014 influenza season. Similarly, influenza vaccination among pregnant women in tropical and subtropical regions has reduced the incidence of laboratory-confirmed influenza by 50% in the mothers and by 49–63% in their infants under six months of age [55].

Pertussis remains a significant global health issue, with around 16 million cases annually, 95% occurring in LMICs in the early 2000s. By 2011, the US ACIP expanded its vaccination strategy from targeting adults and caregivers (the "cocoon" strategy) to include pregnant women who had not previously been vaccinated against pertussis, preferably in their late second or third trimesters. In 2012, due to low vaccination rates among pregnant women and evidence suggesting maternal anti-pertussis antibodies are short-lived, ACIP revised its guidelines to recommend vaccinating all prenatal women at 20 weeks' gestation, regardless of prior vaccination status. This change led to a decrease in pertussis rates across all age groups, most significantly in infants under three months with a vaccine efficacy of 92%. The UK now routinely administers the TDaP/IPV vaccine to pregnant women, while the United States continues with TDaP [59].

Initiated in 2010, the Global Vaccine Action Plan (GVAP) was built on the Global Immunization and Vaccine Strategy (GIVS, 2006–2015) which comprised of discontinuing wild Polio transmission, eradicating neonatal tetanus, and other preventable diseases in pregnant women, achieving 90% national DTP3 treatment and 80% in each district, introducing new vaccines, and reducing child mortality rates. One notable outcome of GVAP for pregnant mothers was the 16% reduction in maternal and neonatal tetanus cases, due to the increased coverage of tetanus toxoid: containing vaccinations (TT-CV) [56]. However, the overall global coverage conceals a highly dynamic situation with some countries like North America making remarkable progress while African regions experiencing concerning declines in coverage due to various challenges including safety incidents, and political, social, and economic instability [59].

Till 2015, 23 million children remained unprotected against diphtheria, pertussis, and tetanus. According to WHO, only about 60% of pregnant women in LMICs regions obtained the suggested TT-CV, leaving 40% unprotected against maternal and neonatal tetanus. The factors contributing to under-immunization included poor access to health facilities and immunization campaigns, inefficient use of resources, and limited technical capacity of under-empowered National Immunization Technical Advisory Groups (NITAGs) [59].

Nutritional Programs

Food distribution programs (FDPs) that incorporate balanced energy protein (BEP) supplementation and dietary interventions have demonstrated significant success in improving maternal and birth outcomes. BEP supplementation has been linked to a 61% reduction in stillbirths, a 50% decrease in perinatal mortality, and an average increase in delivery weight by 107.28 g. Similarly, FDPs have contributed to an increase in average birth weight by 46 g, improved birth length, and substantial reductions in stunting by 18% and wasting by 13%. Additionally, integrating family planning strategies with nutritional services through existing delivery channels has proven to be an effective approach to addressing women's health needs ($P < 0.001$) [57].

Despite the progress, global concerns persist regarding poor nutrition among women, particularly in LMICs. The occurrence of low body mass index (BMI) was in South Asia and sub-Saharan Africa is 24 and 20%, respectively [58]. According to WHO 2021 report, anemia affects 36.5% of pregnant women worldwide [59]. Studies across Ethiopia, India, Bangladesh, and Burkina Faso underscore substantial nutrient deficits during pregnancy due to inadequate anti-natal care (ANC), nutrition service delivery, and counselling on weight gain, with prevalence rates ranging from 74 to 95%. Several factors can impede healthy eating during pregnancy such as hormonal changes that can alter taste preferences and appetite, morning sickness characterized by nausea and vomiting, and limited economic incomes may limit intake of fresh, nutritious diet. Additionally, a lack of nutrition education and awareness can result in poor dietary choices [62].

Policy and Practice Implications

To improve prenatal outcomes, few following steps should be considered for inclusion in future policies.

Research-Based Initiatives

Enhancing prenatal care through research-based initiatives marks a significant advancement in the understanding and monitoring of fetal health. By integrating innovative tools into prenatal practices, healthcare providers can strengthen early intervention strategies, thereby promoting better outcomes for both mothers and their babies and improving the overall quality of prenatal healthcare.

Increase Utilization of Fetal Neuroimaging

Increasing the utilization of fetal neuroimaging in screening prenatal development is crucial for early detection and intervention of neurodevelopmental abnormalities. This advanced imaging technology allows for detailed visualization of the fetal brain, enabling healthcare providers to identify potential issues such as structural defects, abnormal brain growth, and connectivity disorders. For instance, according to a review, lack of serum analytes comprising alpha-fetoprotein, HCG, unconjugated estriol, inhibin A, and pregnancy-associated plasma protein A (PAPP-A) during 20 weeks of gestation neural screening could enhance the risk of DS in the fetus by 60% [34]. Through fetal neuroimaging, researchers can investigate the progression of brain development in the womb, offering crucial insights into the effects of prenatal exposures on various stages of gestation. A study was conducted by utilizing morphometry on fetal MRI, which revealed a substantial variance in anteroposterior span of the fetal cerebellar vermis between fetuses with an average gestational age of 33.67 weeks (28–39 weeks) exposed to opioids in utero and those not exposed ($P = 0.004$) [60]. Similarly, Huang et al. developed a three-dimensional automated segmentation network designed for MRI to explain essential tissues during fetal brain scanning that help in diagnosing the congenital conditions during pregnancy with an average Dice similarity coefficient (DSC) of 83.79%, an average volume similarity (VS) of 84.84%, and an average Hausdorff 95 Distance (HD95) of 35.66 mm [61].

Implementing Machine Learning and Predictive Modeling

Implementing machine learning and predictive modeling in prenatal screening is essential because these technologies can enhance the accuracy and early detection of potential developmental issues in the fetus. Machine learning techniques, capable of managing vast datasets, discerning patterns, and forecasting results, offer a nuanced understanding of the correlation between maternal exposures and brain growth. Husna et al. proposed a novel method to identify ASD by utilizing single-volume brain images derived from Functional (f) MRI data by using enhanced convolutional neural network (CNN), which achieved accuracies of 63.4 and 87.0% in ASD identification [65]. Similarly, another study suggested Functional Near-Infrared Spectroscopy (fNIRS) data could advance ASD etiology research by utilizing a combined Long Short-Term Memory (LSTM) neural network and CNN model. Their analysis focused on the global time-varying activities of hemodynamic oscillations in oxy-hemoglobin (HbO2) and deoxy-hemoglobin (Hb), achieving an accuracy of 95.7%, sensitivity of 97.1%, and specificity of 94.3% [62].

Initiatives to Enhance Prenatal Care Access

Enhancing access to prenatal care involves implementing the following initiatives to foster a more equitable and supportive environment for all expectant mothers.

Supporting Economically Vulnerable Mothers

Supporting economically weak mothers is crucial for improving prenatal development and ensuring healthier outcomes for both the mothers and their babies. Economic hardship can significantly impact a mother's ability to access essential prenatal care, maintain a balanced diet, and manage stress, all of which are vital for fetal development. Providing financial assistance and resources—such as food vouchers, subsidized healthcare, and prenatal vitamins—can effectively reduce barriers to adequate prenatal care [63]. For instance, National Health Insurance Program by the Federal Ministry of Health in Nepal has established a safe motherhood program that facilitates free institutional deliveries and offers incentives to both mothers and healthcare providers. These initiatives have contributed significantly to reducing Nepal's Neonatal Mortality Rate (NMR) from 50 to 21 per 1,000 live births and decreasing the MMR from 539 to 281 per 100,000 live births [64]. Similarly, Special Supplemental Nutrition Program for Women, Infants, and Children (WIC) in the United States provides access to nutritious food, education on healthy eating, and essential prenatal vitamins, which caused an 11% decline in the prevalence of SGB, and enhanced cognitive and physical development in infants [65].

Educational Campaigns

Educational programs for pregnant mothers have greatly enhanced maternal and fetal health outcomes by providing crucial information on prenatal care, nutrition, and lifestyle choices. Healthcare providers serve as primary agents in promoting prenatal development and mitigating adverse maternal outcomes [66]. In a study, women reported that their preferred source of information regarding risks in future pregnancies and potential future health concerns was their healthcare professionals, especially obstetric medicine specialists. This highlights the critical role of healthcare providers in delivering information on healthcare risks associated with the health of the mother, the fetus, and future pregnancies [67]. Other information sources include community centers, and online platforms. Educational interventions have proven highly effective in enhancing the management of HDP. Analysis found that mothers who attended antenatal precaution by self-management mobile phone and tablet apps were 1.26 times more likely to recognize labor risk symptoms compared to those who did not. Additionally, participants who delivered in specialized healthcare facilities were 3.57 times more likely to be aware of prenatal complications than those who gave birth at home, primarily on account of the information provided by the medical supervisors [65]. A randomized trial found that distributing educational pamphlets about HDP significantly improved knowledge scores in the intervention group compared to the control group after one month, achieving an 88.2% increase [67].

Remote Healthcare Monitoring

Remote healthcare monitoring has demonstrated effectiveness in enhancing outcomes for pregnant women and their fetuses by providing continuous, real-time access to medical care and support. A study has revealed that by wearing a wrist-mounted wearable sensor device that captures blood pressure, heart rate, and steps, patients can control and monitor their blood pressure for about 75% of their daily time. This monitoring resulted in a 7% reduction in maternal mortality rates in Lama and Peru [68]. Furthermore, PregCare introduced a novel care model for low-risk pregnancies, empowering expectant mothers, and reducing face-to-face visits by up to 50%, with approximately 6–8 clinic and hospital visits throughout pregnancy [69]. In a meta-analysis, remote fetal monitoring reduced the risk of neonatal asphyxia (risk ratio 0.66, 95% CI 0.45–0.97; $P = 0.04$) compared to a control group [70].

Mental Health Initiatives

Establishing maternal mental health initiatives can reduce stress levels and improve overall pregnancy outcomes, including lower rates of preterm birth and IUGR. Research findings indicate that implementing attachment and relaxation training during pregnancy visits had effectively reduced maternal anxiety and post-partum depression ($P < 0.001$) Similarly, a study in Iran comparing applied relaxation exercise with standard care (routine hospital-based ANC) among primiparous females with elevated anxiety in their second trimester showed a reduction in LBW, cesarean section rates, and instrumental delivery 7 weeks post-intervention ($P = 0.052$) [71].

Conclusion

Prenatal development is a crucial period that shapes lifelong health and well-being, with the germinal, embryonic, and fetal stages being particularly sensitive to environmental, genetic, socioeconomic, and psychological factors. These influences impact fetal brain health, birthweight, and future risk of chronic conditions. Comprehensive prenatal care—encompassing nutrition, psychological support, and avoidance of harmful exposures—is vital for optimizing fetal development and minimizing adverse outcomes. While policies like the CoC framework, immunization, and nutritional programs show promise, their effectiveness is often hindered by disparities in healthcare access and socioeconomic challenges. To enhance prenatal care, future initiatives should prioritize support for vulnerable mothers, expand education and remote healthcare, and advance research through fetal neuroimaging and machine learning for early disease detection. Ensuring comprehensive and equitable prenatal care is a must for promoting long-term health and resilience.

References

1. Nigussie, K., Degu, G., Chanie, H., & Edemealem, H. (2021). Magnitude of Unintended Pregnancy and Associated Factors Among Pregnant Women in Debre Markos Town, East Gojjam Zone, Northwest Ethiopia: A Cross-Sectional Study. *International Journal of Women's Health, 13*, 129–139.
2. Syed, U., et al. (2022). Advancing Maternal and Perinatal Health in Low-and Middle-Income Countries: A Multi-country Review of Policies and Programs. *Frontiers in Global Women's Health, 3*. Retrieved from https://doi.org/10.3389/fgwh.2022.909991
3. McDonald, C. R., Weckman, A. M., Wright, J. K., Conroy, A. L., & Kain, K. C. (2020). Pregnant Women in Low- and Middle-Income Countries Require a Special Focus During the COVID-19 Pandemic. *Frontiers in Global Women's Health, 1*, 1–6. Retrieved from https://doi.org/10.3389/fgwh.2020.564560
4. Merid, M. W., et al. (2024). Women in Low- and Middle-Income Countries Receive Antenatal Care at Health Institutions, Yet Not Delivered There: A Multilevel Analysis of 2016–2021 DHS Data. *The American Journal of Tropical Medicine and Hygiene, 52*(1). Retrieved from https://doi.org/10.1186/s41182-023-00561-5.
5. Ayele, T. B., & Moyehodie, Y. A. (2023). Prevalence of Preterm Birth and Associated Factors Among Mothers Who Gave Birth in Public Hospitals of East Gojjam Zone, Ethiopia. *BMC Pregancy and Childbirth, 23*(1), 204. Retrieved from https://doi.org/10.1186/s12884-023-05517-5
6. Jana, A. (2023). Correlates of Low Birth Weight and Preterm Birth in India. *PloS One, 18*(8), e0287919. Retrieved from https://doi.org/10.1371/journal.pone.0287919.
7. Martin, J. A., et al. (2021). *National Vital Statistics Reports, 70*(2), 1–10.
8. Perin, J., et al. (2023). Systematic Estimates of the Global, Regional and National Under-5 Mortality Burden Table to Birth Defects in 2000–2019: A Summary of Findings from the 2020 WHO Estimates. *BMJ Open, 13*(1), e067033. Retrieved from https://doi.org/10.1136/bmjopen-2022-067033
9. Hall, D. (2024). Meiotic Drive and Sex Chromosome Cycling. *Evolution, 58*(5), 925–931.
10. Paris, J., et al. (2023). *Child Growth and Development*. LibreTexts.

11. Professional, C. C. (2024).*Fetal Development: Week-by-Week Stages of Pregnancy.* Cleveland Clinic. https://my.clevelandclinic.org/health/articles/7247-fetal-development-stages-of-growth
12. Karaca, N. H. (2022). Prenatal Development. In*Research Anthology on Advancements in Women's Health and Reproductive Rights* (pp. 712–731). IGI Global.
13. Mahmood, T. (2020). An Overview of Complications Associated with Obesity During Pregnancy. *Obesity and Obstetrics, 1*, 75–82.
14. Langley-Evans, S. C., Pearce, J., & Ellis, S. (2022). Overweight, Obesity and Excessive Weight Gain in Pregnancy as Risk Factors for Adverse Pregnancy Outcomes: A Narrative Review. *Journal of Human Nutrition and Dietetics, 35*(2), 250–264. Retrieved from https://doi.org/10.1111/jhn.12999.
15. Ye, J., et al. (2023). The Global, Regional and National Burden of Type 2 Diabetes Mellitus in the Past, Present and Future: A Systematic Analysis of the Global Burden of Disease Study 2019. *Frontiers in Endocrinology, 14*, 1–12.
16. Wu, Y., et al. (2020). Association of Maternal Pre-Pregnancy Diabetes and Gestational Diabetes Mellitus with Congenital Anomalies of the Newborn. *Diabetes Care, 43*(12), 2983–2990. Retrieved from https://doi.org/10.2337/dc20-0261.
17. Ornoy, A., Becker, M., Weinstein-Fudim, L., & Ergaz, Z. (2021). Diabetes during Pregnancy: A Maternal Disease Complicating the Course of Pregnancy with Long-Term Deleterious Effects on the Offspring: A Clinical Review. *International Journal of Molecular Sciences, 22*(6), 2965. https://doi.org/10.3390/ijms22062965
18. Ionescu, M. I., et al. (2024). Nurturing Development: How a Mother's Nutrition Shapes Offspring's Brain Through the Gut. *Nutritional Neuroscience, 23*, 1–23. Retrieved from https://doi.org/10.1080/1028415X.2024.2349336
19. Brown, B., & Wright, C. (2020). Safety and Efficacy of Supplements in Pregnancy. *Nutrition Reviews, 78*(10), 813–826. Retrieved from https://doi.org/10.1093/nutrit/nuz101.
20. Walle, B. M., Adekunle, A. O., Arowojolu, A. O., Dugul, T. T., & Mebiratie, A. L. (2020). Micronutrients Deficiency and Their Associations with Pregnancy Outcomes: A Review. *Nutrition and Dietary Supplements*, 237–254. Retrieved from https://doi.org/10.2147/NDS.S274646.
21. Keats, E. C., Haider, B. A., Tam, E., & Bhutta, Z. A. (2019). Multiple-Micronutrient Supplementation for Women During Pregnancy. *Cochrane Database of Systematic Reviews, 3*(3), CD004905. Retrieved from https://doi.org/10.1002/14651858.CD004905.pub6.
22. Kenner, C., Altimier, L. B., & Boykova, M. V. (2019). Fetal Development: Environmental Influences and Critical Periods. *Comprehensive Neon Nurs Care*. Springer Publishing Company, 1–2019.
23. Ruan, J., Zhong, X., Mai, J., Liu, C., & Ding, H. (2024). The Status and Influencing Factors of Abnormal Fetal Pregnancy Outcomes in 265 Cases in China: A Retrospective Study. *PeerJ, 12*, e17284. Retrieved from https://doi.org/10.7717/peerj.17284.
24. Dulek, H., Vural, F., Aka, N., & Zengin, S. (2019). The Prevalence of Thyroid Dysfunction and Its Relationship with Perinatal Outcomes in Pregnant Women in the Third Trimester. *Northern Clinics of Istanbul, 6*(3), 267–272. Retrieved from https://doi.org/10.14744/nci.2018.51422.
25. Tam, W. H., et al. (2017). In Utero Exposure to Maternal Hyperglycemia Increases Childhood Cardiometabolic Risk in Offspring. *Diabetes Care, 40*(5), 679–686. Retrieved from https://doi.org/10.2337/dc16-2397.
26. Dejong, K., Olyaei, A., & Lo, J. O. (2019). Alcohol Use in Pregnancy. *Clin Obsterics and Gynecology, 62*(1), 142–155. Retrieved from https://doi.org/10.1097/GRF.0000000000000414.
27. Margolis, E. T., *et al.* (2024). Longitudinal Effects of Prenatal Alcohol Exposure on Visual Neurodevelopment Over Infancy. *Development Psychology*. Retrieved from https://doi.org/10.1037/dev0001727
28. Almeida, R., Barbosa, C., Pereira, B., Diniz, M., Baena, A., & Conde, A. (2022). Tobacco Smoking During Pregnancy: Women's Perception About the Usefulness of Smoking Cessation Interventions. *International Journal of environmental Research and Public Health, 19*(11), 1–17. Retrieved from https://doi.org/10.3390/ijerph19116595.

29. Liu, B., et al. (2020). Maternal Cigarette Smoking Before and During Pregnancy and the Risk of Preterm Birth: A Dose-Response Analysis of 25 Million Mother-Infant Pairs. *PLoS Medicine, 17*(8), e1003158. Retrieved from https://doi.org/10.1371/journal.pmed.1003158.
30. Sequí-Canet, J. M., Sequí-Sabater, J. M., Marco-Sabater, A., Corpas-Burgos, F., Collar Del Castillo, J. I., & Orta-Sibú, N. (2022). Maternal Factors Associated with Smoking During Gestation and Consequences in Newborns: Results of an 18-Year Study. *Journal of Clinical and Translational Research, 8*(1), 6–19.
31. Forray, A. (2016). Substance Use During Pregnancy. *F1000Research, 5*, 1–9.
32. Dadi, A. F., et al. (2020). Global Burden of Antenatal Depression and Its Association with Adverse Birth Outcomes: An umbrella Review. *BMC Public Health, 20*, 173. Retrieved from https://doi.org/10.1186/s12889-020-8293-9.
33. Jiwani, S. S., et al. (2020). Timing and Number of Antenatal Care Contacts in Low and Middle-Income Countries: Analysis in the Countdown to 2030 Priority Countries. *Global Health, 10*(1), 1–12. Retrieved from https://doi.org/10.7189/jogh.10.010502.
34. Russo, M. L., & Blakemore, K. J. (2014). A Historical and Practical Review of First Trimester Aneuploidy Screening. *Seminars in Fetal Neonatal Medicine, 19*(3), 183–187. Retrieved from https://doi.org/10.1016/j.siny.2013.11.013
35. Roddy Mitchell, A., et al. (2023). Prevalence of Perinatal Anxiety and Related Disorders in Low- and Middle-Income Countries: A Systematic Review and Meta-Analysis. *JAMA Network Open, 6*(11), e2343711. Retrieved from https://doi.org/10.1001/jamanetworkopen.2023.43711.
36. Acosta, H., et al. (2019). Maternal Pregnancy-Related Anxiety Is Associated with Sexually Dimorphic Alterations in Amygdala Volume in 4-Year-Old Children. *Frontiers in Behavioral Neuroscience, 13*, 175. Retrieved from https://doi.org/10.3389/fnbeh.2019.00175.
37. Khan, R. R., et al. (2024). Genetic Polymorphisms Associated with Adverse Pregnancy Outcomes in Nulliparas. *Science Reports, 14*(1), 1–11.
38. Almekkawi, A. K., et al. (2022). Folate Pathway Gene Single Nucleotide Polymorphisms and Neural Tube Defects: A Systematic Review and Meta-Analysis. *Journal of Personalized Medicine, 12*(10), 1–15. Retrieved from https://doi.org/10.3390/jpm12101609.
39. Li, Y. H., Yang, J., Zhang, J. L., Liu, J. Q., Zheng, Z., & Hu, D. H. (2017). BMP4 rs17563 Polymorphism and Non-syndromic Cleft Lip with or Without Cleft Palate: A Meta-Analysis. *Medicine, 96*(31), e7676. Retrieved form https://doi.org/10.1097/MD.0000000000007676.
40. Slavotinek, A., et al. (2023). Diagnostic Yield of Pediatric and Prenatal Exome Sequencing in a Diverse Population. *NPJ Genomic Medicine, 8*(1), 10. Retrieved from https://doi.org/10.1038/s41525-023-00353-0.
41. Wang, H., et al. (2021). Maternal Hypertensive Disorders and Neurodevelopmental Disorders in Offspring: A Population-Based Cohort in Two Nordic Countries. *European Journal of Epidemiology, 36*, 519–530. Retrieved from https://doi.org/10.1007/s10654-021-00756-2
42. Donald K. A., et al. (2019). Risk and Protective Factors for Child Development: An Observational South African Birth Cohort. *PLoS Medicine, 16*(9), 1–20. Retrieved from https://doi.org/10.1371/journal.pmed.1002920
43. Girotra, S., Mohan, N., Malik, M., Roy, S., & Basu, S. (2023). Prevalence and Determinants of Low Birth Weight in India: Findings from a Nationally Representative Cross-Sectional Survey (2019–21). *Cureus, 15*(3), e36717. Retrieved from https://doi.org/10.7759/cureus.36717.
44. Blencowe, H., et al. (2019). National, Regional, and Worldwide Estimates of Low Birthweight in 2015, with Trends from 2000: A Systematic Analysis. *The Lancet Global Health, 7*(7), e849–e860.
45. Naaz, A., & Muneshwar, K. N. (2023). How Maternal Nutritional and Mental Health Affects Child Health During Pregnancy: A Narrative Review. *Cureus, 15*(11), e48763. Retrieved from https://doi.org/10.7759/cureus.48763.
46. Bush, N. R., et al. (2020). Family Environment, Neurodevelopmental Risk, and the Environmental Influences on Child Health Outcomes (ECHO) Initiative: Looking Back and Moving Forward. *Frontiers in Psy*chiatry, *11*, 547. Retrieved from https://doi.org/10.3389/fpsyt.2020.00547

47. Tung I., et al. (2023). Prenatal Stress and Externalizing Behaviors in Childhood and Adolescence: A Systematic Review and Meta-Analysis. *Psychological Bulletin, 150*(2), 107–131. Retrieved from https://doi.org/10.1037/bul0000407.
48. Zelka, M. A., Yalew, A. W., & Debelew, G. T. (2023). Effectiveness of a Continuum of Care in Maternal Health Services on the Reduction of Maternal and Neonatal Mortality: Systematic Review and Meta-Analysis. *Heliyon, 9*(6), e17559. Retrieved from https://doi.org/10.1016/j.heliyon.2023.e17559.
49. Seidu A. A., Ahinkorah B. O., Aboagye R. G., Okyere J., Budu E., & Yaya S. (2022). Continuum of Care for Maternal, Newborn, and Child Health in 17 Sub-Saharan African Countries. *BMC Health Services Research, 22*(1), 1394. Retrieved from https://doi.org/10.1186/s12913-022-08693-w
50. Iqbal, S., et al. (2017). Continuum of Care in Maternal, Newborn and Child Health in Pakistan: Analysis of Trends and Determinants from 2006 to 2012. *BMC Health Services Res*earch, *17*(189), 1–15. Retrieved from https://doi.org/10.1186/s12913-017-2111-9.
51. Kitila, S. B., Feyissa, G. T., Olika, A. K., & Wordofa, M. A. (2022). Maternal Healthcare in Low- and Middle-Income Countries: A Scoping Review. *Health Services Insights, 15*, 1–7. Retrieved from https://doi.org/10.1177/11786329221100310.
52. Khan, R., Vandelaer, J., Yakubu, A., Raza, A. A., & Zulu, F. (2015). Maternal and Neonatal Tetanus Elimination from Protecting Women and Newborns to Protecting All. *International Journal of Women's Health, 7*, 171–180. Retrieved from https://doi.org/10.2147/IJWH.S50539.
53. Dhir, S. K., Dewan, P., & Gupta, P. (2021). Maternal and Neonatal Tetanus Elimination: Where Are We Now?*Research Reports in Tropical Medicine, 12*, 247–261. Retrieved from https://doi.org/10.2147/RRTM.S201989.
54. Gavi, the Vaccine Alliance. (2023). *Vaccine Alliance Reaches More Than One Billion Children.* Gavi, the Vaccine Alliance. Retrieved from https://www.gavi.org/news/media-room/vaccine-alliance-reaches-more-one-billion-children.
55. Raut S., et al. (2022). Determinants of Maternal Influenza Vaccination in the Context of Low- and Middle-Income Countries: A Systematic Review. *PLoS ONE, 17*(1), e0262871. Retrieved from https://doi.org/10.1371/journal.pone.0262871
56. Lindstrand, A., Cherian, T., Chang-Blanc, D., Feikin, D., & O'Brien, K. L. (2021). The World of Immunization: Achievements, Challenges, and Strategic Vision for the Next Decade. *Journal of Infection Diseases, 224*(12), S452–S467. Retrieved from https://doi.org/10.1093/infdis/jiab284
57. Lassi, Z. S., Padhani, Z. A., Rabbani, A., Rind, F., Salam, R. A., & Bhutta, Z. A. (2021). Effects of Nutritional Interventions During Pregnancy on Birth, Child Health and Development Outcomes: A Systematic Review of Evidence from Low- and Middle-Income Countries. *Campbell Systematic Re*views, *17*(2), e1150–e1164. Retrieved from https://doi.org/10.1002/cl2.1150.
58. Victora, C. G., Christian, P., Vidaletti, L. P., Gatica-Domínguez, G., Menon, P., & Black, R. E. (2021). Revisiting Maternal and Child Undernutrition in Low-Income and Middle-Income Countries: Variable Progress Towards an Unfinished Agenda. *The Lancet, 397*(10282), 1388–1399. Retrieved from https://doi.org/10.1016/S0140-6736(21)00394-9.
59. Sanghvi, T., et al. (2022). Gaps in the Implementation and Uptake of Maternal Nutrition Interventions in Antenatal Care Services in Bangladesh, Burkina Faso, Ethiopia and India. *Maternal and Child Nutrition, 18*(2), e13293. Retrieved from https://doi.org/10.1111/mcn.13293.
60. Radhakrishnan, R., Brown, B. P., Haas, D. M., Zang, Y., Sparks, C., & Sadhasivam, S. (2022). Pilot Study of Fetal Brain Development and Morphometry in Prenatal Opioid Exposure and Smoking on Fetal MRI. Journal of Neuroradiology, *49*(1), 53–58. Retrieved from https://doi.org/10.1016/j.neurad.2020.12.004.
61. Huang X., et al. (2023). Deep Learning-Based Multiclass Brain Tissue Segmentation in Fetal MRIs. *Sensors, 23*(2), 655–678. Retrieved from https://doi.org/10.3390/s23020655.
62. Husna, R. N. S., Syafeeza, A. R., Hamid, N. A., Wong, Y. C., & Raihan, R. A. (2021). Functional Magnetic Resonance Imaging for Autism Spectrum Disorder Detection Using Deep Learning. *Journal of Technology, 83*(3), 45–52.

63. Marti-Castaner, M., Pavlenko, T., Engel, R., et al. (2022). Poverty After Birth: How Mothers Experience and Navigate U.S. Safety Net Programs to Address Family Needs. *Journal of Child and Family Studies, 31*(8), 2248–2265. https://doi.org/10.1007/s10826-022-02322-0
64. Khatri, R. B., Assefa, Y., & Durham, J. (2023). Multidomain and Multilevel Strategies to Improve Equity in Maternal and Newborn Health Services in Nepal: Perspectives of Health Managers and Policymakers. *International Journal for Equity in Health, 22*(1), 105.
65. Carlson, S., & Neuberger, Z. (2024). WIC Works: Addressing the Nutrition and Health Needs of Low-Income Families for More Than Four Decades. *Center on Budget and Policy Priorities.* Available from https://www.cbpp.org/research/food-assistance/wic-works-addressing-the-nutrition-and-health-needs-of-low-income-families
66. World Health Organization. (2021, December 7). WHO Recommendations on Antiplatelet Agents for the Prevention of Pre-eclampsia.
67. Parfenova, M., et al. (2021). Impact of an Educational Pamphlet on Knowledge About Health Risks After Hypertensive Disorders of Pregnancy: A Randomized Trial. *Journal of Obstetrics and Gynaecology Canada, 43*(2), 182–190. Retrieved from https://doi.org/10.1016/j.jogc.2020.07.008
68. Masoumian Hosseini, M., Masoumian Hosseini, S. T., Qayumi, K., Hosseinzadeh, S., & Sajadi Tabar, S. S. (2023). Smartwatches in Healthcare Medicine: Assistance and Monitoring: A Scoping Review. *BMC Medical Informatics and Decision Making, 23*(1), 248. Retrieved from https://doi.org/10.1186/s12911-023-02350-w.
69. Hod, M., Divakar, H., Kihara, A. B., & Geary, M. (2023). The Femtech Revolution—A New Approach to Pregnancy Management: Digital Transformation of Maternity Care—The Hybrid E-health Perinatal Clinic Addressing the Unmet Needs of Low-and Middle-Income Countries. *Interntional Journal of Gynecology and Obstetrics, 163*(1), 4–10.
70. Li, S., Yang, Q., Niu, S., & Liu, Y. (2023). Effectiveness of Remote Fetal Monitoring on Maternal-Fetal Outcomes: Systematic Review and Meta-Analysis. *JMIR mHealth and uHealth, 11*, e41508. Retrieved from https://doi.org/10.2196/41508.
71. Abera, M., et al. (2024). Effects of Relaxation Interventions During Pregnancy on Maternal Mental Health, and Pregnancy and Newborn Outcomes: A Systematic Review and meta-Analysis. *PloS One, 19*(1), e0278432. https://doi.org/10.1371/journal.pone.0278432.

Chapter 2
Maternal and Neo-Natal Health in Low- and Middle-Income (LMIC) Countries: The Role for mHealth Interventions

Tejal Barai Jaitly, Anuja Jayaraman, Kruti Dalal, Bhuvaneswari Sunil, and Aparna Hegde

Introduction

"Hundreds of pregnant women, alive at sunset last night never saw the sunrise this morning. Some of them died in labour, some died of haemorrhage in a hospital lacking blood, some died in the painful convulsions of eclampsia, and some died on the table of an unskilled abortionist trying to terminate an unwanted pregnancy" [1].

This statement made decades ago, holds true even today; and more than one million further maternal deaths are likely to occur worldwide by 2030 [2]. LMICs bear more than 90% of the burden of maternal mortality, with India having the highest burden of global maternal deaths, stillbirths, and newborn deaths [2] and highest burden of severe maternal morbidity (SMM), that can lead to higher maternal and neonatal deaths [3]. Worldwide, there is also increasing focus on maternal well-being [4].

Key Intervention Areas

Some of the high-risk pregnancy conditions include severe anaemia (haemoglobin less than 7gm/dl); pregnancy-induced hypertension, pre-eclampsia, pre-eclampsia toxaemia; gestational diabetes; young primi (<20 years) or elderly gravida (>

This chapter is partly based on an unpublished narrative review by ARMMAN.

T. B. Jaitly (✉) · A. Jayaraman · K. Dalal · B. Sunil · A. Hegde
ARMMAN, Mumbai, India
e-mail: tejal@armman.org

S. Suri (ed.), *Child Health and Nutrition from Conception to Age Two*,
https://doi.org/10.1007/978-981-95-7868-9_2

35 years); etc. [5]. There is a chance to improve maternal health during pregnancy as there is a higher likelihood of seeking care [4]. Antenatalcare(ANC),postnatalcare(PNC)alongwithsharinglifesavingpromotive and preventive care information are key strategies to saving the life of the pregnant mother and foetus [5].

The three delays model [6] to explain high maternal mortality remains relevant: decision to seek timely healthcare, reaching the appropriate health facility, and the quality of care. Several factors contribute to these delays; lack of birth preparedness and reliable information on care and danger signs, poor ANC, gender and patriarchy, cultural and social norms, poverty, and a weak referral system [7].

Folic acid supplementation given prior to conception can reduce the risk of neural tube defects by 47% [8]. Focusing on women of reproductive age, pregnant women, and newborns; LMICs can improve healthcare-seeking behaviour for neonatal morbidities by 42% [8]. Incorporating informative elements into maternal and newborn community-based intervention packages can reduce the risk of neonatal mortality by 13% (95% CI 4–20) and perinatal mortality by 17% (CI 9–25) [8].

The present chapter looks at use of mHealth interventions in the context of maternal and neo-natal health in LMICs and India. It highlights the conducive policy environment in India, and ARMMANs (Advancing Reduction in Mortality and Morbidity of Mothers, Children and Neonates) experience in mHealth. ARMMAN is a non-governmental organization that leverages technology and partnerships to save lives of mothers and children. In partnership with the Government of India (GoI), it implements the world's largest mobile-based maternal messaging programme and refresher training programme for frontline workers. The chapter delves into learnings, and how interventions are planned and implemented.

What Is mHealth?

Mobile technologies that are used to address healthcare challenges such as access, quality, affordability, matching of resources to needs, and behavioural changes are referred to as mHealth [9]. These technologies are primarily used to deliver and process information [10]. The adoption of mHealth interventions has been encouraged by the World Health Assembly Resolution on Digital Health, urging governments to utilize them for health-related needs and to work towards their development, evaluation, implementation, and scaling [11]. Their ease of use, easy availability, wide penetration and acceptance have contributed to this development [12].

The Push for mHealth in India

India's Maternal Mortality Ratio (MMR) is 97 per 100,000 live births [13]. According to the National Family Health Survey—5 (NFHS), only 58.5% of women aged 15–49 years had four or more ANC visits, 61% of women who were breastfeeding were anaemic, and 52% of women who are pregnant were anaemic, and only 79.1% of newborns received a PNC check-up within two days of their birth. The neonatal mortality rate (NNMR) was 24.9 deaths per 1000 live births [14]. The target is to reduce the MMR to 70 per 100,000 live births and NNMR to 12 per 1000 live births by 2030.

The policy environment in India is favourable. The National Health Policy (NHP) of India, 2017 [15] recognizes the integral role that technology can play through mobile health. It emphasizes leveraging the potential of digital tools to enhance efficiency and outcomes for the healthcare system.

In 2019, the Ministry of Health and Family Welfare (MOHFW), GoI, released the National Digital Health Blueprint (NDHB) [16]. Accordingly, all digital health services should be designed to be delivered based on the mobile-first principle. This was advocated to be the medium of choice for disseminating appropriate and curated content, information, health-related alerts, and updates on maternal and child health (MCH) to health workers on the ground. Thereby making mobile technologies an integral part of the envisioned ecosystem of digital health in the country. In India, there are more than 1.17 billion wireless subscribers, of which, more than 635 million users are in urban areas and more than 535 million in rural areas [17]. While this shows that India has good mobile penetration even in rural areas, some of the states have poor mobile tele-density. Jharkhand and Bihar have a mobile tele-density of only 57.55 and 50.65, respectively, whereas Delhi and Goa have the highest at 190.61 and 177.45, respectively [18]. The GoI aims to achieve universal access to mobile connectivity by 2030 targeting a mobile density[1] of 100; setting clear potential for mHealth in India [16].

Evidence Around mHealth Interventions in LMICs

Key focus areas for mHealth interventions in LMICs include information delivery, reminders for routine ANC visits, providing a platform for support from healthcare providers (HCPs), data collection by frontline workers (FLWs), improving test result turnaround times, and offering peer and psychological support interventions [19]. mHealth interventions were used by HCPs and health workers (HW) more commonly for communication, data collection, or educational purposes in the context of ANC, deliveries, and post-natal care (PNC) in several African and Asian countries [20]. A systematic review across LMIC countries found that the most reported use of

[1] Number of mobile connections per 100 persons.

mHealth interventions was client education and behaviour change communication (BCC); ANC and PNC registration and tracking of vital events and indicators [21].

mHealth interventions aimed at changing attitudes and addressing cultural norms that resist shifts in health-seeking behaviours have been found to improve the uptake of PNC services and skills, such as cord care, improved breastfeeding practices, and vaccinations [22]. Frontline workers using mHealth during home visits also led to increased involvement from male family members and improved access to PNC [23]. In Afghanistan [24], most women and men believed that including husbands in the programme encouraged joint decision-making. In Ethiopia, mHealth interventions motivated mothers to give birth with trained health workers present and to seek PNC promptly [25]. mHealth interventions are also very effective in overcoming traditional access barriers such as distance from clinic or lack of transport [26].

Too many messages can prove counterproductive and lead to recipient fatigue [26]. Studies from Cambodia, Bangladesh, and Kenya reported improvements in family planning outcomes when the information through mHealth technologies is delivered on a weekly or bi-weekly basis. However, too frequent messaging (0–3 messages per day for 4 months) did not resonate with participants, resulting in poor outcomes [26–29]. Too few messages were also found to not be impactful [30, 31].

In rural Liberia, trained birth attendants (TBA) used text messages for their data collection protocol, which led to 63.6% of them showing evidence of statistically significant increased knowledge as well as skill retention [32]. In studies across some LMICs [20, 33–39], HWs and midwives were able to learn using mobile phones as data collection tools with significant retention of knowledge and skills. HWs were able to update health statuses and thereby improve ANC and vaccinations with reduced delays. There was improved communication between HWs and superiors with respect to reporting emergencies, taking stock, requesting technical support, etc. HWs across LMICs in Africa and Asia were found to be more proactive in locating pregnant women, improved ANC follow-ups, and for updating the mother's ANC status at the healthcare facility [21, 40–44]. Usefulness and task-technology fit, besides ease of use of the Hayat app by HWs; were important considerations in a study in Pakistan and Afghanistan [45]. Thus, the app being in the local language, with a simple interface, made it easy for the HWs to adopt and use it.

A SWOT (strengths, weaknesses, opportunities, and threats) analysis across LMICs [26] found that mHealth interventions provided in the local language using locally developed software, had better chance to reach rural areas. The usefulness of text messages was doubtful when recipients are illiterate, and this factor also affected their success with HWs as well [46]. Lack of ownership or access to mobile phone; and dependence on connectivity and electricity were weaknesses. Opportunities include voice messages to address illiteracy, using women's groups to reach out to women with no access to mobile phone, the likelihood of its integration into the healthcare system, potential for collaboration with the government were the other identified opportunities. It has been noted through other studies [20, 47] that poor network coverage and electricity access were areas of concern. Nevertheless, they were found to be cost-effective than traditional communication methods. They also facilitated the integration of HWs across hierarchies and expedited emergency referrals. However, there is limited evidence regarding the scalability of mHealth interventions, as studies often overlook these aspects [19, 46].

Evidence Around mHealth Interventions in India

In India, efforts towards leveraging mHealth, though widespread, are fragmented and siloed in the context of maternal and neonatal health; leading to an overload and loss in fidelity [48].

Results from a study conducted in Gumballi, Karnataka on the Comprehensive Public Health Management (CPHM) app indicate that the field staff had to maintain and carry three different tablets. Yet they still had to enter data manually and maintain registers because supervisors were more comfortable in reviewing paper-based records. The fidelity of the intervention was thus compromised since the focus of HWs was more on completing the paper-based records [48]. The state of Bihar has seen the passage of several interventions, some simultaneously, often with overlapping functions and modes [49–51].

Several studies have reported improved outcomes. A study examining the Continuum of Care Services mHealth platform for FLWs in Bihar found that, in the intervention area, there were higher rates of pregnancy registrations, completion of three ANC visits, receiving at least 90 iron folic acid (IFA) tablets, facility-based delivery, early initiation of breastfeeding, and PNC visits. These indicators also showed improvement within the same district compared to the previous year. Data capture, which earlier involved an average delay of 72 days, was now possible in real-time. Increased ANC visits were noted in the intervention group, with some women even making six visits. Most women in the intervention group (85%) attended PNC visits, compared to only 21% in the control group [52].

mHealth interventions are also impacted by illiteracy, cultural norms, and gender. For any behaviour change, household relationships and practices steeped in culture must be negotiated. In a study in Uttar Pradesh [53], mothers-in-law were invited to watch mHealth videos. Even husbands were included as peripheral audience. Thus, a household level; community-centred approach was used. It was found that women were able to negotiate and exercise agency for the help they needed. In another study [54], voice messages regarding ANC, PNC, and neonatal care were sent on the husband's phone. These messages were discussed in 16% of the families. There was a significant increase in the possibility of the wives adopting improved health behaviour when husbands got involved in discussing the messages with family members. However, about one-fifth of all husbands shared that they were not interested in such messages as they did not see care during pregnancy as a matter pertaining to them.

Connectivity plays an important role in mHealth. In a study [55] in the tribal areas of Gujarat, four PHCs that covered 10% of villages without internet connectivity were omitted as these areas were less developed. This raises the question on the efficacy of mHealth interventions in reaching out to the poorest in backward regions.

mHealth interventions come with their diverse learnings and implementation challenges [49, 50]. In the implementation of the Common Application Software (CAS) [49] and the Mobile Midwife Platform [56], the research team noted that the Anganwadi workers (AWW) often focused on showing videos to beneficiaries instead of using them to facilitate and enhance counselling. There were also reports of shortened, rushed, and impersonal visits. The videos cannot substitute for interpersonal communication. This issue was also noted in the study on the ImTeCHO job aid [57] where the Accredited Social Health Activists (ASHAs) perceived that the videos were meant to reduce their task of counselling.

ARMMAN's Experience with mHealth

The Programmes

ARMMAN leverages technology to create cost-effective, scalable, equity-based, gender-transformative solutions to reduce maternal and child mortality and morbidity. It uses a "blended tech plus touch" model that leverages the existing FLW network and health infrastructure by building strong and sustainable partnerships with national and state governments, partnering with non-governmental organizations (NGOs) and government health facilities create without creating a parallel infrastructure (Table 2.1).

ARMMAN's programmes address the ground realities of culture and gender. The planned gender transformative *Kilkari* 2.0, in addition to the core offering of IVR calls, will offer beneficiaries with smartphones multimedia content such as videos, digital posters/images, and interactive quizzes via WhatsApp. The content is gender transformative to address the limiting socio-cultural and gender norms. The videos, for instance, depict husband helping with household chores and discussing wife's pregnancy needs with her. Similarly, the *Swasth Kadam* programme recommend foods that are affordable and can easily be weaved into the family's routine. This makes the mother feel empowered, and the approach is also sensitive to the family's meagre resources (intersectionality). In the case of the Arogya Sakhi programme, it was found that the testing of pregnant women in front of their families for blood pressure and haemoglobin etc.; made the families more involved as they got to see the results themselves. This interest was leveraged to involve the husbands and the mothers in law and use this opportunity to show preloaded videos that are functional even in the most backward tribal areas with no connectivity.

Table 2.1 ARMMAN's Programmes

Programme	States/district (as of May 2025) Total beneficiaries reached so far. (All of the programmes are being planned for scale-up)
KILKARI: the largest free mobile-based maternal messaging programme in the world, implemented by ARMMAN in partnership with the MOHFW, GoI. Critical preventive care information is shared in the form of recorded voice calls directly to the phones of pregnant women & mothers, from second trimester of pregnancy till the child is one year old. The planned gender transformative Kilkari 2.0 uses multiple delivery channels to deliver content and facilitate two-way communication	27 States and Union Territories (Kilkari) 60 million women and their children
Mobile Academy: largest free mobile-based training programme for health workers in the world, implemented in partnership with the MoHFW, GoI. Aimed at enhancing knowledge of ASHAs and improve the quality of their interactions. It is accessible by a simple mobile phone handset by dialling a short code. Mobile Academy (2.0) will incorporate multimedia content that will also address equity-based challenges	17 States and Union Territories 506,639 ASHAs trained
Integrated High-Risk Pregnancy Tracking and Management (IHRPTM): Capacity building of ANMs, medical officers and specialists. Provide them with decision-supported management strategies such as management protocols, self-learning apps, referral protocols, and real-time data collection app integrated with the state's data collection system/RCH portal	With State governments and UNICEF -Telangana, Uttar Pradesh, Andhra Pradesh 9647 nurses trained, 4432 Medical officers and 758 Specialist doctors
Swasth Kadam: Identify Moderately Underweight children using the "weight for age" WHO Growth Chart. Their caregivers are supported through live telephonic counselling for 8–12 weeks and dissemination of information via WhatsApp for a period of 6 months	Maharashtra (Select districts). 6483 Caregivers reached

(continued)

Table 2.1 (continued)

Programme	**States/district (as of May 2025) Total beneficiaries reached so far. (All of the programmes are being planned for scale-up)**
Arogya Sakhi (AS): Home-Based Antenatal and Infancy Care programme; trains and equips ASHAs (AS) in underserved rural and tribal areas. HWs are provided with a medical kit for basic diagnostic tests and a tablet encoded with an application-based decision support algorithm that guides them through the process. They enter the results in the application on their tablets that alert them in case of high-risk conditions and prompts them on the next steps	Maharashtra (Select districts) 309 AS trained, 11,061 pregnant women supported, 11,004 children reached
mMitra: Started in 2013 as ARMMAN's pioneering free mobile voice call service sending preventive care messages. The success of mMitra led to an invitation from MoHFW, GoI in 2018 to implement Kilkari	Was previously implemented in 9 states
mMitra + + : is designed to take a "tech + touch," fit-for-purpose approach towards improving the health outcomes for pregnant women and children who are at high risk in these urban and peri-urban slums	Mumbai
MaMitra: In partnership with the Brihanmumbai Municipal Corporation (BMC), it aims to strengthen the public health system by ensuring accurate records of pregnant women and mothers, tracking high-risk pregnancies and providing health information	11 BMC-run hospitals across Mumbai

Source (www.armman.org)

Evidence and Learnings

There were positive findings across several studies. In a 2020 impact assessment of m*Mitra* [58], women in the intervention group performed significantly better on four maternal health practice indicators—-receiving tetanus toxoid (TT) injections, consulting a doctor for spotting or bleeding, birth preparedness, and opting for facility-based delivery. The control group performed significantly better regarding resting regularly and having at-home deliveries attended by a skilled birth attendant (SBA).

An Impact Performance Report for *Kilkari* [59] noted that three in four beneficiaries reported significant improvements in knowledge and behaviour relating to child-related practices, and four in five beneficiaries reported improved breastfeeding for over 6 months. It is important to note that 95% of the beneficiaries in the study did not have previous exposure to any mHealth programme like *Kilkari* (Tables 2.2 and 2.3).

Table 2.2 Insights from the *Kilkari* impact study [59]

Satisfaction/outcomes as reported by beneficiaries	Percentage of beneficiaries
Found the call "very effective"	90
Found calls easy to understand and apply to their lives	80
Increased their uptake of regular check-ups	64
Increase in uptake of emergency care for child	54
Factors identified by beneficiaries that can help to increase in uptake	
Availability of "free services" as a factor to increase the uptake	40
Receiving clearer messages	23
Better support from ASHAs/ANMs	19
How useful was the information received? (% noted for those who reported "very useful")	
Injections and vaccinations	94
Hygiene	92
Diet for the children	89
Family planning	87
How much of information was applied into daily lives?	
Injections and vaccinations	86
Hygiene	82
Diet for the children	78
Family planning	71

Table 2.3 mMitra RCT [61]

Key outcomes ($p < 0.05$)	Baseline (%)	Endline (%)
Proportion of women who sought treatment for complications during pregnancy	72	96
Proportion of women who suffered from pregnancy-related complications	38	9
Proportion of women who were aware of the importance of immunization during pregnancy	61	97
Proportion of women who were aware of immunization schedules during infancy	71	93
Proportion of women who were aware of the period of exclusive breastfeeding	66	83
Proportion of women who were aware of the importance of giving colostrum to the baby	72	91
Proportion of women who were aware of the harmful effects of pre-lacteal feeds	41.35	88

In an impact study on MA [60] two-thirds of ASHAs reported improved MCH knowledge. They felt empowered and found to have improved communication skills.

In a randomized control trial (RCT) to evaluate the impact of m*Mitra* and *Arogya Sakhi* [61], significant improvements ($p < 0.05$) in some of the key women's reproductive and child health knowledge and behaviours were observed.

However, these findings did not align well with other studies [62]. In the *Kilkari* RCT arm of the study, some health indicators like exclusive breastfeeding showed very little difference by socio-economic position. Improvements in other indicators, such as sterilization, were more visible among the economically weaker section. Socio-cultural norms also presented implementation and adoption challenges [63]. Women who did not own a phone themselves were difficult to reach and could not access the messages shared on the husband's phones. Messages received by husbands, were rarely discussed with wives. Thus, patriarchy hindered information from reaching beneficiaries. Cultural norms also play a significant role in influencing behaviour change, while beneficiaries reported trusting *Kilkari,* they continued with the practices contrary to *Kilkari's* recommendations [63]. Findings from another study suggested when husbands listened to *KilKari* messages, it helped in improving father's knowledge, that resulted in likelihood of infants aged 0–12 months to receive birth vaccines on time [64]. However, this did not result in complete and comprehensive immunization.

mHealth has the potential to overcome the existing cultural norms, but the intervention's success may be stunted due to supply chain factors [65]. In a study on the m*Mitra* intervention, many primigravida women shared that it was their in-laws that took decisions such as registration at health facilities, ANC, IFA consumption, etc. HWs have also shared the associated taboos behind IFA, that their consumption would lead to the birth of a dark-skinned child. Women shared they need to have exceptional courage to challenge these cultural norms, particularly when it came to IFA and pregnancy scans; and that *mMitra* has the potential to transform orthodox beliefs, perceptions, and behaviours of their families. Women who never sought early ANC or consumed IFA in their early pregnancies did so after listening to *mMitra* calls. However, consumption of IFA was also determined by its availability at health centres.

Discussion

A public health intervention is defined as "planned actions to prevent or reduce a particular health problem, or the determinants of the problem, in a defined population" [66]. Fundamentally, mHealth interventions are public health interventions, and the impact of mHealth interventions can be attenuated by the same factors that affect conventional interventions, viz., traditional, and structural barriers such as lack of transport, gender, patriarchy, poverty, and literacy; as well as health system constraints [67].

There are several advantages of mHealth that have contributed to its widespread impact and acceptance. They are characterized by flexibility and adaptability, and there are also several innovative ways and modes of using mHealth. mHealth interventions can share the critical and routine care information multiple times in a short span with beneficiaries.

These attributes of mHealth interventions are very important in the Indian context. Overcrowded facilities severely restrict the quality of information being shared during visits, and it is often not possible for women to completely comprehend or remember the information that has been shared, that can be addressed with the help of mHealth. Thus, mHealth also helps overcome traditional barriers in seeking care and information leading to it to facilitating and improving care seeking and outcomes as noted across several studies; oftentimes also contributing in building women's agency [22, 26, 52–54, 58, 59, 61, 65].

Moreover, mHealth has proven to be a valuable educational and capacity-building tool for FLWs that is implementable based on convenience and needs of the HWs. Their roles and tasks in the communities have been guided by mHealth. There are some encouraging evidences supporting this, as several HWs felt that their tasks were simplified by mHealth-enabled systems of identification and referral of critical cases and improved communication with superiors. Additionally, there were improved MCH knowledge and skill retention; and HWs felt empowered with enhanced communication skills. mHealth also facilitated crucial and quick data collection and transfer, leading to improved response times [20, 21, 32–44, 47, 60]. With the mHealth intervention researchers have noted improvement in data capturing speed that earlier took an average of 72 days [52]. Quickerinformationconnectivitywith-healthcentres and data information systems, thus reduced delays to help monitor pregnant women.

There is also evidence of challenges. HWs reported an increased workload, with added responsibilities such as curative care. In fact, there is a threat of increased cognitive load on ASHAs because of mHealth [68]. Also, there is loss in fidelity of interventions due to implementation challenges; and as a result of multiple programmes running in parallel [48].

Involving husbands through mHealth also delivered positive results [24, 54, 58]. Furthermore, women could be empowered with the right information to negotiate with their families for the care that they need [53, 54]. It has also been found that even the most marginalized women have indeed been reached through mHealth messaging [61, 64]. In the context of shared phones in families, studies have also reported that the husband was not likely to share or discuss the content of interventions as maternal health was not seen as their domain [55, 63]. According to NFHS–5 [69], several states have shown a high proportion of women not owning mobile phones, with the worst figures being for the states of Andhra Pradesh, Bihar, Gujarat, and West Bengal where only about 50% of women own and use a mobile phone. It is inevitable that such gender-based digital inequality would affect the ability of mHealth interventions to deliver results equitably. However, at the same time, there is evidence to show that when mHealth interventions if planned to address the cultural norms, they were found to be more effective [22, 26, 63].

Innovations in technology are also used to address challenges, such as those related to equity and distribution. For instance, with a focus on improving listenership through artificial intelligence (AI), it was found [70] that specially designed algorithms could prevent mothers from missing health messages. Another study [71] found that ML (machine learning) can improve the prediction of low listenership from 5% (as obtained through random selection) to 25%.

Aligned with the government programmes, mHealth has an important role to play. When FLWs undergo refresher trainings, have improved skills and communication; it contributes to overall quality of care. Or when ANMs, medical officers, etc. are trained to manage, and track high-risk pregnancy conditions; this would lead to rationalization of load on tertiary care systems. When such mHealth programmes are implemented at scale, they play a role in overall health system strengthening.

Recommendations

1. A key question in planning mHealth interventions is what unique advantages they could offer over conventional interventions, and how best can this advantage be utilized. For example, mHealth can enable low-cost refresher trainings for HWs, quick data capture or swift outreach to large populations. When well-planned, mHealth can help address misinformation, increase awareness, empower women, and reduce cultural and traditional barriers that hinder the adoption of health behaviours. However, mHealth interventions should complement, not replace conventional interventions such as interpersonal counselling by FLWs. This symbiotic relationship strengthens the health system.
2. In India, the approach towards mHealth can be seen as fragmented and siloed [72]. However, through continuous learning evolution of nationwide programmes like *Kilkari* and MA (KMA) are examples that large-scale cost-effective solutions are possible, and fragmentation can be avoided. A key strategy of KMA is the use of the "blended tech plus touch" model i.e. working alongside the government and existing networks and not creating parallel structures.
3. The role and support of governments and the public health system is vital to the success of any mHealth intervention. Countries need to ensure governance and standardization of mHealth for the development of a sound ecosystem based on credible, replicable evidence with regulatory and monitoring mechanisms in place. Government support is also needed for scalability and sustainability of mHealth programmes.
4. Implementation research should aim at addressing equity challenges and strengthening of health system and making use of findings for planning at the policy and programme level. The aim is to have the highest health impact for the majority of people in an equitable manner; and study how and why an innovation works and how best to scale it. It is also important to undertake studies to assess how behaviour change models can be applied to mHealth interventions and to

gauge how they are able to address norms and attitudes at the individual and community levels sustainably [73].
5. Before introducing any new mHealth intervention, complete systemic preparation and training is a must. For example, in making the shift to electronic medical records; supervisors, district officials, and all linked stakeholders should be trained to be intervention ready. Interventions should be closely monitored to ensure fidelity, appropriate use, and implementation.
6. mHealth studies should follow set benchmarks and standardized formats for reporting, across innovations and countries. The WHO mHealth Technical Evidence Review Group developed evidence reporting and assessment (mERA) checklist [74] is one such checklist.
7. Ethics, privacy issues, and data security must be prioritized to ensure that mHealth interventions do not jeopardize people's rights and do more harm than good.

Conclusion

mHealth interventions are here to stay. In India, despite a conducive policy environment and rapid technological growth, that also focuses on making technology accessible and available to the poor, the full potential of mHealth interventions is yet to be realized.

The evidence around mHealth is still emerging and has been varied even in similar contexts. Evidence around mHealth interventions delivered at scale is also in its early stages. To integrate mHealth within countries' health systems, governments must take a leading role in the development of such an ecosystem from the front.

The greatest challenge in improving health lies not in developing new technologies or interventions, but in enhancing how these are implemented, integrated, and delivered within systems [75]. Optimal implementation and integration within health systems require ongoing exploration and evidence generation to leverage their strengths, while addressing the weaknesses.

"Such technologies are no longer a luxury; they are a necessity. A key challenge is to ensure that all people enjoy the benefits of digital technologies for everyone. We must make sure that innovation and technology helps to reduce the inequities in our world, instead of becoming another reason people are left behind. Countries must be guided by evidence to establish sustainable harmonized digital systems, not seduced by every new gadget."—Dr. Tedros Adhanom Ghebreyesus [11].

References

1. Hussein, A. (1998). WHO at Fifty: 4. Highlights of Activities from 1989 to 1998. *World Health Forum, 19(4)*, 441–56.
2. World Health Organization. (2023). *Trends in Maternal Mortality 2000 to 2020: Estimates by WHO, UNICEF, UNFPA, World Bank Group and UNDESA/Population Division.*

3. Geller, S. E., Koch, A. R., Garland, C. E., MacDonald, E. J., Storey, F., & Lawton, B. (2018). A Global View of Severe Maternal Morbidity: Moving Beyond Maternal Mortality. *Reproductive Health, 15*, 31–43.
4. Firoz, T., et al. (2018). A Framework for Healthcare Interventions to Address Maternal Morbidity. *International Journal of Gynecology & Obstetrics, 141*, 61–68.
5. Ministry of Health and Family Welfare. (2016). *Pradhan Mantri Surakshit Matritva Abhiyan*. MOHFW. Retrieved from https://pmsma.mohfw.gov.in/wp-content/uploads/2016/10/High-Risk-Conditions-in-preg-modified-Final.pdf
6. Thaddeus, S., & Maine, D. (1994). Too Far to Walk: Maternal Mortality in Context. *Social Science & Medicine, 38*(8), 1091–1110.
7. Actis Danna, V., Bedwell, C., Wakasiaka, S., & Lavender, T. (2020). Utility of the Three-delays Model and its Potential for Supporting a Solution-based Approach to Accessing Intrapartum Care in Low- and middle-income Countries. A Qualitative Evidence Synthesis. *Global Health Action, 13*(1). Retrieved from https://doi.org/10.1080/16549716.2020.1819052
8. Vaivada, T., et al. (2022). What Can Work and How? An Overview of Evidence-based Interventions and Delivery Strategies to Support Health and Human Development from Before Conception to 20 Years. *The Lancet, 399*(10337), 1810–1829.
9. Kay, M., Santos, J., & Takane, M. (2011). MHealth: New Horizons for Health Through Mobile Technologies. *World Health Organization, 64*(7), 66–71.
10. Hausman, V., Miller, R., Qiang, Z., & Yamamichi, M. (2011). *Mobile Applications for the Health Sector (English)*. World Bank Group. Retrieved from http://documents.worldbank.org/curated/en/751411468157784302/Mobile-applications-for-the-health-sector
11. WHO Guideline: Recommendations on Digital Interventions for Health System Strengthening. World Health Organization, 2019. Licence: CC BY-NC-SA 3.0 IGO.
12. World Health Organization. (2023).*Classification of Digital Interventions, Services and Applications in Health: A Shared Language to Describe the Uses of Digital Technology for Health* (2nd ed.). Licence: CC BY-NC-SA 3.0 IGO.
13. Ministry of Health and Family Welfare. (2021). *Maternal Mortality Rate (MMR)*. Retrieved from https://www.pib.gov.in/PressReleasePage.aspx?PRID=1697441
14. International Institute for Population Sciences (IIPS) and ICF. (2021). *National Family Health Survey (NFHS-5)*, India, 2019–21, IIPS.
15. Ministry of Health and Family Welfare. (2017). *National Health Policy 2017*. Government of India. Retrieved from https://www.nhp.gov.in/nhpfiles/national_health_policy_2017.pdf
16. Ministry of Health and Family Welfare. (2019). *National Digital Health Blueprint*. Government of India. Retrieved from https://main.mohfw.gov.in/sites/default/files/Final%20NDHB%20report_0.pdf
17. Telecom Regulatory Authority of India. (2024). *Highlights of Telecom Subscription Data as on May, 2021* [Press Release]. No. 65/2024. Retrieved from https://www.trai.gov.in/sites/default/files/PR_No.65of2024.pdf
18. NITI Aayog. (2021). *SDG India: Index and Dashboard 2020–21. Partnerships in the Decade of Action*. NITI Ayog and United Nations.
19. Lee, S. H., Nurmatov, U. B., Nwaru, B. I., Mukherjee, M., Grant, L., & Pagliari, C. (2016). Effectiveness of mHealth Interventions for Maternal, Newborn and Child Health in Low- and middle-income Countries: Systematic Review and Meta–Analysis. *Journal of Global Health, 6*(1). Retrieved from https://doi.org/10.7189/jogh.06.010401
20. Amoakoh-Coleman, M., et al. (2016). Effectiveness of mHealth Interventions Targeting Health Care Workers to Improve Pregnancy Outcomes in Low-and middle-income Countries: A Systematic Review. *Journal of Medical Internet Research, 18*(8), Article e226.
21. Feroz, A., Perveen, S., & Aftab, W. (2017). Role of mHealth Applications for Improving Antenatal and Postnatal Care in Low- and middle-income Countries: A Systematic Review. *BMC Health Services Research, 17*, 1–11.
22. Mbuthia, F., Reid, M., & Fichardt, A. (2019). MHealth Communication to Strengthen Postnatal Care in Rural Areas: A Systematic Review. *BMC Pregnancy and Childbirth, 19*, 1–10.

23. Mangwi Ayiasi, R., Atuyambe, L. M., Kiguli, J., Orach, C. G., Kolsteren, P., & Criel, B. (2015). Use of Mobile Phone Consultations During Home Visits by Community Health Workers for Maternal and Newborn Care: Community Experiences from Masindi and Kiryandongo Districts, Uganda. *BMC Public Health, 15*, 1–13.
24. Lebrun, V., et al. (2020). Feasibility and Acceptability of an Adapted Mobile Phone Message Program and Changes in Maternal and Newborn Health Knowledge in Four Provinces of Afghanistan: Single-Group Pre-Post Assessment Study. *JMIR mHealth and uHealth, 8*(7), Article e17535.
25. Atnafu, A., Otto, K., & Herbst, C. H. (2017). The Role of mHealth Intervention on Maternal and Child Health Service Delivery: Findings from a Randomized Controlled Field Trial in Rural Ethiopia. *Mhealth, 3*.
26. Sondaal, S. F. V., et al. (2016). Assessing the Effect of mHealth Interventions in Improving Maternal and Neonatal Care in Low- and Middle-income Countries: A Systematic Review. *PLoS ONE, 11*(5), Article e0154664.
27. Aung, B., Mitchell, J. W., & Braun, K. L. (2020). Effectiveness of mHealth Interventions for Improving Contraceptive Use in Low- and Middle-income Countries: A Systematic Review. *Global Health: Science and Practice, 8*(4), 813–26. Retrieved from https://www.ghspjournal.org/content/ghsp/8/4/813.full.pdf
28. McCarthy, O., et al. (2018). A Randomized Controlled Trial of an Intervention Delivered by Mobile Phone App Instant Messaging to Increase the Acceptability of Effective Contraception Among Young People in Tajikistan. *Reproductive Health, 15*, 1–14.
29. McCarthy, O. L., et al. (2019). A Randomized Controlled Trial of an Intervention Delivered by Mobile Phone Text Message to Increase the Acceptability of Effective Contraception Among Young Women in Palestine. *Trials, 20*, 1–13.
30. Johnson, D., et al. (2017). A Randomized Controlled Trial of the Impact of a Family Planning mHealth Service on Knowledge and Use of Contraception. *Contraception, 95*(1), 90–97.
31. Maslowsky, J., Frost, S., Hendrick, C. E., Cruz, F. O. T., & Merajver, S. D. (2016). Effects of Postpartum Mobile Phone-Based Education on Maternal and Infant Health in Ecuador. *International Journal of Gynecology & Obstetrics, 134*(1), 93–98.
32. Munro, M. L., Lori, J. R., Boyd, C. J., & Andreatta, P. (2014). Knowledge and Skill Retention of a Mobile Phone Data Collection Protocol in Rural Liberia. *Journal of Midwifery & Women's Health, 59*(2), 176–183.
33. Lemay, N. V., Sullivan, T., Jumbe, B., & Perry, C. P. (2012). Reaching Remote Health Workers in Malawi: Baseline Assessment of a Pilot mHealth Intervention. *Journal of Health Communication, 17*(1), 105–117.
34. Little, A., Medhanyie, A., Yebyo, H., Spigt, M., Dinant, G. J., & Blanco, R. (2013). Meeting Community Health Worker Needs for Maternal Health Care Service Delivery Using Appropriate Mobile Technologies in Ethiopia. *PLoS ONE, 8*(10), Article e77563.
35. Lori, J. R., Munro, M. L., Boyd, C. J., & Andreatta, P. (2012). Cell Phones to Collect Pregnancy Data from Remote Areas in Liberia. *Journal of Nursing Scholarship, 44*(3), 294–301.
36. Andreatta, P., Gans-Larty, F., Debpuur, D., Ofosu, A., & Perosky, J. (2011). Evaluation of Simulation-based Training on the Ability of Birth Attendants to Correctly Perform Bimanual Compression as Obstetric First Aid. *International Journal of Nursing Studies, 48*(10), 1275–1280.
37. Ngabo, F., et al. (2012). Designing and Implementing an Innovative SMS-based Alert System (RapidSMS-MCH) to Monitor Pregnancy and Reduce Maternal and Child Deaths in Rwanda. *The Pan African Medical Journal, 13*.
38. McNabb, M., et al. (2015). Assessment of the Quality of Antenatal Care Services Provided by Health Workers using a Mobile Phone Decision Support Application in Northern Nigeria: A Pre/Post-intervention Study. *PLoS ONE, 10*(5), Article e0123940.
39. Seidenberg, P., et al. (2012). Early Infant Diagnosis of HIV Infection in Zambia Through Mobile Phone Texting of Blood Test Results. *Bulletin of the World Health Organization, 90*, 348–356.

40. Entsieh, A. A., Emmelin, M., & Pettersson, K. O. (2015). Learning the ABCs of Pregnancy and Newborn Care Through Mobile Technology. *Global Health Action, 8*(1), 29340.
41. Jennings, L., Omoni, A., Akerele, A., Ibrahim, Y., & Ekanem, E. (2015). Disparities in Mobile Phone Access and Maternal Health Service Utilization in Nigeria: A Population-Based Survey. *International Journal of Medical Informatics, 84*(5), 341–348.
42. Lau, Y. K., Cassidy, T., Hacking, D., Brittain, K., Haricharan, H. J., & Heap, M. (2014). Antenatal Health Promotion Via Short Message Service at a Midwife Obstetrics Unit in South Africa: A Mixed Methods Study. *BMC Pregnancy and Childbirth, 14*, 1–8.
43. Lund, S., et al. (2014). Mobile Phones Improve Antenatal Care Attendance in Zanzibar: A Cluster Randomized Controlled Trial. *BMC Pregnancy and Childbirth, 14*, 1–10.
44. Adanikin, A. I., Awoleke, J. O., & Adeyiolu, A. (2014). *Role of Reminder by Text Message in Enhancing Postnatal Clinic Attendance.*
45. Zaidi, S., et al. (2020). Operability, Usefulness, and Task-technology Fit of an mhealth app for Delivering Primary Health Care Services by Community Health Workers in Underserved Areas of Pakistan and Afghanistan: Qualitative Study. *Journal of Medical Internet Research, 22*(9), Article e18414.
46. Ahmed, M. A. A., Gagnon, M. P., Hamelin-Brabant, L., Mbemba, G. I. C., & Alami, H. (2017). A Mixed Methods Systematic Review of Success Factors of mhealth and Telehealth for Maternal Health in Sub-Saharan Africa. *Mhealth, 3*, 22.
47. Colaci, D., Chaudhri, S., & Vasan, A. (2016). MHealth Interventions in Low-income Countries to Address Maternal Health: A Systematic Review. *Annals of Global Health, 82*(5), 922–935.
48. Shilpa, D. M., Naik, P. R., Shewade, H. D., & Sudarshan, H. (2020). Assessing the Implementation of a Mobile App-based Electronic Health Record: A Mixed-Method Study from South India. *Journal of Education and Health Promotion, 9*, 48.
49. Gopalakrishnan, L., Buback, L., Fernald, L., Walker, D., Diamond-Smith, N., & in addition to The CAS Evaluation Consortium. (2020). Using mHealth to Improve Health Care Delivery in India: A Qualitative Examination of the Perspectives of Community Health Workers and Beneficiaries. *PloS One, 15*(1), e0227451.
50. Borkum, E., et al. (2015). Evaluation of the Information and Communication Technology (ICT) Continuum of Care Services (CCS) Intervention in Bihar. *Mathematica Policy Research.*
51. Ward, V., et al. (2021). Implementing Health Communication Tools at Scale: Mobile Audio Messaging and Paper-based Job Aids for Front-line Workers Providing Community Health Education to Mothers in Bihar India. *BMJ Global Health, 6*(5), Article e005538.
52. Balakrishnan, R., Gopichandran, V., Chaturvedi, S., Chatterjee, R., Mahapatra, T., & Chaudhuri, I. (2016). Continuum of Care Services for Maternal and Child Health Using Mobile Technology–A Health System Strengthening Strategy in Low- and middle-income Countries. *BMC Medical Informatics and Decision Making, 16*, 1–8.
53. Kumar, N. & Anderson, R. J. (2015). Mobile Phones for Maternal Health in Rural India. In *Proceedings of the 33rd Annual ACM Conference on Human Factors in Computing Systems*, pp. 427–36.
54. Hazra, A., Khan, M. E., & Mondal, S. K. (2018). Mobile Phone Messaging to Husbands to Improve Maternal and Child Health Behavior in India. *Journal of Health Communication, 23*(6), 542–549.
55. Modi, D., et al. (2019). MHealth Intervention "ImTeCHO" to Improve Delivery of Maternal, Neonatal, and Child Care Services—A Cluster-Randomized Trial in Tribal Areas of Gujarat India. *PLoS Medicine, 16*(10), Article e1002939.
56. Fiore-Silfvast, B., et al. (2013). Mobile Video for Patient Education: The Midwives' Perspective. In *Proceedings of the 3rd ACM Symposium on Computing for Development*, pp. 1–10.
57. Shah, P., et al. (2019). High Uptake of An Innovative Mobile Phone Application Among Community Health Workers in Rural India: An Implementation Study. *The National Medical Journal of India, 32*(5), 262–269.
58. Murthy, N., et al. (2020). Effects of An mHealth Voice Message Service (mMitra) on Maternal Health Knowledge and Practices of Low-Income Women in India: Findings from a Pseudo-Randomized CONTROLLED Trial. *BMC Public Health, 20*, 1–10.

59. Decibels. (2023). *ARMMAN Kilkari Impact Performance Report*. www.armman.org
60. Decibels. (2023). *ARMMAN Mobile Academy Impact Performance Report*. www.armman.org
61. ARMMAN. (2016). *Randomised Cluster Trial: mMitra and Arogya Sakhi*. www.armman.org
62. Mohan, D., et al. (2021). Can Health Information Through Mobile Phones Close the Divide in Health Behaviours Among the Marginalised? An Equity Analysis of Kilkari in Madhya Pradesh India. *BMJ Global Health, 6*(5), Article e005512.
63. Scott, K., et al. (2021). Another Voice in the Crowd: The Challenge of Changing Family Planning and Child Feeding Practices Through mHealth Messaging in Rural Central India. *BMJ Global Health, 6*(5), Article e005868.
64. Chakraborty, A., et al. (2021). Does Exposure to Health Information Through Mobile Phones Increase Immunisation Knowledge, Completeness and Timeliness in Rural India? *BMJ Global Health, 6*(5), Article e005489.
65. Hegde, A., et al. Opportunities to Augment the Maternal and Infant Health Services Using mHealth: Qualitative Evidence of Narratives from the Recipients of mMitra Services and Health Care Providers in Mumbai, India. ARMMAN.
66. Wight, D., Wimbush, E., Jepson, R., & Doi, L. (2016). Six Steps in Quality Intervention Development (6SQuID). *Journal of Epidemiology and Community Health, 70*(5), 520–525.
67. Campbell, N. C., et al. (2007). Designing and Evaluating Complex Interventions to Improve Health Care. *BMJ, 334*(7591), 455–459.
68. DeRenzi, B., et al. (2016). Closing the Feedback Loop: A 12-month Evaluation of ASTA, A Self-tracking Application for ASHAs. In *Proceedings of the Eighth International Conference on Information and Communication Technologies and Development*, pp. 1–10.
69. International Institute for Population Sciences (IIPS) and ICF. (2021). *National Family Health Survey (NFHS-5), 2019*. Retrieved from https://dhsprogram.com/pubs/pdf/FR375/FR375.pdf
70. Killian, J. A., et al. (2023). Robust Planning Over Restless Groups: Engagement Interventions for a Large-scale Maternal Telehealth Program. In *Proceedings of the AAAI Conference on Artificial Intelligence*, vol. 37, no. 12, pp. 14295–303.
71. Shah S., et al. (2023). Preliminary Results in Low-listenership Prediction in One of the Largest Mobile Health Programs in the World. In AAMAS 2023 Workshop on *Autonomous Agents for Social Good*.
72. Kodali, P. B., & Das, S. (2021). Acceptance of mHealth Technologies Among Auxiliary Nurse Midwives in Andhra Pradesh, India: A Mixed Method Study. *Medical Science, 25*(111), 1052–1060.
73. United States Agency for International Development. (2020). *Changing Health Seeking Behaviour*. Retrieved from https://www.usaid.gov/global-health/health-systems-innovation/healthsystems/changing-health-seeking-behavior
74. Agarwal, S., et al. (2016). Guidelines for Reporting of Health Interventions Using Mobile Phones: Mobile Health (mHealth) EVIDENCE Reporting and Assessment (mERA) Checklist. *BMJ, 352*.
75. Hoffman, S. J., Røttingen, J. A., Bennett, S., Lavis, J. N., Edge, J. S., & Frenk, J. (2012). Background Paper on Conceptual Issues Related to Health Systems Research to Inform a WHO Global Strategy on Health Systems Research. *Health Systems Alliance*.

Part II
Critical Interventions to Promote Child Nutrition

Chapter 3
Infant and Young Child Feeding (IYCF) Practices: Significance, Policies, Programmes, Key Learnings and Way Forward

Sheila Vir, Shoba Suri, and Rupal Dalal

IYCF: An Immediate Determinant of Child Nutritional Status

The conceptual framework of child undernutrition indicates that most immediate causes of malnutrition comprise inadequate diet and poor nutrient intake as well as occurrence of infections and other diseases (Fig. 3.1). Moreover, insufficient and inadequate dietary intake and infections create a vicious cycle responsible for poor physical growth and cognitive development, child undernutrition, poor immune response, high morbidity, and mortality among children in the developing countries. Appropriate infant and young child feeding (IYCF) practice is a critical determinant of child nutrition, survival, growth, and development.

Interventions for promoting appropriate IYCF practices are globally accepted important evidence-based interventions which require special attention for prevention of child undernutrition [1]. Additionally, as presented in Fig. 3.1, the context-specific nutrition sensitive interventions need to be addressed for overcoming food insecurity, improving diet diversity, health services, water-sanitation-hygiene (WASH) practices, and women's health care and status. Child health services such as ensuring universal coverage of routine immunization, care practices for prevention and management of diseases such as diarrhoea, worm infestation play a crucial role.

S. Vir (✉)
Public Health Nutrition and Development Centre (PHNDC), New Delhi, India
e-mail: sheila.vir@gmail.com

S. Suri
Observer Research Foundation, New Delhi, India

R. Dalal
Centre for Technology Alternatives in Rural Areas, IIT Bombay, Mumbai, India

S. Suri (ed.), *Child Health and Nutrition from Conception to Age Two*,
https://doi.org/10.1007/978-981-95-7868-9_3

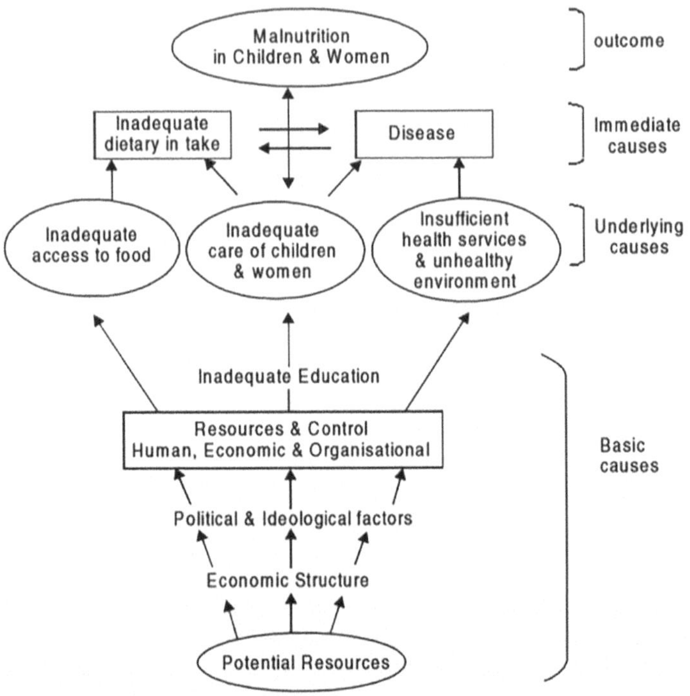

Fig. 3.1 Conceptual framework of malnutrition in children and women. *Source* UNICEF (1998) State of the World's Children Report

First 1000 Days: IYCF an Essential Nutrition Intervention

Inappropriate IYCF practices combined with a high incidence of low birth weight contribute to growth retardation in under two years of age with a higher chance of a child being undernourished at 24 months [2]. It is well established that interventions for nutrition care in the first 1000 days of life (270 days of pregnancy and 730 days of first two years of life of a child) are the most critical intervention to prevent child undernutrition since substantial growth faltering occurs during the pregnancy in place of prenatal period and the first 6 months of life with faltering continuing till 2 years of age, in many low middle-income countries (LMICs) [3, 4].

In 2001, Shrimpton et al. [5] presented the global evidence that undernutrition in children increases steadily in the first 24 months of life (Fig. 3.2). A nutrition survey conducted in the largest state of India, Uttar Pradesh (UP) state in 2000 reported that percentage of underweight children increases between 0 and 24 months [6]. In 2006, WHO presented with child growth standards for under six months, Using the WHO standards, child undernutrition was assessed in under 6 months infants [7], and it was confirmed that the prevalence of stunting and underweight increased steadily up to 24 months, reached its peak at about two years of age and then stabilized. India's large National Family Health Survey (NFHS) 2005–2006 and the subsequent two surveys confirmed that between 0 and 24 months of age, the prevalence rate of both underweight and stunting increased with age [8–10]. As per 2015–2016 NFHS 4, the rate of underweight being almost 30% at 6 months and increasing to 32.7% at 9–11 months, followed by a sharp increase to almost 40% by 23 months (Fig. 3.3) [9]. Such trend in rapid increase in prevalence of stunting between 6 months and 2 years of age is attributed to failure of higher nutrient needs keeping pace with the rapid growth and considerably high requirement for nutrients [11]. These findings confirm that by the age of two years most growth retardation takes place and the "trajectory of length growth after birth seems to be largely set-in uterus" [12]. Region-wise analysis of stunting prevalence rate is also reported to be highest in under the age of two [13]. It is also reported that most growth retardation that occurs in the first two years of life is largely irreversible [14].

In India, growth faltering trend in the critical period of under 24 months, as measured by decline in length-for-age, is noted across the wealth quintiles (Fig. 3.4). Such a trend is also reported in the last National Family Health Survey 5 (NFHS 5) of 2019–2021 with almost a fifth of highest (17%) and 37% in lowest wealth quintile noted to be stunted [10]. Such a trend in the high wealth index group is primarily attributed to inappropriate breastfeeding, poor selection of food items, and inappropriate feeding practices at the time of complementary feeding [15].

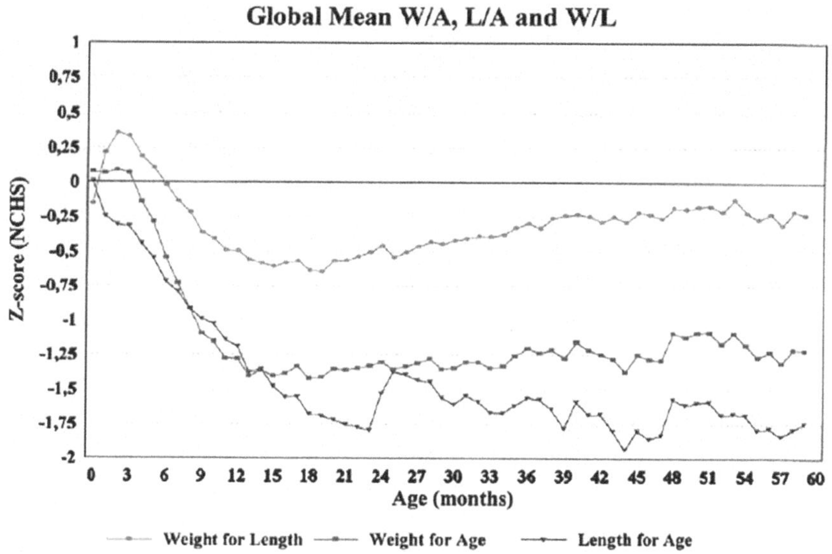

Fig. 3.2 Mean Anthropometric *Z*-scores by age for all 39 studies (children 0–59 months) relative to National Center for Health Statistics (NCHS) reference. *Source* Shrimpton JR et al., 2001. Paediatrics, 107, pp. 1–7

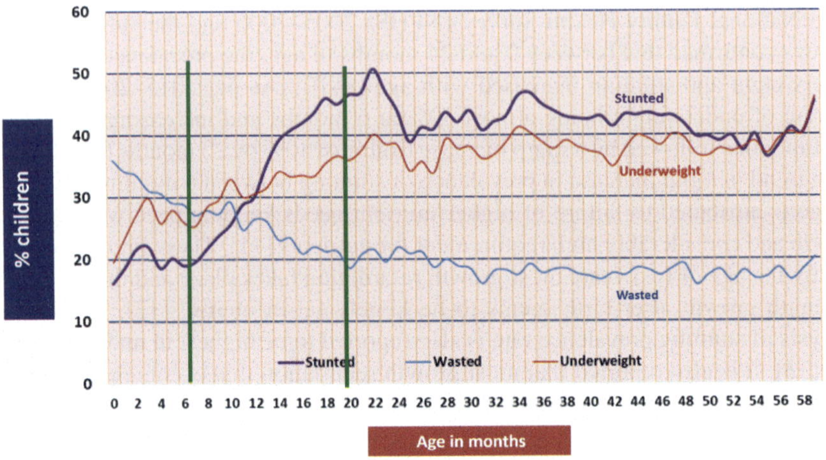

Fig. 3.3 Analysis of NFHS 4, 2015–2016 data, on undernutrition trend with an increase in age. *Source* IIPS (2016) National Family Health Survey 4 India Report (2015–2016)

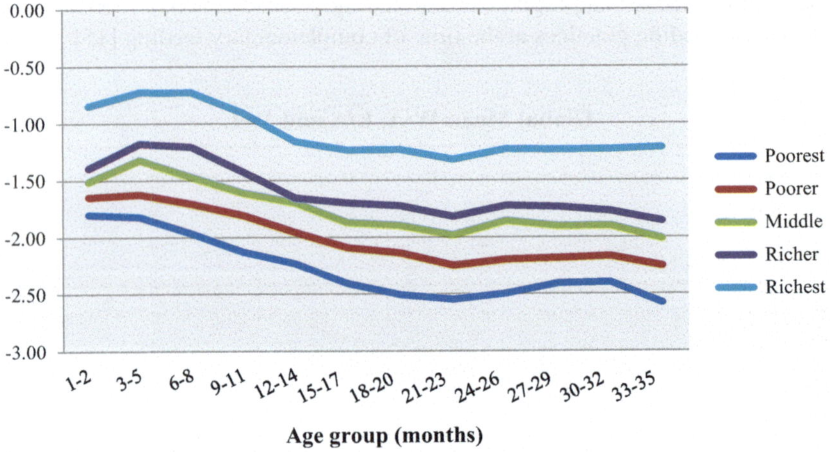

Fig. 3.4 Trends in mean HAZ scores by asset quintiles across age-groups. *Source* IIPS (2016) National Family Health Survey 4 India report (2015–2016)

The significance of first 1000 days is further established with trends in under 5 years mortality. Under-five deaths are also highest in the first two years (Fig. 3.5) with over 80% of child deaths occurring in this period.

Besides rapid physical growth in the first 2 years of life, most of the growth in the nervous system and brain also occurs during this period. A child's brain is reported to grow 75% of adult size and over 1 million new neural connections are formed every second [11, 16]. The nutrient needs of children under two years are therefore exceptionally high [6]. Appropriate feeding of young children under two years is crucial

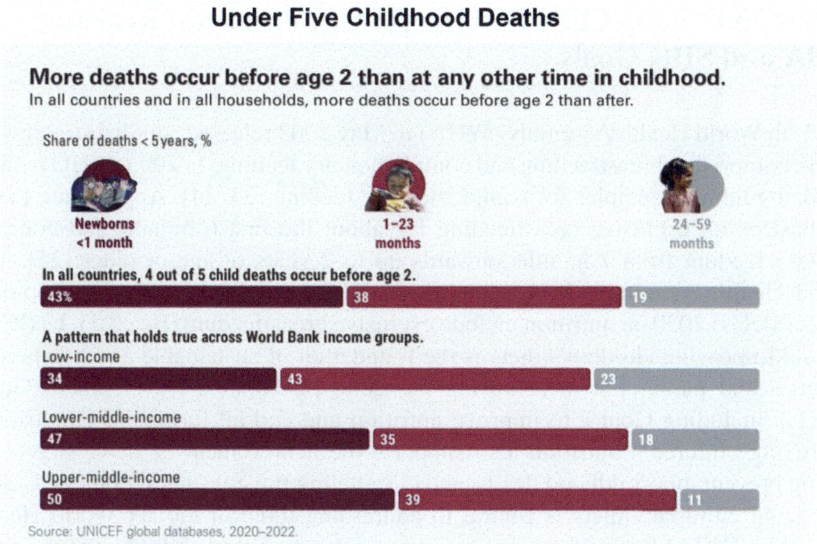

Fig. 3.5 Child death percentage in under 5 years children. *Source* United Nations Children's Fund (2024). When it Matters Most: Improving Nutrition and Survival for the Youngest and Most Vulnerable Children

not only to promote optimum physical growth but to nourish developing brains, build strong immune systems, and enjoy healthy lives [11]. According to Victoria et al. "Children from low- and middle-income countries are born with weights and lengths below WHO growth standards, and early growth faltering is even faster than currently assumed [17]". The window of opportunity for preventing undernutrition crucial below 2 years of age. The consequences of poor feeding practices in early life are visible in the age trend of stunting and wasting [18], and high prevalence rate of anaemia also peaks at 24 months of age [19].

Establishment of appropriate IYCF feeding practice in under-twos is an essential direct nutrition intervention to prevent the undernutrition [20]. Findings of UP state, India study concluded in late 90s "there is a need to accord highest priority to care and feeding (breastfeeding and complementary feeding) below one year. Intervention measures, if delayed beyond this critical period of infancy, may be too late for effective prevention of malnutrition in children" [21, 22]. In early life, "there is clear evidence that poor diets and feeding practices play a major role" [11].

Infant and Young Child Feeding (IYCF) Practices: Reaching WHA and SDG Goals

The 55th World Health Assembly (WHA) in May 2002 released a global strategy for IYCF, comprising breastfeeding and complementary feeding. In 2003, WHO recommended guiding principles for complementary feeding [23, 24]. Appropriate IYCF emphasizes on exclusive breastfeeding for about the first 6 months and complementary feeding from 7 months onwards up to 2 years of age or older [25]. The World Health Assembly (WHA) targets for 2025 and Sustainable Development Goals (SDGs) 2030 on nutrition include exclusive breastfeeding (Box 3.1). UNICEF states, "Improving children's diets is the foundation of sustainable and prosperous societies and paramount to achieving the 2030 Sustainable Development Goals (SDGs), including Goal 2 to improve nutrition and end all forms of malnutrition. Improving children's nutrition also supports the achievement of SDG targets on ending preventable childhood deaths and eliminating poverty, among others. Lastly, improving children's diets is central to addressing three of the six World Health Assembly (WHA) targets for reducing stunting, wasting, and childhood overweight by 2025" [26].

Box 3.1: Targets: World Health Assembly (WHA) and Sustainable Development Goals (SDGs)

WHA: Six Global Maternal, Infant and Child Nutrition targets to be Achieved by 2025 endorsed by the World Health Assembly (WHA) [27]

- 40% reduction in the number of children under 5 who are stunted*
- 50% reduction of anaemia in women of reproductive age
- 30% reduction in low birth weight, no increase in childhood overweight
- Increase the rate of exclusive breastfeeding in the first six months up to at least 50%**
- Reduce and maintain childhood wasting to less than 5%
- No increase in overweight, obesity and diabetes (in adults and adolescents).

(* increased to 50% in case of SDG, ** increased to 70% in case of SDG)

Sustainable Development Goals (SDG) 2030 that pertain to food and nutrition, state 'to end hunger, achieve food security, and improved nutrition and promote sustainable agriculture'. The Goal 2.2 includes the WHA targets (2025). WHA targets now, as indicated above, have been aligned to SDGs goals of 2030 [28].

- 50% reduction in the number of children under 5 who are stunted
- 50% reduction of anaemia in women of reproductive age
- 30% reduction in low birth weight
- Reduce and maintain childhood overweight to less than 3%

- Increase the rate of exclusive breastfeeding in the first 6 months up to at least 70%
- Reduce and maintain childhood wasting to less than 3%

Breastfeeding

Optimal breastfeeding can prevent 13% of all child deaths which is higher than any other preventive intervention [29]. It is estimated that annually breastfeeding could save 8, 20,000 lives. Infants are not breastfed are 15 times higher chances to die from pneumonia and 11 times higher possibility to die from diarrhoea than children who are exclusively breastfed [30, 31]. A meta-analysis reports that early initiation of breastfeeding that is recommended to be within one hour of birth, can prevent a significant number of neonatal deaths. This is evident from studies that report new-borns, who starts breastfeeding 24 h or more after birth, are twice as higher risk of neonatal mortality [32, 33]. A systematic study presents evidence that the risk of all-cause mortality is higher in predominantly partially and non-breastfed infants compared to exclusively breastfed infants 0–5 months of age [34]. In low- and middle-income countries, breastfeeding reduces the incidence of respiratory infections by one-third and diarrhoea episodes by almost half. With reference to India, it is estimated that appropriate BF could reduce 1,56,000 child deaths each year, reduce a minimum of 3,436,560 respiratory infections, and 3,900,000 episodes of diarrhoea, particularly in young children [35, 36]. Analysis of NFHS 3 data indicate sub-optimal IYCF practices that are associated with poor nutrition outcomes in children [37]. The relationship of breastfeeding and higher intelligence is also well established. According to Lancet, children who are breastfed longer are reported to have higher intelligence than those who are breastfed for shorter periods [35]. On an average, the crucial difference is estimated to be 3 points across all income levels, in rich or poor. This implies impact on improved academic performance, increased long-term earnings, and productivity; it is also noted that breastfeeding is beneficial to mothers' health and is protective against breast and ovarian carcinoma, and exclusive breastfeeding and predominant breastfeeding increase the duration of lactational amenorrhoea [38]. Appropriate breastfeeding includes adoption of the following three practices:

Early Initiation of Breastfeeding (EIBF)

Initiating breastfeeding immediately after birth and within an hour is referred to as EIBF. EIBF results in early skin to skin contact and brings closeness between mother and baby, benefits in regulating body temperature of new-born, and receipt of beneficial bacteria from their mother's skin and increasing chances of mothers of following the practice of exclusive breastfeeding [39]. According to WHO and UNICEF, EIBF does not require that the infant suckled at the breast and that milk was transferred from breast to infant.

With increasing trend in institutional deliveries, breastfeeding journey by caregivers/mothers is expected to often begin in the institution set up. However, the opportunity of contacts with mothers in the institution is not being used optimally for EIBF. This is evident from India data that the percentage of mothers following EIBF practice is 42% as compared to 89% institutional delivery [10]. The findings reveal that training institutional staff and mothers on early initiation and appropriate breastfeeding techniques, especially by mothers who undergo caesarean delivery, needs special attention.

Exclusive Breastfeeding (EBF) up to Six Months of Age

In the first six months of life, nutrition needs of infants are fully met if an infant is exclusively breastfed (EBF) [40, 41]. EBF implies no other foods or fluids, not even water, while infants can receive ORS, drops of syrups of vitamins, minerals, and medicines when required. Breastfeeding by a wet nurse, feeding using expressed breastmilk, and feeding donor human milk are included as being breastfed. EBF protects against diarrhoea, lower respiratory infections, as well as childhood obesity and overweight [39].

WHO Global Strategy for Infant and Young Child Feeding recommends that infants be exclusively breastfed until they turn six months of age. Exclusive breastfeeding is recognized to be the safest and healthiest option for children everywhere, "guaranteeing infants a food source that is uniquely adapted to their needs while also being safe, clean, healthy and accessible" [39]. WHO definition of indicator EBF is "percentage of infants 0–5 months of age who were fed exclusively with breast milk during the previous day". The recommended numerator is "infants 0–5 months of age who were fed only breast milk during the previous day", while the recommended denominator is "infants 0–5 months of age".

For establishing EBF, breastfeeding rates should be prevented from dropping consistently following moving to home after institutional delivery. This also includes supportive policies and supportive environment for mothers working in formal or informal sector or those who had caesarean deliveries. Intensive home-level breastfeeding counselling is convincing to mothers when coupled with frequent monitoring and sharing of information of infants' progress in weight gain [42].

In case of low birth weight "at risk" babies (<2.5 kg), special care in EIBF and EBF is essential for reducing wasting rate in infants. It is also reported that all new-borns babies who are in fact less than the WHO 2006 median birth weight (<3.2 kg for female babies and 3.3 kg for male babies) [7] should ideally be exclusive breastfed with appropriate cross cradle hold techniques, effective latching to breast as well as feeding hind milk by following the technique of emptying one breast for feeding before shifting to another one [43]. A community set up study from India demonstrates that "effective" exclusive breastfeeding in infants 0–6 months, using "cross-cradle hold with U support", has significant positive impact on optimum transfer of breastmilk and in contributing to "catch up" growth in low birth weight (LBW) infants and in reducing wasting. Use of such appropriate breastfeeding technique by mothers in the first 14 weeks of life is reported to have resulted in a substantial increase in weight of the growing baby—30 g per day as compared to the earlier estimate of average accepted rate of 17 g per day [44].

Continued Breastfeeding (CBF) Beyond 6 Months

It is recommended that children should continue to be breastfed for two years or beyond, i.e. beyond the recommended exclusive period of the first 6 months of life along with introduction of feeding of semi-solid feeds. CBF contributes to a substantial portion of energy and other essential nutrients to children who are in transition from EBF to adoption of complementary feeding practices. Moreover, CBF practice is of immense value in the feeding of sick children who have loss of appetite or are disinterested in being fed during illness or could suffer from dehydration despite being provided nutrient dense food for recovery [39, 45]. Additionally, CBF is reported to be associated with higher performance in intelligence tests among children and adolescents [39]. It is also reported that children breastfed longer than 12 months benefit the maximum. CBF is recommended for at least 2 years [39]. The indicator is defined as percentage of children 12–23 months of age who were fed breast milk during the previous day. The recommended numerator is "children 12–23 months of age who were fed breast milk during the previous day" and the denominator is "children 12–23 months of age". It is also recommended that whenever the sample size is large enough, the CBF indicator be disaggregated further and presented separately for the following age groups: 12–15, 16–19, and 20–23 months.

The practice of continued breastfeeding is much better in LMIC countries as compared to developed countries (Fig. 3.6). The following are some primary factors that adversely influence the duration of breastfeeding [46].

- Concerns about infant nutrition and weight.
- Mother's concern about taking medications while breastfeeding.
- Unsupportive work policies and lack of parental leave.
- Cultural norms and lack of family support.
- Unsupportive hospital practices and policies.

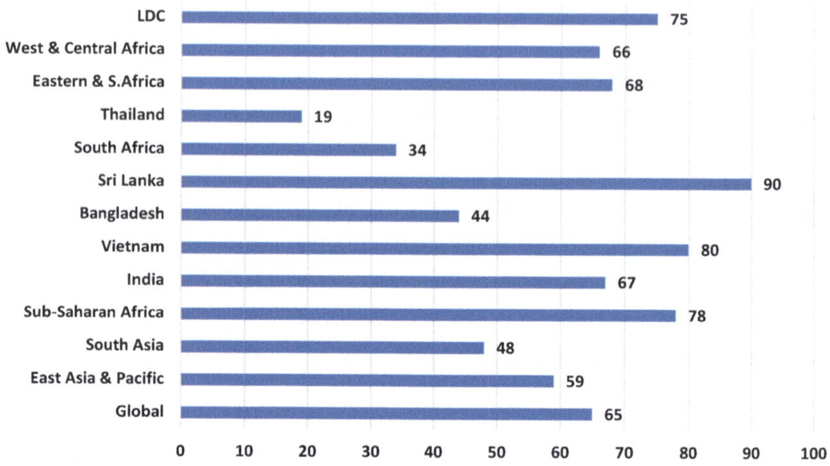

Fig. 3.6 Percentage prevalence rate of Continued Breastfeeding (CBF). *Source* UNICEF (2023) The State of the World's Children

Complementary Feeding

Complementary feeding (CF) is a period of transition when a baby is introduced to eat family foods while still being breastfed. CF is defined "as the process starting when breast milk alone is no longer sufficient to meet the nutritional requirements of infants, and therefore other foods and liquids are needed to complement breast milk" [11]. CF is recommended to follow the EBF period of completion of 6 months. In this period of accelerated growth rate of infants, appropriate CF is crucial for meeting higher demands not only for energy and protein but also for various micronutrients or minerals and vitamins. Additionally, ensuring use of safe, potable water for drinking and washing hands with soap and water while handling food prior to cooking and while feeding a child are extremely important practices to be followed as part of appropriate CF.

The three essential components of complementary feeding (CF) are described below, along with details of the term minimum acceptable diet (MAD) and the issue of feeding during illness.

- Timely introduction of complementary foods (semi-solid or soft foods, solid foods along with the continuation of breastfeeding) after completing 6 months or 180 days of EBF.
- Age-appropriate complementary foods: Diet diversity and feeding adequate in quality as well as quantity. It should be ensured that the food items selected for CF are from a range of food groups. CF should not be only energy dense but also contain adequate amount of good quality proteins and various micronutrients. Additionally, CF should is of right consistency. Pulses and milk, often diluted with water and incorrectly considered required for ease in swallowing food by a

child, is not a correct practice. Such dilution of CF should be actively discouraged and a child should be fed food items that are manually (not thinned by machine or electric liquidizer) mashed.
- Age-appropriate frequency of feeding CF is essential to enhance quantity of CF.

Timely Introduction of CF

From 7 months onwards, breast milk alone is not sufficient to meet the energy and other nutritional requirements of 7–23 months [39]. Nutrient requirements increase significantly with accelerated growth-birth weight doubles by 6 months and are estimated to triple by 1 year while body length increases by 1.5 times by the first year. Most of the organs of the body also grow rapidly, both structurally and functionally, during the early years with a slower growth rate later. Children under two years, in the period of accelerated growth, have a much higher nutrient requirements per kilogram of body weight than at any other time in life. Maximum growth faltering is noted in the period of over 6 months which coincides with the transition from exclusive breastfeeding to consuming a wide range of family foods while continuing with breastfeed [47, 48].

Breastfeeding alone is not able to meet the higher requirements in the period of accelerated growth since the volume of breast milk as well as nutrient concentrations of breast milk get reduced from 6 months onwards [49]. The total energy and protein requirements for an infant 6–12 months range from 650–720 kcal/day and 9–10.5 g protein/day while on an average after six months of age breastmilk provides 500 kcal and 5 g protein per day. The significance of shifting from EBF to CF is essential to meet the requirements for various nutrients and make infants less vulnerable to all forms of malnutrition including stunting, wasting, micronutrient deficiencies, overweight and obesity as well as diet related non-communicable diseases and optimum cognitive development [47, 48, 50]. A lower risk of stunting or underweight is reported in children aged 6 to 8 months in 14 countries who ate solid or semi-solid foods [51].

Feeding the first food or the first bite is viewed as an important milestone in child's life since it marks a new phase of exploring with new tastes, textures, and smells [11]. This turning point in a child's life is celebrated by different names that are inherent in the tradition, such as "annaprasan" in India. The guiding principle for diversified food for CF implies selecting and feeding foods from at least five out of eight defined food groups (breast milk, grains/tubers/plantains, pulses/nuts/seeds, dairy products comprising milk, infant formula, yoghurt, and cheese, flesh foods, eggs, vitamin A rich fruits and vegetables, and other fruits and vegetables).

Usage of Diversified Diet

Adequate and regular consumption of diverse range of foods containing quality protein and micronutrients along with intake of carbohydrates and oil is essential [52, 53]. Little or no consumption of nutrient dense foods such as eggs, dairy products, fruits, and vegetables between 6 and 23 months of age has been reported to be associated with stunting [54]. The guiding principle for diversified food selection is complementary feed which should have daily food items from five of the eight defined groups (breast milk, grains/tubers/plantains, pulses/nuts/seeds, dairy products (milk, infant formula milk, yoghurt, cheese), flesh foods, eggs, vitamin A rich fruits and vegetables and other fruits and vegetables). Diet diversity score and achieving minimum dietary diversity for children 6–23 months of age were significantly associated stunting and underweight [37].

Breastfeeding is advised to be continued more than 6 months since BF enhances CF quality and contributes to attaining optimal growth [11]. Additionally, daily consumption of eggs as a part of CF needs to be promoted since egg consumption results in increasing intake of not only protein and energy but also contributes to higher consumption of essential fatty acids, vitamin B6, vitamin D, phosphorous, and selenium [52]. In a randomized controlled trial in Ecuador, daily consumption of eggs by children aged 6–9 months significantly improved growth and reduced prevalence of stunting by 47% and underweight by 74% [55].

For meeting nutrient needs, selection of appropriate food items is crucial. In such a situation, it is important to ensure inclusion of foods in CF from both Type 1 and Type 2 nutrients (Box 3.2). Moreover, appropriate selection and consumption of these food items in a child's early life also influence food habits in future [52].

For improving quality of CF food, another alternative is preparation of home level dense nutrition mix powder or nutri-mixtures with good shelf life by using food items from both Type 1 and 2 nutrients and daily incorporation of these in feed for CF. Regular incorporation of such nutri-mixtures as food supplements in CF of children has demonstrated positive effects on nutritional status of children [42].

Box 3.2: Use Both Type 1 and Type 2 Nutrients in CF

Complementary feeding for children requires both Type 1 and Type 2 nutrients as recommended by Dr. Michael Golden and the Indian Academy of Pediatrics [56]. Type 1 nutrients, known as "Functional Nutrients," include vitamins and minerals like iodine, calcium, and iron. These have specific roles and are stored in body. Deficiencies can be identified through clinical signs or biochemical tests and are often addressed by public health measures such as specific nutrient supplements or fortified foods.

Type 2 nutrients, or "growth nutrients," such as essential amino acids, essential fatty acids, zinc, and magnesium, are crucial for tissue building and metabolic functions. These nutrients are not stored in the body and must be consumed daily for lean body mass building and linear growth in children. Deficiency in Type 2 nutrients lead to growth stagnation, weight loss, and wasting as the body conserves these nutrients for essential functions. Prolonged deficiency can result in chronic malnutrition, stunted growth, and impaired cognitive development.

In India, most complementary feeding programs focus on Type 1 nutrients, neglecting Type 2 nutrients needed for growth and for preventing malnutrition. Animal-source foods like dairy, eggs, fish, and meat are rich in Type 2 nutrients. For vegetarian families, provision of Type 2 nutrients is a challenge. Home-made nutrient dense mixture supplements, prepared and incorporated in CF by trained mothers using locally available food items such as peanut, sesame seed, and sprouted bean powders has shown significant improvement in child growth, making it a viable strategy for combating malnutrition in vegetarian communities.

Frequency of Feeding-Minimal Meal Frequency (MMF)

Children under two years cannot eat by themselves and need to be appropriately fed. Frequent feeding of meals is advised since children at a young stage have small stomach size and cannot consume the entire quantity of food at one time. However, the total amount of food offered at each of the meals needs to be increased with increase in age [11]. Additionally, the consistency of food offered at each meal should be increasingly thickened—from dropping consistency to family food consistency. Feeding watery food items such as watery pulses (dals) or watery rice should be totally avoided right from the initiation of CF. The belief that a child cannot swallow mashed food of dropping consistency is a myth.

As per WHO guidelines, frequency of feeding measured as minimal meal frequency (MMF) of CF differs for breastfed children and non-breastfed children [26].

MMF for Breastfed Children

Infants >6–8 months are recommended to be provided food other than breast milk two to three times per day while at 9–23 months, three to four times per day with additional nutritious snacks offered one to two times [57]. Feeding meals/snacks less frequently than recommended can compromise total energy. Protein and micronutrient intake contributing to growth faltering, stunting, and micronutrient deficiencies.

MMF for Non-Breastfed Children

The recommended frequency for non-breastfed children is four to five meals per day [57].

For assessing MMF, the following factors should be taken into consideration:

- "Feedings" include both meals and snacks other than trivial amounts.
- Milk feeds include any formula (e.g. infant formula, follow-on formula, "toddler milk") or any animal milk other than human breast milk, (e.g. cow milk, goat milk, evaporated milk, or reconstituted powdered milk) as well as semi-solid and fluid/drinkable yoghurt and other fluid/drinkable fermented products made with animal milk.
- Milk feeds are not included for breastfed children because the minimum meal frequencies for this indicator assume average breast milk intake: if a substantial amount of energy is derived from other milk feeds, breast milk intake is likely to be considerably lower than average.

Minimum Acceptable Diet (MAD)

MAD, an indicator to measure CF status, combines information on minimum dietary diversity (MDD) and MMF [57, 58] and is measured as percentage of children >6–23 months of age who consumed MAD during the previous day [39]. It is important to note that in case of non-breastfed children, children should have received milk at least twice on the previous day.

In summary, recommended MAD is as follows:

- *For breastfed children*: receiving at least the minimum dietary diversity and minimum meal frequency for their age during the previous day.
- *For non-breastfed children*: receiving at least the minimum dietary diversity and minimum meal frequency for their age during the previous day as well as at least two milk feeds.

For MAD assessment, denominator is taken as children >6–23 months of age while numerator includes children >6–23 months of age who consumed a minimum acceptable diet during the previous day. One of the limitations of measure of MDM is that the amount of a particular food item is not taken into consideration, and this may be misleading in case the CF practice in a community primarily uses milk, pulses, and rice in diluted or watery form.

Feeding During Illness

Active feeding and adequate complementary is recommended during and after any illness since young children are at a high risk of losing muscle mass while ill and not consuming adequate quantity of quality food. Prevalent beliefs of withholding feeding during diarrhoea or other illnesses are noted in India [8, 9, 40]. A young child in the post-illness period needs special care of being fed nutrient dense diet high in protein and micronutrients along with feeding of breast milk.

Indicators for Assessing IYCF Practices

The 2008 WHO indicators for IYCF were revised in 2021 [39]. It is now recommended to assess the IYCF status using the full set of indictors for any given population and make no distinction between core and optional indicators. A number of indicators are recommended for usage at population-level or for large surveys and not for screening or assessment of individuals. The purpose of the indicators is assessing and describing trends over time; targeting and strategizing interventions and programme designing; and undertaking monitoring and evaluation.

An Overview of IYCF Situation: Global, South Asia, and India

Global Scenario of IYCF Situation

Analysis of data on various indicators of IYCF reported by UNICEF in 2023, for both breastfeeding and complementary feeding, is presented below for selected regions and countries (Fig. 3.6 and Table 3.1).

As presented in Table 3.1, global percentage for two indicators of breastfeeding (EIBF and EBF) is below 50%. EIBF percentage region wise shows a wide range –39% in South Asia and 65% in Eastern and South Africa. On the other hand, EBF percentage is highest in South Asia (61%) and lowest in West and Central Africa (38%). In 43 out of 122 countries, EBF is over 50% while EBF is over 70% in only on 6 countries (Sri Lanka 81%, Rwanda 81%, Solomon Islands 76%, Vanuatu 73%, Burundi 72%, and Zambia 70%) [59].

Within South Asia, though the EBF rate is reported to be highest, but only one of the countries in the region (Sri Lanka) is reaching the SDG target of over 70% [59]. The percentage rate of continued breastfeeding (CBF) beyond 6 months is also highest in South Asia region (78%) followed by LDC (75%) and Africa regions. CBF practice is rather low in East Asia and Pacific (59%) and Latin American and Caribbean countries (48%) and could be attributed to a great extent due to mothers being out of home on work as well as influence of aggressive marketing of breast milk substitutes. The latter is also reflected in increase in the practice of the feeding infant formula in East Asia and Pacific (28%) as compared to 6% in South Asia and 11% globally.

Table 3.1 Infant and Young Child Feeding practices (%) across regions

	EIBF	EBF	CF >6–8 months	Contd. BF
Global	47	48	72	65
East Asia & Pacific	41	42	84	59
LAC	55	43	88	48
South Asia	39	61	56	78
Sub-Saharan Africa	54	45	76	67
India	41	64	49	80
Vietnam	23	45	86	44
Bangladesh	47	63	75	90
Sri Lanka	90	81	94	90
South Africa	67	32	83	34
Thailand	34	14	92	19
Eastern & S. Africa	65	55	79	68
West & Central Africa	46	38	74	66
Least Developed Countries (LDC)	57	54	76	75

Source UNICEF (2023) The State of the World's Children

Data on CF shows over 7 out of 10 children are fed semi-solid feed between >6–8 months of age. CF practices are complex since the feeding practice as well as choice of food is driven by a few misunderstanding, myths, and traditional practices of the influencers that act as barriers. These barriers are very context specific. In addition to income and cost constraint, the other factors contributing to poor MAD scenario are lack of knowledge on selection of food items and feeding practices, traditional beliefs, convenience, lack of land, low agricultural production, seasonality influencing unavailability of vegetables and fruit production, low availability of legumes and low acceptability of animal source food items due to cultural reasons, participation of women in workforce, time availability, increasing urbanization, desirability and increased dependency on aggressively marketed commercial food items or processed food items. Some of these factors are clear from a survey finding from India that reports that within the same households where adults are consuming over 70% of recommended energy and protein, a much lower percentage of children are in this category [60]. Moreover, common myths in India often result in feeding diluted food and discouraging consumption of eggs.

The global percentage for minimal acceptable diet (MAD) is rather low at 18% with a wide MAD percentage range of 3% in Liberia and 74% in Serbia with 16 countries reporting MAD percentage of over 50%. The poor MAD percentage reveals that the state of young children's diets remains a persistent bottleneck to greater progress on nutrition. Poor buying power, however, is not the mere problem of low MAD percentage. Interestingly, even in the wealthiest population group within India have low MAD of only 25% [40]. In the last decade, the following 10 countries (Bangladesh, Burkina Faso, Cambodia, Côte d'Ivoire, the Gambia,

Kyrgyzstan, Maldives, Nepal, Sierra Leone, and Timor-Leste), though poor, have reported at least 10%points increase in MAD [11, 59]. High MAD score in the countries is possibly influenced by the recommended practice of continuing breastfeeding practice together with feeding of diversified food items.

On the other hand, MAD in many countries is noted to be adversely influenced by frequent and increased consumption of ultra-processed foods (UPF) that is noted to be rapidly replacing family level prepared food items in LMICs [49]. With good marketing strategy, UPF are sold in attractive colourful packages and are tasty, ready to eat or quick to prepare and consume. These are often available in low-cost small packets. Such UPF items are source of energy/calories that fill stomach, contribute to satiety but do not meet the nutritional needs, especially of quality protein and of micronutrients [11, 39]. Moreover, UPF are generally unhealthy since contents of saturated fats/trans fatty acids, sugar, salt, and carbohydrates are often rather high.

Consumption of UPF food items is reported to be continuously on a rise in Asia, Africa, Latin America, and Middle East [11]. A recent household food item expenditure report of India shows highest food percentage expenditure on beverages and processed food items—27.2% on beverages and processed food items compared to 18.84% on milk and milk products and 9.7% on vegetables [60]. A study of children 12–13 months in Nepal reports consumption of unhealthy snack food and beverages (USFB) results in poor growth outcomes such as lower length for age at one year of age [61]. UNICEF 2021 reports "three in five children worldwide were not fed nutrient-rich eggs, fish, or meat during the previous day, and two in five children were not fed any vegetables or fruit. At the same time, many young children were consuming unhealthy processed snacks and drinks that displace healthier alternatives and set children on a path to overweight" [11].

*World Breastfeeding Trends Initiative (WBT*i*)*

It assists countries to assess the IYCF status and benchmark the progress in implementation of global strategy for IYCF with a view to bridge the gaps noted in policy and programmes [62]. In South Asia, as per WBT*i* data, only Afghanistan, Bangladesh, and Sri Lanka have shown positive results over the last decade [63].

IYCF Strategies, Policies, and Programmes: Making a Difference

In the last five decades, a wide range of measures have been undertaken by many LMICs towards the establishment of appropriate IYCF practices. These include legal measures, issuing national policies on IYCF including mother supportive maternity leave and other government policies for breastfeeding working mothers, mainstreaming promotion of IYCF with antenatal, delivery and post-delivery services, provision of free supplementary food to 7–24 months, undertaking trials on incorporation of home level produced nutrient-rich food mixtures in CF feed and experimenting with community-based projects.

Legal Measures-International Code for Marketing of Breastmilk Substitute (Code)

The Code, a legal measure to prevent open marketing of milk formula, discourages marketing and use of industrially produced milk as a substitute for breast milk and for establishing measures for monitoring the implementation of the code. Estimated 136 out of 194 countries have country level legal measure in place with some or all provisions of the International Code [64]. Inadequate monitoring mechanism remains a serious concern. In India, the legal measure is the IMS Act (The Infant Milk Substitutes, Feeding Bottles, and Infant Foods: Regulation of Production, Supply and Distribution Act 1992 and Amendment Act 2003) [65] but the monitoring remains weak [63].

Support to Working Mothers

Cessation of EBF is primarily attributed to mothers returning to work. Inability of mothers to feed expressed milk, lack of family support, lack of enabling working environment for feeding, economic constraints at home and availability of alternatives such as formula feeds in an active marketing environment.

With an increase in urbanization and continuous increase in mothers working away from home, evidence indicates policy on maternity leave helps in EBF. The International Labour Organisation's (ILO) "Maternity Protection Convention" guarantees a minimum of 14 weeks of maternity leave paid at 66% of previous earning and allows women the right to one or more daily breaks to breastfeed [66]. The informal sector is not covered under the Convention, or the country-based legal framework of most countries. In India, Maternity Benefit Act (MBA), amended in 2017, offers paid leave policy to women employees (employed in factories, mines and shops or commercial establishments employing 10 or more employees) for 26 weeks—increased from the earlier leave policy of only 12 weeks. The Act also includes policy of establishing crèches with a minimum of 50 employees.

Baby-Friendly Hospital Initiative (BFHI)

A global programme actively promotes breastfeeding practices in institutional setup in response to the Innocenti Declaration of 1990 of WHO-UNICEF breastfeeding meeting. BFHI strategy was revised in 2005 and 2018 to implement 10 short-listed institutional based practices that protect, promote, and support breastfeeding [67, 68]. The BFHI strategy "helped to transform health care policies by restoring breastfeeding as the natural and normal practice for nurturing babies" but requires sustained commitment at multiple levels with adequate financial and human resources [63].

Home and Community-Centred Trials and Programmes in LMICs

In the last three decades, a few projects were launched focusing on training frontline workers to undertake effective counselling for equipping mothers and caregivers as well as community leaders to promote appropriate breastfeeding techniques and complementary feeding practices. These projects focused on education, guidance, and support mothers before after delivery, including after discharge from the hospital [63]. Special programmes were launched in many countries for building an enabling environment for breastfeeding through generation of awareness of family members and society with the aim to promote optimal breastfeeding practices.

In 2016, the Ministry of Health and Family Welfare, Government of India launched a nationwide programme "Mothers' Absolute Affection (MAA)", literally meaning "mother", to further strengthen ten steps to breastfeeding [69] and mobilize family members and at health facilities to breastfeed successfully.

Human Milk Banks (HMBs)

Established under the WHO guidelines at secondary and tertiary levels of public health facilities to provide breastfeeding support to mothers who cannot or may eventually, breastfeed. About 600 HMBs have been rolled out in 50 countries [70]. Beneficial effects on EBF practices upon discharge from hospital or intensive newborn care unit have been reported [70, 71].

Innovative IYCF Projects and Programme Experiences

A range of IYCF programme experiences are reported from various countries. For example, in India, community-based IYCF projects with UNICEF support were launched such as DULAR with focus on EBF in Bihar, Positive Deviance Programme in West Bengal, Mitanin in Chhattisgarh state, Maternal Child Health Nutrition (MCHN) Project in UP. Additionally, other well documented and externally evaluated projects implemented during this period include CARE supported large RACHANA programme UNICEF supported Lalitpur Project in a western district of UP state and World Bank supported ISSNIP (ICDS System Strengthening and Nutrition Improvement Project) Project in eight states of India [6, 72–77]. Most of these projects emphasized on the strategy of community mobilization through trained community women or working with "Mother support groups", home level counselling or use of fixed day strategy at ICDS for group discussion on IYCF themes. The key lessons emerging from these experiences have been built in 2018 in the Nutrition Mission Strategy of India (POSHAN Abhiyaan) [78].

A recently reported successful project on promotion of "effective" EBF in West India emphasized on the use of appropriate techniques, such as "cross cradle hold technique" (CCT) for breastfeeding by well-trained healthcare workers [43]. The results were alarming—daily average weight gain of 30 g per day in first 14 weeks compared to generally acceptable norm in India of 17 g.

Global documents on successful implementation of complementary feeding projects are relatively very few. In India's Uttar Pradesh state, with support of UNICEF, a successful viable model was implemented through the government systems in five districts of the state. The key factors that substantially improved CF practices applied the principles of Triple A (Assess, Analyse and Act) for individual counselling on timely introduction of semi-solid feed, appropriate frequency of feeding and increasing consumption of diversified diets in adequate quantity and consistency. The interventions concentrated on effective training of frontline workers, group discussion with mothers on a fixed day per month, institutionalization of monitoring growth of under twos and demonstrating CF technique using recommended size bowl and spoon [79].

The success was attributed to creating a team of well-trained skilful healthcare workers who as part of training worked with adopted mother–child dyad for practical experience on face-to-face counselling on maternal nutrition and IYCF, and linking the counselling with monitoring of status of child's weight and preparation and incorporation of home prepared nutrition dense food supplement mixtures, rich in protein and micronutrients with good shelf life in CF [80]. A package of Health Spoken Tutorials (HSTs) developed in local language in India have proved to be effective training and communication tool in establishing appropriate IYCF practices [43].

In addition to the above, an interesting block level trial in promoting eggs as a part of complementary feed was also experimented. The trial focused on support in form of hens and chickens for poultry keeping to only those selected families who had history of having moderately or severely undernourished child under five years [42]. There was a substantial impact on nutritional status of the children who regularly consumed eggs. These findings concur with the report of Ecuador trial on early introduction of eggs at 6–9 months in CF which significantly improved child growth [55]. These trials present evidence that nutrition counselling for behavioural change in CF should be accompanied with inputs for increasing access to quality protein food items such as eggs.

Another successful IYCF project with positive impact on child nutrition is reported from Sri Lanka, South Asia. The Family Health Bureau of the Ministry of Health, Nutrition, and Indigenous Medicine (MoHNIM) implemented an integrated package of MCH services comprising IYCF promotion, growth monitoring, and provision of nutrition supplement and protocol for management of undernourished children [81]. The IYCF Programme design concentrated on imparting skills on IYCF by in-service trained health staff on standardized integrated training packages and lactation management training to the hospital staff.

Conclusion

The current situation and trend of IYCF and child undernutrition reveals that the current progress is not sufficient to achieve the WHA nutrition targets (2025) and the global Sustainable Development Agenda (SDG) by 2030. For accelerating progress in reducing undernutrition, urgent and intensive actions are needed to ensure proper IYCF practices cum maternal feeding care is an integral part of "aspirational" care in the first 1000 days. It is crucial for a country to invest in implementation research to ensure that the contacts during antenatal services, institutional deliveries, routine child immunization and referral during illness in the first 1000 days are used to the optimum for establishing appropriate IYCF practices as well as interventions for maternal nutrition care. In this context, the first and second measles immunization contacts need to view as suitable opportunities to check CF practices and nutritional status. For effective IYCF counselling at these contacts by frontline workers, there is a need to invest in the recruitment, practical training, and motivation of these workers. Training and communication support materials such as training handbook, digitalized visuals, and HSTs are available that could be effectively used for establishment of appropriate IYCF practices [7, 11, 82]. Additionally, it is critical that senior school curriculum includes subject on IYCF and nutrition care of self, family, and young children so that future parents are sensitized about IYCF and incorporate the correct principles in nutrition care practices.

References

1. Victora, C. G. et al. (2008). Maternal and Child Undernutrition: Consequences for Adult Health and Human Capital. *The Lancet, 371*(9609), 340–57. Retrieved from https://doi.org/10.1016/S0140-6736(07)61692-4.
2. Bégin, F., & Aguayo, V. M. (2017). First Foods: Why Improving Young Children's Diets Matter. *Maternal & Child Nutrition, 13*(2), e12528. Retrieved from https://doi.org/10.1111/mcn.12528.
3. Gragnolati, M., Bredenkamp, C., Shekar, M., Das Gupta, M., & Lee, Y. -K. (2006). *India's Undernourished Children: A Call for Reform and Action.* The World Bank. Retrieved from https://doi.org/10.1596/978-0-8213-6587-8.
4. Leroy, J. L., Ruel, M., Habicht, J. -P., & Frongillo, E. A. (2015). Using Height-for-Age Differences (HAD) Instead of Height-for-Age Z-Scores (HAZ) for the Meaningful Measurement of Population-Level Catch-Up in Linear Growth in Children Less Than 5 Years of Age. *BMC Pediatrics, 15*(1), 145. Retrieved from https://doi.org/10.1186/s12887-015-0458-9.
5. Shrimpton, R., Victora, C., Onis, M., Lima, R., Blössner, M., & Clugston, G. (2001). Worldwide Timing of Growth Faltering: Implications for Nutritional Interventions. *Pediatrics, 107*, e75. Retrieved from https://doi.org/10.1542/peds.107.5.e75.
6. Vir, S. C. (2013). Community Based Maternal and Child Health Nutrition Project, Uttar Pradesh: An Innovative Strategy Focusing on "At Risk" Families. *Indian Journal of Community Medicine: Official Publication of Indian Association of Preventive & Social Medicine, 38*(4), 234–239. Retrieved from https://doi.org/10.4103/0970-0218.120159.
7. *The WHO Child Growth Standards.* (n.d.). Retrieved from https://www.who.int/tools/child-growth-standards.
8. International Institute for Population Sciences (IIPS) & Macro International. (2007). *National Family Health Survey (NFHS-3), 2005–06: India: Volume I.* IIPS.
9. International Institute for Population Sciences (IIPS) & Macro International. (2017). *National Family Health Survey (NFHS-4), 2015–16: India: Volume I.* IIPS.
10. International Institute for Population Sciences (IIPS) & Macro International. (2021). *National Family Health Survey (NFHS-5), 2019–21: India: Volume I.* IIPS.
11. UNICEF. (2021). *Fed to Fail: The Crisis of Child Nutrition.* UNICEF.
12. Shrimpton, R. (2012). Global Policy and Programme Guidance on Maternal Nutrition: What Exists, the Mechanisms for Providing It, and How to Improve Them? *Paediatric and Perinatal Epidemiology, 26*(s1), 315–325. Retrieved from https://doi.org/10.1111/j.1365-3016.2012.01279.x.
13. United Nations Children's Fund (UNICEF). (2024). *When It Matters Most: Improving Nutrition and Survival for the Youngest and Most Vulnerable Children.* UNICEF.
14. ACC/SCN. (2004). *Fifth Report on The World Nutrition Situation: Nutrition for Improved Development Outcomes.* United Nations Administrative Committee on Coordination/Standing Committee on Nutrition, Geneva.
15. Petrikova, I. (2021). The Role of Complementary Feeding in India's High Child Malnutrition Rates: Findings From a Comprehensive Analysis of NFHS IV (2015–2016) Data. *Food Security, 14*(1), 39–66. https://doi.org/10.1007/s12571-021-01202-7
16. O'Sullivan, A. J., & Monk, C. (2020). Maternal and Environmental Influences on Perinatal and Infant Development. *Future of Children, 30*(2), 11–34.
17. Victora, G. C., de Onis, M., Pedro, H. C., Blössner, M., DiplOec, T., & Shrimpton, R. (2010). Worldwide Timing of Growth Faltering: Revisiting Implications for Interventions. *Pediatrics, 125*(3), e473–e489. Retrieved from https://doi.org/10.1542/peds.2009-1519.
18. Andersen, C. T. et al. (2024). Maternal and Child Nutrition Services Associated with Nutritional Knowledge and Practices, India. *Bulletin of the World Health Organization, 102*(1), 9–21. Retrieved from https://doi.org/10.2471/BLT.22.289129.
19. Kotecha, P., & Vir, S. C. (2011). Iron Deficiency and Iron Deficiency Anemia in Young Children. In S. C. Vir (Ed.), *Public Health Nutrition in Developing Countries* (1st ed., pp. 638–662). Woodhead Publishers.

20. Vir, S. C. & Suri, S. (2023). Young Child Undernutrition: Crucial to Prioritize Nutrition Intervention in the First 1000 Days of Life. *Indian Journal of Pediatrics, 90*(1).
21. Vir, S. C., & Nigam, A. K. (2001). Nutritional Status of Children in Uttar Pradesh. *Nutrition Foundation of India Bulletin, 22*(1), 4–6. NFI Bulletin.
22. Vir, S. C. (2013). Community Based Maternal and Child Health Nutrition Project, Uttar Pradesh: An Innovative Strategy Focusing on "At Risk" Families. *Indian Journal of Community Medicine, 38*(4), 234. Retrieved from https://doi.org/10.4103/0970-0218.120159.
23. *Global Strategy for Infant and Young Child Feeding*. (n.d.). Retrieved from https://www.who.int/publications/i/item/9241562218.
24. *Guiding Principles for Complementary Feeding of the Breastfed Child—PAHO/WHO | Pan American Health Organization*. (2011). Retrieved from https://www.paho.org/en/documents/guiding-principles-complementary-feeding-breastfed-child-0.
25. Meek, J. Y., Noble, L., & Section on Breastfeeding. (2022). Policy Statement: Breastfeeding and the Use of Human Milk. *Pediatrics, 150*(1), e2022057988. https://doi.org/10.1542/peds.2022-057988
26. United Nations Children's Fund (UNICEF). (2020). *Improving Young Children's Diets During the Complementary Feeding Period: UNICEF Programming Guidance*. UNICEF.
27. World Health Organization. (2012). *Maternal, Infant and Young Child Nutrition* (WHA 65.5). World Health Organization.
28. Arora, A. (2019). *WHO/UNICEF Discussion Paper: The Extension of the 2025 Maternal, Infant and Young Child Nutrition Targets to 2030*. UNICEF DATA. Retrieved from https://data.unicef.org/resources/who-unicef-discussion-paper-nutrition-targets/.
29. Bryce, J., el Arifeen, S., Pariyo, G., Lanata, C. F., Gwatkin, D., & Habicht, J.-P. (2003). Reducing Child Mortality: Can Public Health Deliver? *The Lancet, 362*(9378), 159–164. Retrieved from https://doi.org/10.1016/S0140-6736(03)13870-6.
30. León-Cava, N., Pan American Health Organization & LINKAGES Project (Eds.). (2002). *Quantifying the Benefits of Breastfeeding: A Summary of the Evidence*. Food and Nutrition Program, Pan American Health Organization: LINKAGES Project, Academy for Educational Development.
31. Black, R. E. et al. (2008). Maternal and Child Undernutrition: Global and Regional Exposures and Health Consequences. *The Lancet, 371*(9608), 243–260. Retrieved from https://doi.org/10.1016/S0140-6736(07)61690-0.
32. Smith, E. R. et al. (2017). Delayed Breastfeeding Initiation and Infant Survival: A Systematic Review and Meta-Analysis. *PLOS ONE, 12*(7), e0180722. Retrieved from https://doi.org/10.1371/journal.pone.0180722.
33. Pandey, R. S., & Vir, S. C. (2021). Essential Newborn and Health Care: Emerging and Evolving Interventions and Program Scenario: Global and India. In S. C. Vir (ed.), *Public Health Nutrition in Developing Countries* (2nd ed., Chapter 6). Woodhead Publishers.
34. Sankar, M. J. et al. (2015). Optimal Breastfeeding Practices and Infant and Child Mortality: A Systematic Review and Meta-Analysis. *Acta Paediatrica, 104*(S467), 3–13. Retrieved from https://doi.org/10.1111/apa.13147.
35. Victora, C. G. et al. (2016). Breastfeeding in the 21st Century: Epidemiology, Mechanisms, and Lifelong Effect. *The Lancet, 387*(10017), 475–490. Retrieved from https://doi.org/10.1016/S0140-6736(15)01024-7.
36. Rollins, N. C. et al. (2016). Why Invest, and What It Will Take to Improve Breastfeeding Practices? *The Lancet, 387*(10017), 491–504. Retrieved from https://doi.org/10.1016/S0140-6736(15)01044-2.
37. *Age-Appropriate Infant and Young Child Feeding Practices Are Associated with Child Nutrition in India: Insights from Nationally Representative Data*. (n.d.). Retrieved from https://doi.org/10.1111/mcn.12036
38. Chowdhury, R. et al. (2015). Breastfeeding and Maternal Health Outcomes: A Systematic Review and Meta-analysis. *Acta Paediatrica, 104*(S467), 96–113. Retrieved from https://doi.org/10.1111/apa.13102.
39. WHO-UNICEF. (2021). *Indicators for Assessing Infant and Young Child Feeding Practices*.

40. Sachdeva, R. C., & Kundu, P. (2021). Optimal Neonatal Nutrition and Care: Early and Exclusive Breastfeeding and Human Milk Banking Support System. In S. C. Vir (Ed.), *Public Health Nutrition in Developing Countries* (2nd ed., pp. 361–419). Woodhead Publishers.
41. Dalal, R. M. & Agnihotri, S. B. (2021). Nutrition Care in the First Year of Life: Significance, Key Experiences, and Emerging Lessons in Preventing Growth Faltering and Promoting "Catch Up" Growth. In S. C. Vir (Ed.), *Public Health Nutrition in Developing Countries* (2nd ed., pp. 499–562). Woodhead Publishers.
42. Dalal, R., & Vir, S. C. (2024). Innovative Intervention Spearhead Substantial Improvement in Maternal Nutrition Care and Young Child Feeding Practices and Contribute to the Reduction in Child Undernutrition: Key learnings. *Under Publication.*
43. Dalal, R., Fancy, M. K., Chaudhary, S., Abraham, M., Vir, S. C., & Gaurav, S. (2023). Establishment of Cross-Cradle Hold Technique Combined with Intensive Breastfeeding Counselling Positively Impacts the Weight Gain Rate in Early Infancy. *Maternal & Child Nutrition, 19*(4), e13529. Retrieved from https://doi.org/10.1111/mcn.13529
44. Brown, K., Stallings, R., de Kanashiro, H., Lopez de Romaña, G., & Black, R. (1990). Effects of Common Illnesses on Infants' Energy Intakes from Breast Milk and Other Foods During Longitudinal Community-Based Studies in Huascar (Lima), Peru. *The American Journal of Clinical Nutrition, 52*(6), 1005–1013. Retrieved from https://doi.org/10.1093/ajcn/52.6.1005.
45. Odom, E. C., Li, R., Scanlon, K. S., Perrine, C. G., & Grummer-Strawn, L. (2013). Reasons for Earlier Than Desired Cessation of Breastfeeding. *Pediatrics, 131*(3), e726–e732. Retrieved from https://doi.org/10.1542/peds.2012-1295.
46. Garg, A. (2021). Complementary Feeding: Programme Design Framework, Implementation, and Measuring Progress. In S. C. Vir (Ed.), *Public Health Nutrition in Developing Countries* (2nd ed., pp. 420–449). Woodhead Publishers.
47. Michaelsen, K. F., Grummer-Strawn, L., & Bégin, F. (2017). Emerging Issues in Complementary Feeding: Global Aspects. *Maternal & Child Nutrition, 13*(S2), e12444. Retrieved from https://doi.org/10.1111/mcn.12444.
48. ICMR-National Institute of Nutrition (NIN). (2024). *Dietary guidelines for Indians.* ICMR-National Institute of Nutrition.
49. Nutrition W. P. (1998). *Complementary Feeding of Young Children in Developing Countries: A Review of Current Scientific Knowledge* (WHO/NUT/98.1). Article WHO/NUT/98.1. Retrieved from https://iris.who.int/handle/10665/65932.
50. Marriott, B. P., White, A., Hadden, L., Davies, J. C., & Wallingford, J. C. (2012). World Health Organization (WHO) Infant and Young Child Feeding Indicators: Associations with Growth Measures in 14 Low-income Countries. *Maternal & Child Nutrition, 8*(3), 354–370. Retrieved from https://doi.org/10.1111/j.1740-8709.2011.00380.x.
51. Prado, E. L., & Dewey, K. G. (2014). Nutrition and Brain Development in Early Life. *Nutrition Reviews, 72*(4), 267–84. Retrieved from https://doi.org/10.1111/nure.12102.
52. Lanigan, J. A., Bishop, J. A., Kimber, A. C., & Morgan, J. (2001). Systematic Review Concerning the Age of Introduction of Complementary Foods to the Healthy Full-Term Infant. *European Journal of Clinical Nutrition, 55*(5), 309–320. Retrieved from https://doi.org/10.1038/sj.ejcn.1601168.
53. Aguayo, V. M., Nair, R., Badgaiyan, N., & Krishna, V. (2016). Determinants of Stunting and Poor Linear Growth in Children Under 2 Years of Age in India: An In-depth Analysis of Maharashtra's Comprehensive Nutrition Survey. *Maternal & Child Nutrition, 12*(S1), 121–140. Retrieved from https://doi.org/10.1111/mcn.12259.
54. Papanikolaou, Y., & Fulgoni, V. L. (2018). Egg Consumption in Infants is Associated with Longer Recumbent Length and Greater Intake of Several Nutrients Essential in Growth and Development. *Nutrients, 10*(6), Article 6. Retrieved from https://doi.org/10.3390/nu10060719.
55. Iannotti, L. L. et al. (2017). Eggs in Early Complementary Feeding and Child Growth: A Randomized Controlled Trial. *Pediatrics, 140*(1), e20163459. Retrieved from https://doi.org/10.1542/peds.2016-3459.
56. Dalwai, S. et al. (2013). Consensus Statement of the Indian Academy of Pediatrics on Integrated Management of Severe Acute Malnutrition. *Indian Pediatrics, 50*(4), 399–404. Retrieved from https://doi.org/10.1007/s13312-013-0111-3.

57. World Health Organization. (2005). *Guiding Principles for Feeding Non-breastfed Children 6–24 Months of Age*. World Health Organization.
58. World Health Organization. (2003). *Guiding Principles for Complementary Feeding of the Breastfed Child*. Pan American Health Organization-World Health Organization.
59. United Nations Children's Fund (UNICEF). (2023). *The State of the World's Children Report 2023*. UNICEF, SWORC 2023, New York, NY: UNICEF.
60. National Sample Survey Office (NSSO). (2024). *Survey on Household Consumption Expenditure: August 2022 to July 2023* (NSS Report No. 591, HCES 2022-23). Ministry of Statistics and Programme Implementation, Government of India.
61. Pries, A. M., Rehman, A. M., Filteau, S., Sharma, N., Upadhyay, A., & Ferguson, E. L. (2019). Unhealthy Snack Food and Beverage Consumption Is Associated with Lower Dietary Adequacy and Length-for-Age *z*-Scores among 12–23-month-olds in Kathmandu Valley, Nepal. *The Journal of Nutrition, 149*(10), 1843–1851. Retrieved from https://doi.org/10.1093/jn/nxz140.
62. World Breastfeeding Trends Initiative (WBTi). (2004). *Breastfeeding Promotion Network of India/International Baby Food Action Network*. Retrieved from http://worldbreastfeedingtrends.org/.
63. Gupta, A., & Suri, S. (2021). Protection, Promotion, and Support to Breastfeeding. In S. C. Vir (Ed.), *Public Health Nutrition in Developing Countries* (2nd ed., Vol. 1, pp. 322–360), Woodhead Publishers India.
64. World Health Organization, & United Nations Children's Fund (UNICEF). (2018). *Marketing of Breast-Milk Substitutes: National Implementation of the International Code, Status Report*. World Health Organization.
65. Government of India. (2003). *The Infant Milk Substitutes, Feeding Bottles and Infant Foods (Regulation of Production, Supply and Distribution) Act, 1992 as amended in 2003 (IMS Act)*. Retrieved from http://www.bpni.org/docments/IMS-act.pdf.
66. International Labour Organization (ILO). (2000). *Maternity Protection Convention, 2000 (C183)*.
67. United Nations Children's Fund (UNICEF). (2015). *UNICEF 1990–2005: Innocenti Declaration on the Protection, Promotion and Support of Breastfeeding*. Retrieved from https://waba.org.my/innocenti15/Innocenti15finalpink.pdf.
68. *Implementation Guidance: Protecting, Promoting, and Supporting Breastfeeding in Facilities Providing Maternity and Newborn Services: The Revised Baby-friendly Hospital Initiative 2018*. Retrieved from https://www.who.int/publications/i/item/9789241513807.
69. Government of India. (2016). *Mothers Absolute Affection (MAA): Programme for Promotion of Breastfeeding–Operational Guidelines 2016*. Ministry of Health & Family Welfare. Retrieved from http://nhm.gov.in/MAA/Operational_Guidelines.pdf.
70. Sachdeva, R. C. & Kundu, P. (2021). Optimal Neonatal Nutrition and Care: Early and Exclusive Breastfeeding and Human Milk Banking Support System. In S. C. Vir (Ed.), *Public Health Nutrition in Developing Countries* (2nd ed., vol. 1, pp. 361–419). Woodhead Publishers India.
71. PATH. (2019). *Strengthening Human Milk Banking: A Resource Toolkit for Establishing & Integrating Human Milk Bank Programs, A Global Implementation Framework*. Retrieved from https://www.path.org/who-we-are/programs/maternal-newborn-child-health-and-nutrition/strengthening-human-milk-banking-resource-toolkit/.
72. Abott, S., Barney, J., & Bassett, R. D. (2005). *Dular Project Bihar: Final Evaluation Report*.
73. Vir, S. C., Kalita, A., Mondal, S., & Malik, R. (2014). Impact of Community-Based Mitanin Programme on Undernutrition in Rural Chhattisgarh State, India. *Food and Nutrition Bulletin, 35*(1), 83–91. Retrieved from https://doi.org/10.1177/156482651403500110.
74. ORG Centre for Social Research. (2006). *Community Based Maternal Child Health Project Evaluation*. Division of AC Nielsen ORG-MARG Pvt Ltd, Lucknow.
75. Indian Council of Medical Research (ICMR). (2007). *Positive Deviance Programme in West Bengal*. National Institute of Nutrition, Hyderabad.
76. Dreyfus, M., Li, Y., Chaudhery, D., & Singh, V. (2006). *Evaluation Research of Nutrition Interventions in INHP I Areas of CARE India: Final Evaluation Report*. CARE India, King George Medical University, & Johns Hopkins Bloomberg School of Public Health.

77. CARE. (2007). *Reproductive & Child Health & Nutrition and HIV/AIDS (RACHANA) Programme 2001–2006: Summary of Approaches and Results.*
78. NITI Aayog. (2020). *POSHAN Abhiyaan and NITI Aayog: Accelerating Progress on Nutrition in India: What Will it Take?* Third Progress Report. WCD Division, NITI Aayog..
79. Vir, S. C. (2023). Maternal and Child Nutrition. In S. C. Vir (Ed.), *Child, Adolescent, and Woman Nutrition in India: Public Policies, Programmes, and Progress* (pp. 174–247). KW Publishers.
80. Dalal, R., & Thar, R. (2022). Growth Promoting Recipes. In S. Banapurmath, K. Tiwari, A. Bharadva, E. K. Bang, & S. Mishra (Eds.), *Essentials of Maternal, Infant, Young Child, and Adolescent Nutrition* (Review of IAP–IYCF). Tree Life Media (a division of Kothari Medical).
81. *Addressing-Critical-Failures-of-Infant-and-Young-Child-Nutrition-IYCN-in-South-Asia-IYCN-Challenges-Faced-by-Working-Women-in-Urban-Areas-in-India-and-Sri-Lanka.pdf*. Retrieved from https://documents1.worldbank.org/curated/en/180421573111860339/pdf/Addressing-Critical-Failures-of-Infant-and-Young-Child-Nutrition-IYCN-in-South-Asia-IYCN-Challenges-Faced-by-Working-Women-in-Urban-Areas-in-India-and-Sri-Lanka.pdf.
82. CORD & PHNDC (2026). Utthan: Maternal—Child Health and Nutrition Improvement. *First 1000 Days of Life: A Training Handbook* (Hindi version). CORD Training Centre, Sidhbari, HP 176215.

Chapter 4
Importance of Growth Monitoring and Assessment in Early Childhood

Rajesh Kumar Sinha and Praveen Kumar

Introduction

Undernutrition during the first thousand days in life of children is a significant public health problem in low- and middle-income countries (LMICs). The effects of undernutrition in children aged less than five years are wide ranging, and include increased vulnerability to infections, which lead to high childhood morbidity and mortality [1, 2]. It also causes impaired physical and cognitive development resulting in diminished educational and career performance in the future [3]. Globally in 2022, around 149 million children aged less than five years were stunted, around 45 million wasted, and another 37 million overweight [4]. According to the Global Burden of Disease Study, nearly 70% of deaths among children aged less than five years can be attributed to underlying malnutrition in India. World Health Organization (WHO) has also identified childhood malnutrition as one of the health problems that need special attention in terms of its management and control.

The most cost-effective approach to address this public health problem is by regularly tracking, early identification, and prevention of growth faltering [5]. Growth monitoring involves the systematic tracking of a child's physical growth and development. This includes regular measurements and recording of the child's weight and height or length and their plotting on growth charts to assess the nutritional status and compare with the standard population-based growth curves. Regular growth monitoring and assessment identifies any growth faltering which helps in detecting early state complications [6]. Alongside assessment of physical growth, growth monitoring

R. K. Sinha (✉)
Jaipuria Institute of Management, Jaipur, India
e-mail: cmarajesh@gmail.com

P. Kumar
Lady Hardinge Medical College and Associated Kalawati Saran Children's Hospital, New Delhi, India

S. Suri (ed.), *Child Health and Nutrition from Conception to Age Two*,
https://doi.org/10.1007/978-981-95-7868-9_4

may also involve assessing the child's developmental milestones and cognitive abilities. This helps healthcare providers assess nutritional status and detect any development delays or potential issues, enabling appropriate interventions and referrals for optimal child well-being.

Growth monitoring can lead to early identification and management of growth-related issues like stunting, wasting, and obesity, which respectively affect about 22, 8, and 6% of children globally [6]. The WHO also recognized it as a fundamental strategy to prevent malnutrition and emphasized its inclusion as an integral part of child health and nutrition programs [7]. Other benefits of growth monitoring and assessment include improvements in maternal nutritional knowledge, better infant and young child feeding practices, and increased participation of caregivers in nutrition clinics [8].

Early identification and management of growth failure, through effective growth monitoring and promotion, not only save many lives but also save costs of the health system [9].

Historical Perspective

The evolution of growth monitoring for childcare gained recognition in the early twentieth century with the introduction of growth charts to track the growth patterns of children. In the mid-twentieth century, the WHO and the Center for Disease Control and Prevention started developing standard growth charts based on large-scale population-based studies to track growth patterns in children. In the early twenty-first century, growth monitoring and assessment evolved as a scientific approach to evaluate child health and development. It was also integrated into broader frameworks of early childhood development, assessing feeding practices, and addressing social determinants of health that impact growth. The present growth standards being used to compare a child's growth were developed by the WHO based on the data collected from sampled children from six countries: Brazil, Ghana, India, Norway, Oman, and the United States of America under the WHO Multicentre Growth Reference Study (MGRS) [10]. As per the WHO, these standards can be used as a global benchmark for children as the growth pattern of children is similar when their nutritional, health, and other childcare-related needs are fulfilled. International initiatives like the Sustainable Development Goals (SDGs) have accentuated the importance of growth monitoring as a key strategy of child healthcare programs. Several countries have included growth monitoring and assessment as part of their integrated public health policies to promote optimal growth and development in children.

Steps of Conducting Growth Monitoring and Assessment

Determining the Correct Age of the Child

The child's age is an important parameter to assess the growth of the child and to have an accurate plotting of weight or length/height for the age of the child on the growth chart. Correct plotting of a child's growth will help doing the correct nutritional classification of the child.

Accurate Weight and Height/Length Measurements of a Child

Taking accurate weight and height/length of a child on a regular interval is necessary for growth monitoring and assessment. Length is taken for children less than two years of age or who cannot stand on their own, and height is taken for children aged more than two years. Both weight and height/length should be recorded up to one decimal point in the growth monitoring record. These measurements are essential for assessing growth patterns over time and are easy to perform in clinical and community settings [10].

Plotting the Weight and Height/Length Accurately on Different Growth Charts of Appropriate Gender

In 2006 as per WHO Child Growth Standards after taking the weight and height/length measurements, growth monitoring of children aged up to 5 years is to be done by using weight-for-age, weight-for-height/length, and height/length-for-age-based criteria [10]. Different growth charts are used for girls and boys since they differ in birthweight and attain different sizes relative to their age.

A growth chart is a tool used to assess and monitor a child's growth over time. Pink-bordered charts are for girls and blue-bordered charts are for boys, with two types: weight-for-age and weight-for-length/height.

Weight-for-Age Chart:

- In the weight-for-age growth chart, the horizontal line at the bottom represents the *X*-axis, also called the "month axis", which is used to record the child's age. The vertical line on the left is the *Y*-axis or "weight axis", used to record the child's weight from birth onward (Figs. 4.1 and 4.2).
- The month axis spans five large boxes, each representing one year, with 12 smaller squares inside each box indicating months. Thus, each small square equals one month. The weight axis is marked in kilograms and each line shows 1 kg.
- At each visit, the child's current weight is recorded under the corresponding date.

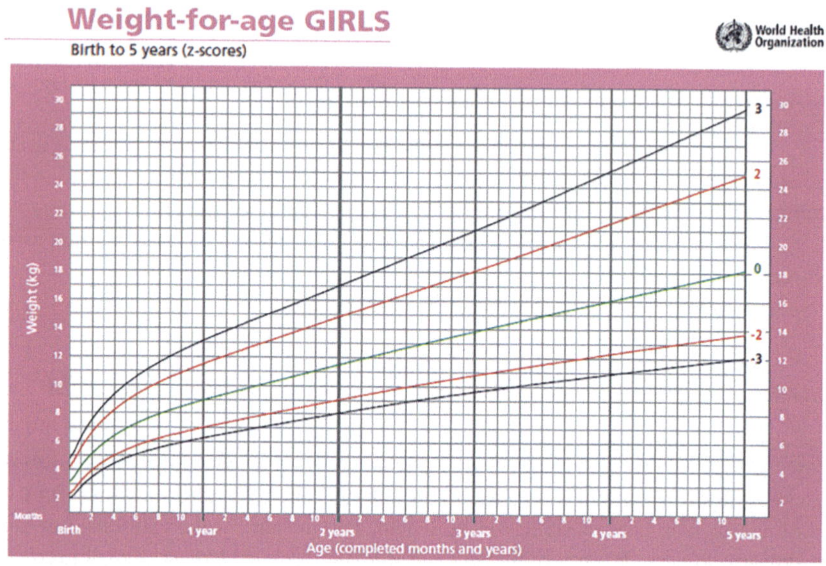

Fig. 4.1 Weight-for-age chart (girls)

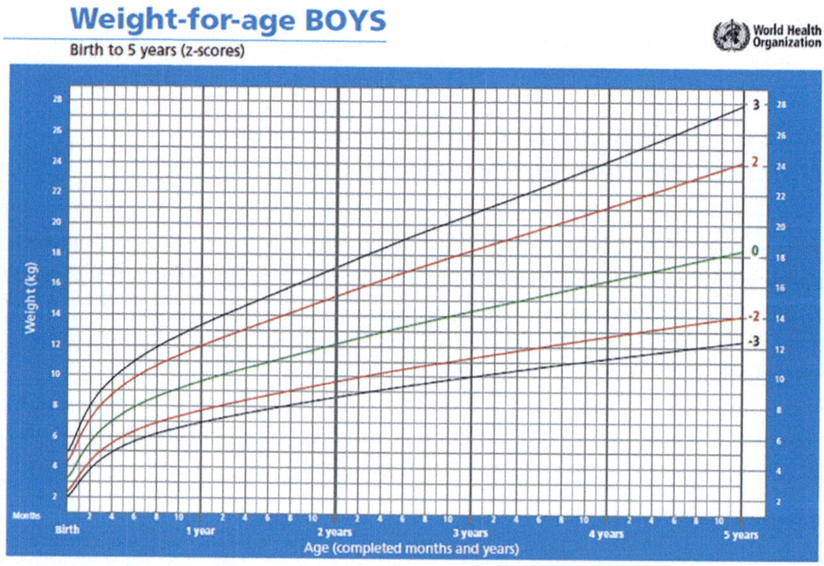

Fig. 4.2 Weight-for-age chart (boys)

- A plotted point is the intersection on the chart where the line from the child's age (*X*-axis) meets the line from their weight (*Y*-axis). Connecting these points over time forms the growth curve, which reflects the child's growth trend. The direction of the curve is more important than any single weight measurement, as it shows whether the child is progressing normally.
- Each growth chart includes five pre-printed reference curves, known as Z-score lines, which serve as benchmarks to interpret growth and assess nutritional status:
  - The middle curve represents the median, indicating the average growth pattern.
  - Children exhibiting normal growth typically have their weight plotted between the second and fourth curves above the lowest curve.
  - Moderately underweight children have their weight plotted between the second curve and the bottommost curve.
  - Severely underweight children have their weight below the bottommost curve on the chart.

Weight-for-Length/Height Chart:

- Low weight in a child may happen due to wasting or stunting or both together. Plotting parameters on a weight-for-length/height chart helps us to differentiate wasted and stunted children whose weight-for-age alone is not able to differentiate.
- The horizontal line at the bottom of the chart represents the *X*-axis, which is used to record the child's length/height up to five years. The vertical line on the left side is the *Y*-axis, referred to as the weight axis, used to record the child's weight from birth onward (Figs. 4.3 and 4.4).

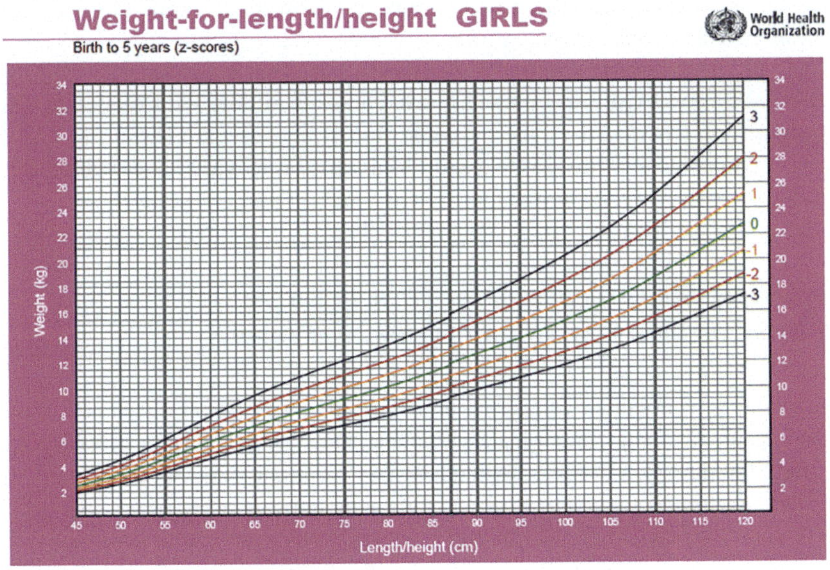

Fig. 4.3 Weight-for-length/height chart (girls)

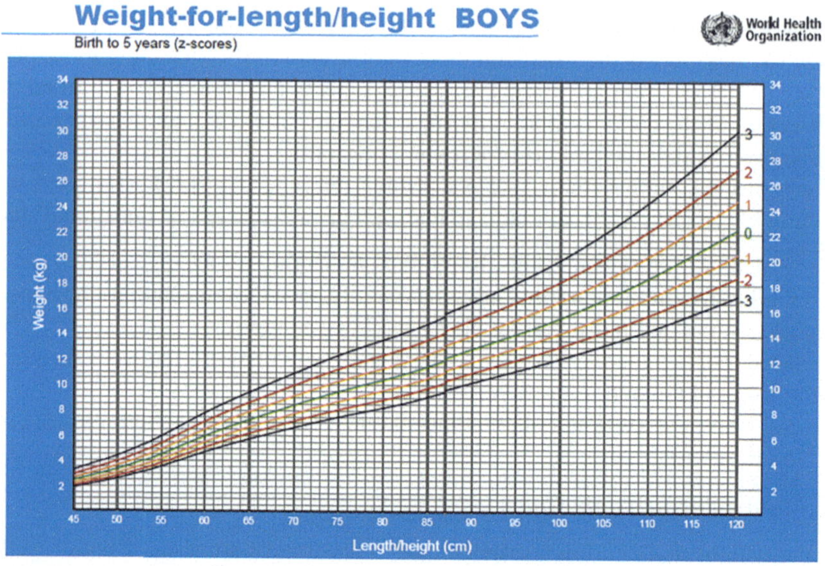

Fig. 4.4 Weight-for-length/height chart (boys)

- Each growth chart includes five pre-printed reference curves, also known as Z-score lines, which help evaluate and interpret a child's growth pattern and assess nutritional status.
- The middle curve on the chart denotes the median, or average growth. The two curves above the median represent values above average, while the two curves below indicate values below average.
- The weight of normal and healthy children, based on their length/height, typically falls between the second and fourth curves. Children with Moderate Acute Malnutrition (MAM) have their weight plotted between the second and lowest curve, while those with Severe Acute Malnutrition (SAM) have weight values below the bottommost curve.

Interpreting the Direction of the Growth Curve and Recognizing If the Child Is Growing Properly

A growth curve is obtained when growth measurements (e.g. weight) of two or more time points are available, and joined with a line. Depending upon the growth pattern of a child, the direction of the growth curve may be flat, upward, or downward. This helps in determining whether the child is growing appropriately or not. An upward growth curve indicates that the child is growing healthy and gaining weight. When the weight gain of the child as per the age is not sufficient, then the growth curve is either flat or downward. A flat curve or a curve moving downwards for two successive months calls for healthcare provider and caregiver's attention.

Discussing the Child's Growth with the Caregiver and Follow-up Actions: Discussing a child's growth with the caregiver, based on the growth curve, is a critical element of growth monitoring. Thus, the growth chart serves as an educational and a promotional tool for both health workers and caregivers. It also initiates a communication process related to a child's growth and guides the caregiver when the child's growth is unfavorable.

Classification of Nutritional Status Using Measured Anthropometric Parameters

After taking the anthropometric measurements of the child and computing *z*-scores or standard deviation (SD) scores (using the WHO charts), the next step is to classify the child's nutritional status based on the WHO classification table (Table 4.1). A well-growing child will have his nutritional parameters (length/height for age, weight for age, and weight for length/height) within ±2 *z*-scores (SD scores) of the median expected for the age and sex. Individuals lying outside this range are malnourished and should therefore be carefully evaluated and managed. If the child's nutritional parameters are less than the –2 *z*-score, it indicates the presence of stunting, underweight, and wasting, respectively.

Stunting

Stunting, or shortness, is an indicator of chronic (long term) malnutrition and sets during the early years of life. Failure to achieve expected length/height compared to a healthy, well-nourished child of the same age and sex is a sign of stunting. As shown in Table 4.1, if the child's height-for-age *z* (SD) score is between median to –2SD, then the nutritional status of the child is said to be "normal". If it is between –2SD and –3SD, then the nutritional status of the child is said to be "moderately stunted" and if it is below –3SD, the nutritional status of the child is said to be "severely stunted". Stunting impacts both the physical and cognitive development of the child, and adversely impacts their learning abilities and adult life productivity [11].

Table 4.1 WHO classification of malnutrition

Anthropometric indicator and condition	Age		Z-Score						
	0–23 months	24–60 months	< −3	> −3 to < −2	> −2 to < −1	> −1 to < +1	> +1 to < +2	> +2 to < +3	> +3
Length-for-age Stunting	√		Severe stunting	Moderate stunting	Normal				Extreme tallness is not usually a nutrition issue. May indicate endocrine disorder
Height-for-age Stunting		√							
Weight-for-age Underweight	√	√	Severe underweight	Moderate underweight	Normal		Do not use weight-for-age to determine overweight. Weight-for-length/height (0–60 months) and BMI-for-age (all ages) are better for assessing overweight in children		
Weight-for-length Wasting, overweight/ obesity	√		Severe wasting/severe acute malnutrition (SAM)	Moderate wasting/ moderate acute malnutrition (MAM)	Normal		Possible risk of overweight	Overweight	Obesity
Weight-for-height Wasting, overweight/ obesity		√							
BMI-for-age Wasting, overweight/ obesity	√	√	Severe wasting/SAM	Moderate wasting/MAM	Normal		Possible risk of overweight	Overweight	Obesity

Underweight

Underweight is defined as not reaching the expected weight for a healthy, well-nourished child of the same age and sex. If the child's weight-for-age SD-score is between median to –2SD, then the nutritional status of the child is said to be "normal". If it falls between –2SD to –3SD, then the nutritional status of the child is said to be "moderately underweight" and if it is below –3SD, then the nutritional status of the child is said to be "severely underweight". Being underweight could be due to either stunting or wasting or both and is a primary indicator of heightened risk of illnesses [11].

Wasting

Wasting, or thinness, is an indicator of acute (short term) undernutrition or low weight for corresponding length/height. If the child's weight for length/height lies between median to –2SD, then the nutritional status of the child is said to be "normal". If it falls between –2SD to –3SD, then the nutritional status of the child is said to be "moderately wasted" and if it is below –3SD, then the nutritional status of the child is said to be "severely wasted". Wasting is an acute form of malnutrition, resulting from loss of muscle mass, often caused due to illness or inadequate food intake. A child with wasting has lower immunity and is more prone to illness.

Children under five years of age, with any level of anthropometric deficits are at a higher risk of morbidity and mortality. Multiple anthropometric deficits further aggravate this risk.

- **Weight for Length/Height**: Weight for length/height is a measure of weight compared to the reference weight for that gender and length/height. This index is used to assess nutritional status of children under five years and is also useful when age is not known or unreliable.
- **Body Mass Index**: It is calculated as [weight in kilogram (kg)/(height in meter)^2]. It is a recommended index to assess nutritional status of children who are five years or above. Age and gender-specific BMI percentile curves are available for reference.
- **Head Circumference**: The head circumference should be recorded between birth and six years when maximum brain growth occurs. Head circumference should be plotted on Head Circumference Growth Chart to identify abnormalities.
- **Waist Circumference**: The waist circumference helps to identify overweight and obese children and adolescents. This should be measured for children above five years.

Importance of Growth Monitoring and Assessment in Early Childhood

Growth monitoring and assessment help in the early detection of abnormal growth among children. Early identification of growth faltering facilitates early treatment and management of conditions causing abnormal growth. It also provides opportunities to educate caregivers on childhood care and feeding. Several pieces of evidence suggest that regular growth monitoring and assessment help reduce childhood malnutrition, morbidity, mortality, while also increases the uptake of child health and nutrition services. In addition, it also helps in the early identification of underlying diseases like turner's syndrome, celiac disease, tuberculosis, gastroesophageal reflux diseases (GERD), etc.

Evidence of Growth Monitoring on Reducing Childhood Malnutrition, Morbidity, Mortality, and Uptake of Other Services

Several studies have reported the benefits of monitoring growth in children. Studies suggest that growth monitoring in the first 1000 days of a child's life, starting from conception till the end of the second year is crucial to ensure good health, development, and long-term benefits [12]. A study conducted in South Trelawny, Jamaica, noted a decrease in the prevalence of underweight and a decrease in childhood morbidity [13]. An experimental study conducted in India with growth monitoring combined with individual counseling and targeted supplementation found significantly lower childhood mortality, higher weight and length gains, and higher hemoglobin concentration. The findings were also found equitable with a greater proportional benefit to children from the disadvantaged groups [14]. Two other growth monitoring programs in India found better nutritional status and survival of children [15, 16]. The Joint Nutrition Support Programme (JNSP) in Tanzania, led by WHO and UNICEF [17, 18], used aggregated growth monitoring data to assess child malnutrition at the community level. This approach, which also included actions to promote maternal and child health, improve water and sanitation practices, enhance household food security, and support livelihoods, resulted in reduced rates of underweight among children and improved immunization coverage. The Tamil Nadu Integrated Nutrition Project (TINP) included growth monitoring, targeted nutrition counseling, supplementary feeding for growth faltering, immunization, and deworming. This approach led to improved weight gain and a higher likelihood of receiving immunization, deworming, and vitamin A supplementation [19, 20]. Another study in Tamil Nadu, India found that growth monitoring in conjunction with an intensive nutrition education intervention achieved better weight and height gains [21]. An evaluation of India's Integrated Child Development Services (ICDS) scheme, launched in 1975, revealed that the program—offering monthly growth monitoring for children, ready-to-eat meals or take-home rations, iron and folic acid, vitamin A every six months, and pre-school education—resulted in significantly fewer cases of moderate and severe malnutrition compared to non-ICDS area [22, 23]. A study conducted in Honduras on growth monitoring and promotion found improvements in childcare knowledge, attitudes, and practices among caregivers [24].

Community-based growth monitoring programs significantly improve nutritional outcomes among children, especially in LMICs. Countries like Brazil and Kenya have demonstrated significant improvements in child health outcomes with diligent growth tracking by the network of community health workers [25]. Growth monitoring programs, when implemented effectively, have a profound public health impact. Early identification and immediate action to address malnutrition help in reducing child mortality, improving recovery and rehabilitation [26].

Evidence of Growth Monitoring on Improving Utilization of Health Services

Evidence of growth monitoring was also linked to increased utilization of health services. The study in Bangladesh found that the growth monitoring program had higher immunization rates, oral rehydration solutions (ORS), and vitamin A supplementation in the intervention arm [27]. Similarly in India, Avsm et al. (1995) found that uptake in ICDS such as vitamin A, iron, and folate supplementation proved to be more effective than non-ICDS blocks [22]. Other studies conducted in India [15], and Haiti [16] also observed an increase in health service utilization, immunizations, ORS, deworming, family planning services, and vitamin A supplementation. A study conducted in Casamance, the southern part of rural Senegal, revealed that growth monitoring and promotion sessions elevated the participation of mothers in bringing their children to health centers for routine health checkups, and in nutrition and health education sessions [28]. The evidence indicates that growth monitoring can improve utilization of healthcare services to achieve greater nutritional status and survival of children. Several studies have found that utilization of services leads to enhanced nutritional status of children. A study conducted in India found that growth monitoring and nutrition education led to increased service uptake, resulting in better linear growth, improved breastfeeding and complementary feeding practices [29].

Growth monitoring and promotion is essential not just for individual child health but also to provide insights for public health policy and programming [30]. It provides valuable data for allocation of public health resources and evaluates the effectiveness of current health strategies. Growth monitoring also led to community mobilization and social action to address the problem of child malnutrition. It helps in improving the knowledge and awareness of caregivers, community members, and leaders leading to collective and effective action to address the social determinants of child malnutrition and promote good health.

Challenges of Growth Monitoring in Children

Inadequate Resources

In spite of its significance, the growth monitoring program faces several challenges that can hinder its effectiveness. One of the critical challenges is the lack of adequate resources, inadequate infrastructure, shortage of trained manpower, and insufficient or non-functional equipment, especially in the LMICs. Limited access to such resources can severely impact the quality and frequency of growth monitoring [31, 32]. Additionally, inadequate infrastructural support for data collection, storage, and analysis can also lead to incomplete or inaccurate growth tracking [33].

Lack of Skilled Health Workers

Well-trained manpower, who can accurately measure, record, and interpret the data, is critical for any growth monitoring program. Gaps in training and providing handholding support to healthcare workers lead to inaccurate measurements and misinterpretations in the growth data which results in incorrect diagnoses and inappropriate interventions [34]. Experience from large-scale programs found inaccuracy in growth data due to errors in taking weight and length/height and plotting. Interpreting growth charts is another technical aspect where inaccuracies were often reported. These studies have also found unsatisfactory levels of precision by health workers [35–39]. Lack of supportive supervision and feedback mechanism was also found to be the shortcoming of a community-based growth monitoring and promotion program [40, 41]. Several studies have shown that growth monitoring and promotion programs achieved good outcomes where considerable time was spent on training and supervision of health workers [21, 41]. It is important to provide adequate training to community health workers, provide ongoing support, and equip them with the necessary resources needed for effective growth monitoring.

Emerging technologies like mobile health (mHealth) solutions have shown promise in enhancing the scope and accuracy of growth monitoring. Mobile health applications and portable devices enable more frequent data collection and real-time educating the caregivers for potentially increasing the reach and impact of growth monitoring and promotion programs [30]. Furthermore, the integration of technology in growth monitoring helps in effectively tracking child's growth and provides timely alerts of any deviations from normal patterns [42].

Cultural Beliefs Hindering Growth Monitoring

Cultural beliefs and practices were also found to be influencing the effectiveness of growth monitoring programs [43]. A significant challenge in implementing effective growth monitoring programs is the level of awareness and understanding among the caregivers of young children. Black et al. highlighted the need for community education and awareness campaigns to improve the uptake and success of growth monitoring programs [1].

Disconnect Between Growth Monitoring Linked Counseling and Other Activities

The WHO defines growth monitoring and promotion as nutrition interventions that not only measure and plot the weight of children but also use the information to counsel caregiver on children's physical growth and motivate them to enhance development [6]. Ideally, the counseling should address the specific needs of each mother and her child, and hence, health workers should be trained in providing need-based counseling and support to each caregiver [44]. Numerous studies have also found that the skills of health workers on anthropometric measurements were fairly good but they were lacking in nutritional and interpersonal communication skills [27, 45].

In the studies conducted in Ghana, Lesotho, and Thailand, growth monitoring alone, without additional linked activities such as nutrition education and supplementation, did not show a clear pattern of improved nutritional status [46–49]. Bhandari & Bahl, found that growth monitoring services, especially in the low-resource settings, are fragmented and require integration of growth monitoring with broader child health services to maximize its impact [29]. An integrated package that includes growth monitoring, health and nutrition education, nutritional supplementation, and referral for high-risk cases is found to be effective in achieving nutritional goals [12, 50]. Hence, it is also important to prioritize building the nutrition knowledge and counseling skills of healthcare providers alongside improving their growth monitoring skills. There is a clear association between weight gain velocity and childhood mortality [51] so, it would be important to organize regular growth monitoring of children, which will help in reducing the burden of childhood morbidity and mortality. It is very difficult to treat severe malnutrition and evidences also indicates that case-fatality rates remain high in most settings [52].

Sub-optimal Coverage of the Growth Monitoring Programs

The success of the growth monitoring also depends on its optimal coverage. However, several studies have found that the coverage or participation of regular growth monitoring is not optimal [44, 53]. Challenges such as geographical barriers, lack of transportation, and financial constraints can affect regular attendance to growth monitoring sessions, impacting early detection and treatment of growth abnormalities [54]. As growth monitoring and promotion includes a full package of preventive care services, sub-optimal coverage will limit its impact [55, 56]. Several studies showed that many caregivers fail to attend the growth monitoring sessions due to high opportunity costs or other family commitments [35, 57]. Other reasons were found to be high waiting time or very brief and ineffective nutritional counseling [44]. A review of large-scale programs supported by UNICEF [58], including the ICDS program in India [26], and the BRAC [59] program in Bangladesh observed low coverage and attendance as major weaknesses that prevented the achievement of desired outcomes. In India, the ICDS program has been universalized to maximize outreach; however, data from the national survey NFHS-5 (2019–2021) reported that only 60% of children received growth monitoring services [60].

These challenges demand a comprehensive approach involving infrastructure enhancement, policy adjustments, community engagement, and enhanced training programs. Overcoming these hurdles is crucial to harness the full potential of growth monitoring in effectively promoting child health and development. Jones et al. recommended that community involvement, political will, and a multi-sectoral approach involving health, education, and nutrition will help achieve the desired outcome from the growth monitoring program [61].

Policy and Public Health: How Different Countries Integrate Growth Monitoring into Public Health Policy

Many countries have included regular growth monitoring as a critical part of their public health policies to improve the overall health and nutritional status of children. For example, the USA has introduced growth monitoring as a standard practice in pediatric healthcare. In India, a large-scale ICDS program includes monthly growth monitoring and promotion activities where the nutritional status of children enrolled in these centers is tracked using monthly growth monitoring activities in addition to other nutrition promotion activities. Similarly, in Bangladesh, community-based programs such as the Community Clinic Health Assistance Project regularly track growth of the children aged less than five years and additionally provide counseling to caregivers on nutrition and feeding practices, and refer children with severe malnutrition to health facilities for treatment. In Brazil, growth monitoring has been introduced as one of the core activities in the public health program called the Family Health Strategy (FHS). In this, regular growth monitoring sessions are held whereby community health workers (CHWs) visit households to assess the growth of children, to provide health and nutrition counseling to caregivers, and to refer children with growth faltering to inpatient facilities for further evaluation and treatment. The program has shown significant improvements in child health outcomes, and this is directly associated with regular growth monitoring sessions [62].

For effective implementation of the growth monitoring and assessment program, the governments should set guidelines, ensure ethical technology use, and support device procurement for CHWs. Public awareness campaigns and community feedback are essential for program success and participation.

Growing Debate on Using the Who Growth Standards Versus Regional Growth Reference

Growth standards represent a healthy pattern of growth based on a selected reference sample of healthy children. This tells how the children ought to grow rather than how they grow. On the other hand, growth reference tells how the children grow and may be applied to other children to see whether their growth follows the growth of the reference group [63]. The WHO MGRS growth standards of 2006 are intended to provide a universal metric for assessing the growth and development of children. These standards are based on the growth patterns of healthy children from diverse ethnic backgrounds who were raised in environments that support their optimal growth potential. This provides a common platform for cross country comparison and a comparison of the growth of children from various ethnicities and races. As MGRS study was conducted among healthy children living in optimal conditions, it provides an aspirational growth standard for children living in different countries to reach their full genetic potential by providing them with appropriate nutritional interventions. Many countries adopted these standards for monitoring the growth of their children. After the introduction of growth standards of WHO, there is an ongoing debate regarding the use of WHO growth standards versus using the country-specific growth reference, which is considered to account for genetic factors. Many studies have found that the WHO growth standards over-diagnose stunting, wasting, and underweight in many countries and eventually increase the perceived disease burden in children. These studies did not show the growth trajectories like the WHO growth standards. The studies also found regional differences in child growth patterns when compared with the WHO standard. This suggests adopting region-specific growth reference to increase the sensitivity in identifying children with adverse nutritional outcomes. This concern is particularly relevant for Asian countries, where children tend to be thinner and lighter compared to the WHO reference population. Several countries have now started using their growth reference instead of the WHO standards to provide a more accurate growth assessment of their children. For example, the UK uses the WHO growth standard for children only up to four years of age while the USA only uses it for children up to two years of age. Even countries like India,

Malawi, and Indonesia are prompted to use their own growth reference for better representation and providing appropriate nutritional interventions [64–67]. However, despite these concerns, the WHO-MGRS standards should continue to be used, given their aspirational nature and the comprehensive data they provide for tracking and improving child health outcomes. Evidence shows that Indian states and other developing countries such as Vietnam, Bangladesh, and China have successfully reduced stunting using WHO-MGRS growth standards [64]. This suggests the WHO MGRS growth standards offer a valuable tool for global health monitoring, however, their application requires careful consideration of local contexts and continuous evaluation to ensure they meet the diverse needs of populations worldwide. Moreover, a universal growth standard is crucial for assessing compliance with the United Nations Convention on the Rights of the Child, ensuring every child's right to healthy growth and development. A balanced approach is needed, where the WHO growth standards are used for global comparison, while regional growth references are also incorporated to formulate more effective child nutrition policies and programs in developing countries.

Conclusion

Malnutrition among children is an important health problem in developing countries due to its high prevalence and associated risks. Regular growth screening can be beneficial to assess the extent of the problem. The body of evidence shows that regular, quality growth monitoring and nutrition education help prevent malnutrition.

Understanding a child's nutritional status is an essential component of a broader analysis of their overall health. The integration of regular growth monitoring and assessment into the existing health systems helps in safeguarding children's overall health and development, which, in turn, supports stronger communities and economies. Continued research, adequate funding, and global cooperation are essential to address the challenges faced by growth monitoring programs and to ensure their effectiveness and sustainability. While growth monitoring and assessment are essential to promote children's health, their efficacy heavily relies on community participation, adequate skills of health workers, effective counseling to the parents, and linkage with other nutrition and health services. It is also important to address barriers such as resource limitations and cultural resistance to enhance its effectiveness. Its integration within the larger health systems can provide enough resources for training healthcare workers, technological enhancements, and public awareness to foster a supportive environment for growth monitoring. The use of technologies, such as mobile applications for comparing growth patterns against standards, can provide timely alerts on growth-related issues. The use of image analysis technology can easily detect abnormalities or trends that might not be immediately apparent. Future research can be conducted to enhance the effectiveness, accessibility, and ethical use of these technologies in growth monitoring and assessment of children.

Growth monitoring is pivotal in advancing the SDGs, particularly SDG 2, which targets hunger eradication, food security, nutrition enhancement, and sustainable agriculture. It enables healthcare providers to evaluate children's nutritional status, detect early signs of malnutrition, and deliver tailored interventions, aligning with SDG 3's emphasis on universal health and well-being. The early detection of health or developmental delays supports SDG 4's mission of inclusive education and lifelong learning, as it aids children in reaching cognitive milestones and excel academically. Moreover, growth monitoring fosters collaboration (SDG 17) by uniting healthcare providers, policymakers, community workers, and families to enhance child's health and well-being. This underscores the critical role of growth monitoring in achieving international health objectives like the SDGs, and in significantly enhancing child health, nutrition, and overall well-being.

References

1. Baguune, B., Aminu, D. M., Bekyieriya, E., & Adokiya, M. N. (2023). Utilization of Growth Monitoring and Promotion Services and Undernutrition of Children Less Than Two Years of Age in Northern Ghana. *BMC Nutrition, 9*(1), 70. Retrieved from https://doi.org/10.1186/s40795-023-00729-6
2. Swaminathan, S., et al. (2019). The Burden of Child and Maternal Malnutrition and Trends in Its Indicators in the States of India: The Global Burden of Disease Study 1990–2017. *The Lancet Child & Adolescent Health, 3*(12), 855–870.
3. Black, R. E., et al. & Maternal and Child Nutrition Study Group. (2013). Maternal and Child Undernutrition and Overweight in Low-Income and Middle-Income Countries. *The Lancet, 382*(9890), 427–51. Retrieved from https://doi.org/10.1016/S0140-6736(13)60937-X
4. World Health Organization. (2024). *Malnutrition.* Retrieved from https://www.who.int/news-room/fact-sheets/detail/malnutrition#:~:text=Globally%20in%202022%2C%20149%20million,age%20are%20linked%20to%20undernutrition.
5. Griffiths, M. & Rosso, J. D. (n.d.). *Growth Monitoring and the Promotion of Healthy Young Child Growth: Evidence of Effectiveness and Potential to Prevent Malnutrition.* The Manoff Group. Retrieved from http://www.manoffgroup.com/documents/GMP_UNICEF_Nov_1608.pdf
6. United Nations Children's Fund. (2013). *Improving Child Nutrition: The Achievable Imperative for Global Progress.* UNICEF.
7. World Health Organization. (2009). *WHO Child Growth Standards.* Retrieved from https://doi.org/10.1111/j.1469-8749.2009.03503.x
8. Hossain, S. M. M., Duffield, A., & Taylor, A. (2005). An Evaluation of the Impact of a US$60 Million Nutrition Programme in Bangladesh. *Health Policy and Planning, 20,* 35–40.
9. Bern, C., Zucker, J. R., Perkins, B. A., Otieno, J., Oloo, A. J., & Yip, R. (1997). Assessment of Potential Indicators for Protein-Energy Malnutrition in the Algorithm for Integrated Management of Childhood Illness. *Bulletin of the World Health Organization, 75*(1), 87–96.
10. Multicentre Growth Reference Study Group. (2006). WHO Child Growth Standards Based on Length/Height, Weight and Age. *Acta Paediatrica Supplement.*
11. Olofin, I., et al. & Nutrition Impact Model Study. (2013). Associations of Suboptimal Growth with All-Cause and Cause-Specific Mortality in Children Under Five Years: A Pooled Analysis of Ten Prospective Studies. *PLOS ONE, 8*(5), https://doi.org/10.1371/journal.pone.0064636.
12. Garner, P., Panpanich, R., & Logan, S. (2000). Is Routine Growth Monitoring Effective? A Systematic Review of Trials. *Archives of Disease in Childhood, 82,* 197–201.

13. Melville, B., Fidler, T., Mehan, D., Bernard, E., & Mullings, J. (1995). Growth Monitoring: The Role of Community Health Volunteers. *Public Health, 109*, 111–116.
14. Kielmann, A. A., Taylor, C. E., & Parker, R. L. (1978). The Narangwal Nutrition Study: A Summary Review. *American Journal of Clinical Nutrition, 31*, 2040–2052.
15. Chaudhuri, S. N. (1988). Growth Monitoring in the Evolution of Clinic-Based Health Care Through a Community-Based Action Program. *Indian Journal of Pediatrics, 55*(1), S84–S87.
16. Genece, E., & Rohde, J. E. (1988). Growth Monitoring as an Entry Point for Primary Health Care. *Indian Journal of Pediatrics, 55*(1), S78–S83.
17. Government of the United Republic of Tanzania, World Health Organization, & United Nations Children's Fund. (1989). *The Joint WHO/UNICEF Nutrition Support Programme in Iringa, Tanzania 1983–1988 Evaluation Report*. Dar es Salaam.
18. United Nations Children's Fund (1993). *We will Never Go Back*. UNICEF.
19. Shekar, M. (1991). *The Tamil Nadu Integrated Nutrition Project: A Review of the Project with Special Emphasis on the Monitoring and Information System* (Cornell Food and Nutrition Policy Program Working Paper).
20. Shekar, M., & Latham, M. C. (1992). Growth Monitoring Can and Does Work! An Example from the Tamil Nadu Integrated Nutrition Project in Rural South India. *Journal of Pediatrics, 59*, 5–15.
21. George, S. M., Latham, M. C., Abel, R., Ethirajan, N., & Frongillo, E. A. (1993). Evaluation of Effectiveness of Good Growth Monitoring in South Indian Villages. *The Lancet, 342*, 348–352.
22. Avsm, Y. S., Gandhi, N., Tandon, B. N., & Krishnamurthy, K. S. (1995). Integrated Child Development Services Scheme and Nutritional Status of Indian Children. *Journal of Tropical Paediatrics, 41*, 123–128.
23. Kapil, U., & Pradhan, R. (1999). Integrated Child Development Services (ICDS) Scheme and Its Impact on Nutritional Status of Children in India and Recent Initiatives. *Indian Journal of Public Health, 43*, 21–25.
24. Van Roekel, K., Plowman, B., Griffiths, M., de Alvarado, V. V., Matute, J., & Calderón, M. (2002). BASICS II Midterm Evaluation of the AIN Program in Honduras, 2000. *Survey report*, BASICS II/USAID.
25. Griffin, J. B., et al. (2016). Effectiveness of Community Health Workers Delivering Preventive Interventions for Maternal and Child Health in Low- and Middle-Income Countries: A Systematic Review. *BMC Public Health, 13*, 847. Retrieved from https://doi.org/10.1186/1471-2458-13-847
26. Ashworth, A., *et al.* (2006). Effectiveness of Community-Based Treatment of Severe Malnutrition. *Food and Nutrition Bulletin.*
27. Karim, F., Huq, N., Brown, L., & Chowdhury, A. M. R. (1994). Growth Monitoring in the Context of a Primary Health Care Programme. *Food and Nutrition Bulletin, 15*, 192–199.
28. Pinchinat, S., et al. (2004). No Improvement in Weight-for-Age of Young Children in Southern Senegal, 1969–1992, Despite a Drastic Reduction in Mortality: Evidence from a Growth Monitoring Programme. *International Journal of Epidemiology, 33*, 1202–1208.
29. Bhandari, N., Mazumder, S., Bahl, R., Martines, J., Black, R. E., & Bhan, M. K. (2005). Use of Multiple Opportunities for Improving Feeding Practices in Under-Twos within Child Health Programmes. *Health Policy and Planning, 20*, 328–336.
30. Taylor, M., Tapkigen, J., Ali, I., Liu, Q., Long, Q., & Nabwera, H. (2023). The Impact of Growth Monitoring and Promotion on Health Indicators in Children Under Five Years of Age in Low- and Middle-Income Countries. *The Cochrane Database of Systematic Reviews, 10*(10), CD014785. Retrieved from https://doi.org/10.1002/14651858.CD014785.
31. Victora, C., et al. (2016). Breastfeeding in the 21st Century: Epidemiology, Mechanisms, and Lifelong Effect. *The Lancet, 387*(10017), 475–490. Retrieved from https://doi.org/10.1016/S0140-6736(15)01024-7.
32. Belew, A. K., et al. (2024). Utilisation of Growth Monitoring and Promotion Services and Associated Factors Among Mothers of Children Younger Than 2 Years in Gondar Zuria District, Northwest Ethiopia: A Community-Based, Cross-Sectional Study. *BMJ Open, 14*, e076147. Retrieved from https://doi.org/10.1136/bmjopen-2023-076147.

33. Ashworth, A., Shrimpton, R., & Jamil, K. (2008). Growth Monitoring and Promotion: Review of Evidence of Impact. *Maternal & Child Nutrition, 4*(1), 86–117. Retrieved from https://doi.org/10.1111/j.1740-8709.2007.00125.x.
34. Ashworth, A., & Millward, D. J. (1986). Catch-Up Growth in Children. *Nutrition Reviews, 44*(5), 157–163. Retrieved from https://doi.org/10.1111/j.1753-4887.1986.tb07613.x.
35. Gopaldas, T., Christian, P. S., Abbi, R. D., & Gujral, S. (1990). Does Growth Monitoring Work as It Ought to in Countries of Low Literacy? *Journal of Tropical Pediatrics, 36*, 322–327.
36. Kuhn, L., & Zwarenstein, M. F. (1990). Weight Information on the 'Road to Health' Card Inadequate for Growth Monitoring. *South African Medical Journal, 78*, 495–496.
37. Dixon, R. A. (1993). Cost-Effectiveness of Growth Monitoring and Promotion. *The Lancet, 342*, 317.
38. Dixon, R. A., & Sutton, P. (1994). Child Growth Monitoring: Errors of Measurement with the TALC Direct Recording Scale. *Journal of Tropical Pediatrics, 40*, 376–378.
39. Valadez, J. J., Brown, L. D., Vargas, W. V., & Morley, D. C. (1996). Using Lot Quality Assurance Sampling to Assess Measurements for Growth Monitoring in a Developing Country's Primary Health Care System. *International Journal of Epidemiology, 25*, 381–387.
40. Hendrata, L., & Rohde, J. E. (1988). Ten Pitfalls of Growth Monitoring and Promotion. *Indian Journal of Pediatrics, 55*(1), S9–S15.
41. Alderman, M. H., Wise, P. H., Ferguson, R. P., Laverde, H. T., & d'Souza, A. J. (1978). Reduction of Young Child Malnutrition and Mortality in Rural Jamaica. *Journal of Tropical Pediatrics, 24*, 7–11.
42. Rollins, N. C., et al. (2016). Why Invest, and What It Will Take to Improve Breastfeeding Practices? *The Lancet, 387*(10017), 491–504. Retrieved from https://doi.org/10.1016/S0140-6736(15)01044-2.
43. Charlton, K. E., Kawana, B. M., & Hendricks, M. K. (2009). An Assessment of the Effectiveness of Growth Monitoring and Promotion Practices in the Lusaka District of Zambia. *Nutrition (Burbank, Los Angeles County, California), 25*(10), 1035–46. Retrieved from https://doi.org/10.1016/j.nut.2009.03.008.
44. Gerein, N. M., & Ross, D. A. (1991). Is Growth Monitoring Worthwhile? An Evaluation of Its Use in Three Child Health Programs in Zaire. *Social Science & Medicine, 32*, 667–675.
45. Kapil, U., Saxena, N., Nayar, D., & Gnanasekaran, N. (1996). Status of Growth Monitoring Activities in Selected ICDS Projects of Rajasthan. *Indian Pediatrics, 33*, 949–952.
46. Pielemeier, N. R. (1978). *Use of the Child's Growth Chart as an Educational Tool*. Office of Nutrition Development Support Bureau Agency for International Development.
47. Viravaidhya, K. V., Tima, K. N., & Merrill, H. D. (1981). *Impact of Age/Weight Charts Maintained in the Home and Nutrition Education on Nutritional Status of Infants and Pre-school Children*. Nutrition Division, Ministry of Public Health, Royal Thai Government.
48. Hampshire, R. D., Aguayo, V. M., Harouna, H., Roley, J. A., Tarini, A., & Baker, S. K. (2004). Delivery of Nutrition Services in Health Systems in Sub-Saharan Africa: Opportunities in Burkina Faso, Mozambique, and Niger. *Public Health Nutrition, 7*, 1047–1053.
49. Roberfroid, D., Lefèvre, P., Hoerée, T., & Kolsteren, P. (2005). Perceptions of Growth Monitoring and Promotion Among an International Panel of District Medical Officers. *Journal of Health, Population, and Nutrition, 23*, 207–214.
50. Tonglet, R., et al. (1999). How Useful Are Anthropometric, Clinical, and Dietary Measurements of Nutritional Status as Predictors of Morbidity of Young Children in Central Africa? *Tropical Medicine and International Health, 4*, 120–130.
51. Ross, A., & English, M. (2005). Early Infant Growth Monitoring: Time Well Spent? *Tropical Medicine and International Health, 10*, 404–411.
52. Waterlow, J. (1999). Treatment of Children with Malnutrition and Diarrhoea. *The Lancet, 354*, 1142.
53. Coetzee, D. J., & Ferrinho, P. (1994). Nutritional Status of Children in Alexandra Township: Clinic-Based Data and a Community Survey. *South African Medical Journal, 84*, 413–415.
54. Owais, A., Hanif, B., Siddiqui, A. R., Agha, A., & Zaidi, A. K. (2011). Does Improving Maternal Knowledge of Vaccines Impact Infant Immunization Rates? A Community-Based Randomized-Controlled Trial in Karachi, Pakistan. *BMC Public Health*.

55. Rasheed, P., Sunbul, T. J., Ahmed, B. E., & Al Saleh, A. M. (1996). The Growth Chart: Its Use and Perception Among Mothers Visiting Primary Health Care Centers of Al Khobar, Saudi Arabia. *Saudi Medical Journal, 17*, 195–203.
56. Mapatano, M. A., Lusamba, D., & Banea, M. (1997). Evaluation of Growth Monitoring Programme in Children in Kinshasa. *East African Medical Journal, 74*, 96–99.
57. Faber, M., Oelofse, A., & Benade, A. J. S. (1998). A Model for Community-Based Growth Monitoring System. *African Journal of Health Sciences, 5*, 72–78.
58. Pearson, R. (1995). *Thematic Evaluation of UNICEF Support to Growth Monitoring*. (Evaluation and Research Working Paper Series No. 2). New York: UNICEF.
59. Karim, R., Lamstein, S. A., Akhtaruzzaman, M., Rahman, K. M., & Alam, N. (2003). The Bangladesh Integrated Nutrition Project: Endline Evaluation of the Community-Based Nutrition Component. Institute of Nutrition and Food Sciences, University of Dhaka, Bangladesh, and the Friedman School of Nutrition Science and Policy, Tufts University, USA.
60. Ministry of Health and Family Welfare, Government of India. (2021). *National Family Health Survey (NFHS-5), 2019–21, India Report*. Retrieved from https://dhsprogram.com/pubs/pdf/FR375/FR375.pdf.
61. Jones, G., et al. (2015). How Many Child Deaths Can We Prevent This Year? *The Lancet, 362*(9377), 65–71. Retrieved from https://doi.org/10.1016/S0140-6736(03)13811-1.
62. Victora, C. G., et al. (2011). Health Conditions and Health-Policy Innovations in Brazil: The Way Forward. *The Lancet, 377*(9782), 2042–2053. Retrieved from https://doi.org/10.1016/S0140-6736(11)60055-X.
63. Prasad, V., Sinha, D., & Joseph, R. J. (2024). Global Relevance of MGRS Growth Standards: The Case of India. *BMJ Paediatrics Open, 8*, e002472. Retrieved from https://doi.org/10.1136/bmjpo-2023-002472.
64. Marume, A., Archary, M., & Mahomed, S. (2022). Validation of Growth Standards and Growth References: A Review of Literature. *Journal of Child Health Care, 26*(3), 498–510. Retrieved from https://doi.org/10.1177/13674935211024816
65. Ahmad, U. N. (2011). A Randomised Controlled Trial Exploring How New WHO Growth Charts Influence Healthcare Workers' Clinical Decisions and Recommendations About Exclusive Breastfeeding for Infants Aged <6 Months. *Archives of Disease in Childhood, 96*, A73. Retrieved from https://doi.org/10.1136/adc.2011.212563.170.
66. Marko, K., et al. (2011). Prevalence of Wasting Among Under 6-Month-Old Infants in Developing Countries and Implications of New Case Definitions Using WHO Growth Standards: A Secondary Data Analysis. *Archives of Disease in Childhood, 96*, 1008–1013.
67. Khadilkar, V. (2013). The Growing Controversy About Growth Charts: WHO or Regional? *International Journal of Pediatric Endocrinology, 2013*(1), O6.

Chapter 5
Leaving No One Behind: Progress in Child Immunization Among the Disadvantaged Populations in India, 1992–93 to 2020–21

William Joe, Saroj Kumar, and Ishika Pahuja

Introduction

By the age of three, more than 80% of a child's brain is already formed (WHO, 2023), making the quality of early experiences critically influential for lifelong health, learning, and behavior. The rapid and foundational nature of brain development during early childhood implies that any significant disruption, such as severe illness, can have disproportionately profound and lasting negative impacts across all developmental domains. This highlights the critical importance of protective health interventions, such as immunization, which act to preserve this sensitive developmental window, thereby safeguarding optimal brain development and subsequent developmental trajectories. The various domains of ECD i.e. physical (e.g., reaching, crawling, walking), cognitive (e.g., thinking, learning, problem-solving), communication/linguistic (e.g., listening, understanding, talking), and social and emotional (e.g., playing, exploring, interacting, regulating emotions)—are deeply interconnected. This interconnectedness means that an intervention positively impacting one domain, such as physical health through immunization, is likely to have cascading benefits across others. For instance, frequent or recurring infections during childhood can hinder growth and cause stunting. This can negatively impact adult health, cognitive abilities, and economic productivity. Vaccines offer broad advantages that go beyond preventing illness, positively impacting cognition, schooling, economic productivity, and even fertility.

Vaccines rank among the most significant scientific achievement of the 20th century [11]. Over the past few decades, vaccines have saved millions of lives worldwide and proffered wide-ranging health and economic benefits [8, 27]. Globally, since

W. Joe (✉) · S. Kumar · I. Pahuja
Institute of Economic Growth, Delhi, India
e-mail: william@iegindia.org

S. Suri (ed.), *Child Health and Nutrition from Conception to Age Two*,
https://doi.org/10.1007/978-981-95-7868-9_5

the launch of the Expanded Programme on Immunization (EPI) in 1974, vaccines have prevented 101 million infant deaths and 146 million under-five deaths [36]. In the last two decades (2001–2020), investments worth USD 34 billion in immunization programs across 94 low-and middle-income countries (LMICs) have yielded USD 1.53 trillion in economic benefits [26, 28]. The 2030 Agenda for Sustainable Development adopted by the United Nations (UN) General Assembly vide resolution (A/RES/70/1) takes cognizance of the role of vaccines [38]. The Sustainable Development Goal (SDG 3) to ensure healthy lives and to promote well-being for all at all ages has specifically listed SDG target 3.8 for achieving universal health coverage in various essential health care services including vaccines. The SDGs Global Indicator Framework (A/RES/71/313) has defined indicator 3.b.1 on vaccination coverage and calls for tracking the proportion of the target population covered by all vaccines included in the respective national programs [39]. The hallmark of the 2030 Agenda, however, is the cardinal promise that no one will be left behind while implementing the 2030 Agenda for Sustainable Development.

The concept of no-one-left-behind is central to the philosophy of the Government of India about "*Sabka Sath, Sabka Vikas, Sabka Vishwas, Sabka Prayaas*" that ensures that the development journey of the nation is universal, inclusive, and progressive [21–23]. Primary health care in India predominantly follows the government-led public health framework involving a vast network of frontline workers and community health workers. The universal approach to public health in India calls for reaching out to all the vulnerable and marginalized sections of the population through surveys, surveillance, and active outreach through special drives for service delivery. The recently launched *Ayushman Bharat* (Healthy India) initiative has rejuvenated the primary health care sector in India with specific designs to achieve the SDG targets along with its emphasizing the commitment to ensuring no one is left behind. This policy stance has accorded significant importance at the G20 Health Ministers meeting (August, 2023) with the G20 nations reaffirming that the "*need of the hour is to converge, consolidate, and create a healthier future and the importance of strengthening national health systems including through effective community involvement and the underlying principle of 'Leave No One Behind' and considering vulnerable populations living in crises affected settings*" [23]. The joint document by the NITI Aayog and the United Nations (India) also emphasize on the need to design special surveys to ensure that no one is left behind. This would also support strengthening the monitoring system with disaggregated information on various vulnerable groups such that the farthest are reached first [2].

Motivation

Despite such relevance, universal coverage in childhood vaccination remains an agenda yet to be finished for the LMICs. The UN resolutions (A/RES/70/1; A/RES/71/313) emphasize that such intricate concerns should be routinely examined through reliable disaggregated data to measure the progress and comprehend the magnitude of inequities and exclusions of the disadvantaged populations. The central role of data in decision-making has intensified the policy focus on identification of the vulnerable sections through disaggregated analysis by age, sex, disability, ethnicity, poverty, geography, migratory status, and other nationally relevant dichotomies and categories. Accordingly, under immunization programs, the outcome focus is now inverted from full immunization to zero-dose, i.e., children who have not received any routine vaccinations [9]. The global patterns in vaccination progress review are also evolving accordingly [40]. With the SDGs promise of leaving no one behind, global assessments have re-conceptualized vaccination coverage from the lens of zero-dose which refers to a case where the child was consistently missed and has failed to receive any routine vaccine [40]. Globally, in 2023, 14.5 million children are estimated to be zero-dose children. The magnitude has decreased since the COVID-19 pandemic levels of 18.2 million children in 2021 but are yet to reach the pre-pandemic level of 12.8 million in 2019. The zero-dose children also account for 70% of all under-immunized children who are not only spread across vulnerable geographies but are also disadvantaged because of socioeconomic deprivations as well societal biases including barriers related to gender, ethnicity, and religion [15].

Objectives

Since inception, the national immunization program of India has followed the principle of universal coverage and is guided by rigorous monitoring to address shortcomings and inequities in vaccination coverage [12–14]. Systematic review of process and outcome indicators have provided valuable insights for policy guidelines and on the state-of-the-affairs in national vaccination coverage [33]. For instance, historical neglects and inequities in child immunization often manifest across the axes of gender, caste, religion, income, education, and geographical barriers [20]. Notwithstanding wealth-related inequalities in receipt of all basic vaccines, further intensification of such inequalities is apparent when such identities intersect with gender biases and historical neglects in development [6, 17, 29]. Besides, despite a DPT1 (first dose of Diphtheria, Pertussis, and Tetanus vaccine) coverage of above 90%, India is estimated to have 1.6 million zero-dose children who comprise of more than 11% share in the global count of zero-dose children [40]. It is apparent that global progress in several of the SDGs is closely tied to India's achievements, including its vaccination targets.

This chapter reviews the progress in child immunization coverage in India using five rounds of the National Family Health Survey (NFHS) data. The NFHS surveys are conducted by the International Institute for Population Sciences (IIPS) under the stewardship of Ministry of Health and Family Welfare (MoHFW), Government of India. This analysis draws information on childhood vaccination available in the NFHS rounds conducted in 1992–93, 1998–99, 2005–06, 2015–16, and 2019–21. The details regarding the sampling design and survey implementation are available in the national reports [16].

Evolution of National Immunization Program

Global Context

National immunization programs worldwide have developed alongside the global initiatives [31, 36]. In 1974, the benchmark 27th World Health Assembly resolution led to the EPI program across countries with focus on tuberculosis, smallpox, poliomyelitis, diphtheria, pertussis, tetanus, and measles. In 1982, UNICEF led the child survival and development revolution with focus on improving GOBI (growth monitoring, oral rehydration therapy, breastfeeding promotion) indicators. In 1984, the first standard schedule for the basic vaccines was finalized. Following the Manhattan Declaration in 1990, the Children's Vaccine Initiative (CVI) was launched with UNICEF, the WHO, the World Bank, the United Nations Development Program (UNDP), and the Rockefeller Foundation as the core members.

In 1999, WHO established the Strategic Advisory Group of Experts (SAGE) on immunization, and it was followed up by the establishment of Global Alliance on Vaccines and Immunization (GAVI) in 2000 (now referred to as GAVI, The Vaccine Alliance). The latter is a culmination of long due challenges in public-private partnership in vaccine development and system strengthening under the Children's Vaccine Initiative [24]. The core members of GAVI (viz. WHO, UNICEF, the World Bank, and the Bill & Melinda Gates Foundation, BMGF) collaborated with various national governments, national and international donors (including private sector), vaccine research and industry partners as well as various other stakeholders to strengthen national immunization programs.

Ever since, GAVI has been instrumental in providing alternative solutions to country-specific challenges through public-private partnerships and introduction of new vaccines in the national immunization programs [31]. In recent years, vaccine development has expanded for several population-wide epidemics and infections. As of 2024, the EPI covers 13 vaccines across countries along with 17 vaccines to address context-specific requirements that is governed by the respected National Technical Advisory Group on Immunization [36]. However, the progress assessment is guided by the Immunization Agenda 2030 that was endorsed by the 73rd WHA in 2020 for accelerating progress toward the SDGs through system strengthening for delivery of EPI. The IA2030 is now focused on post-pandemic recovery and consolidation in immunization gains across countries [41].

Indian Context

The major landmarks under the national immunization program in India aligns well with the global developments in the field [7, 36]. In 1978, the Government of India rolled out the Expanded Programme for Immunization (EPI) which was subsequently scaled up as the Universal Immunization Program in 1985. The focus on immunization further unfolded through Child Survival Safe Motherhood (1992) and Reproductive Child Health (1997) initiatives. Meanwhile, the program on National Immunization Day for Polio Eradication was launched in 1995. Following the stagnancy in completed immunization rates, a specific Immunization Strengthening Project (2000–03) and a Multi-Year Plan (2005–10) was developed within the Universal Immunization Program.

The immunization strategy received a major fillip with National Rural Health Mission (NRHM, 2005) that leveraged the federal structure for resource sharing in the health sector to bring successful changes in infrastructure, human resources, and service delivery for child immunization [30, 32]. New vaccines such as 2nd dose of measles and pentavalent were introduced in 2010 and 2011, respectively. The strategy toward intensification of routine immunization was introduced in 2012 with subsequent introduction of open vaccine vial policy to avoid waiting lists and wastages. In 2014, the efforts were intensified through Mission Indradhanush (MI), and India achieved the milestone of being certified as Polio Free in 2014. Gradually, vaccines such as Rubella and Rotavirus were also introduced in the national immunization program. The NFHS 2015–16 estimates, however, persistent in demonstrating a slow progress in immunization and to expedite progress, the strategies were further reinforced in 2017 under the Intensified Mission Indradhanush (IMI) program. The IMI adopts a target prioritization approach whereby districts with low coverage receive additional engagements from the frontline workers.

Trends in Immunization Coverage

All India Coverage, 1993–2021

The NFHS provides information on receipt of all basic vaccines (birth dose of BCG, three doses of DPT and poliomyelitis each at specified intervals, and measles vaccination). Full immunization is defined as cases of children (12–23 months) who have received all the eight basic vaccines irrespective of the specified schedule. While timeliness in the receipt of vaccination is an important concern, the coverage assessment exercise largely focuses on status of receipt of all the mandated vaccines. Figure 5.1 shows the trends in coverage of full immunization in India along with the prevalence patterns of vaccine-specific dose, partial immunization as well as zero-dose children. In the last three decades, the full immunization coverage at the national level shows a two-fold increase from 35.4% in 1992–93 to 76.2% in 2019–21 (Tables S1 and S2). Bulk of the coverage improvements in full immunization have occurred since the launch of the NRHM in 2005 and have accelerated since the introduction of the intensified Mission Indradhanush in 2017. Although coverage levels have not yet achieved the desired targets, it is noteworthy that post-NRHM, the rural-urban disparities in full immunization coverage have been eliminated (Table S3). In 1992–93, the full vaccination coverage in rural and urban India was 30.9% and 50.7%, respectively. In 2019–21 with programmatic efforts, the full immunization coverage is estimated to be 76.6% and 75.2%, respectively, with narrowing rural-urban differentials (Table S4). While rural India has marched ahead of their urban counterparts in full immunization but such lagging estimates for urban areas is of concern for policymaking.

The improvements in full immunization are accompanied with consistent reductions in prevalence of zero-dose children. Zero-dose is defined as a case where a child was consistently missed and has failed to receive any routine vaccine [40]. However, there can be two alternative approaches to define zero-dose children as follows: first, we follow the definition adopted by Immunization Agenda 2030 (IA2030) to estimate the prevalence of zero-dose children as non-receipt of DPT1 vaccine [40]; and second, we define zero-dose children as those who have not received any basic vaccine. The prevalence of zero-dose children (no DPT1) was 31.7% in 1992–93 and has declined to 7.0% in 2019–21. The alternative definition shows the reduction of zero-dose (no vaccine) from prevalence level of 30.0% in 1992–93 to 3.6% in 2019–21. Both rural and urban areas have shown similar trends in the reduction of zero-dose prevalence in recent years. Given the large birth cohorts in India, the prevalence of zero-dose is rather huge and a major concern for achieving the SDG targets. The vaccine-specific dose information suggests that in the 1990s lowest coverage used to be in receipt of measles vaccine (42.2% in 1992–93) but in 2019–21 the lowest coverage is noted for OPV3 (81.1% in 2019–21). The regular efforts in the

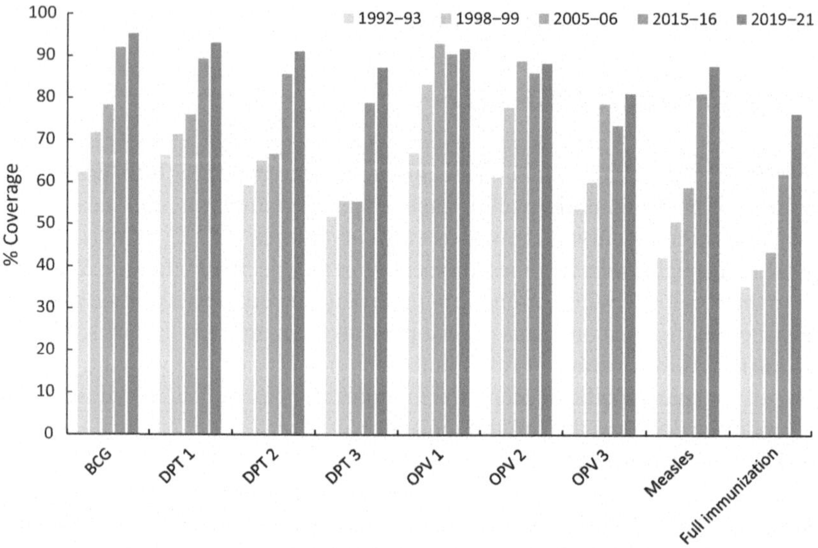

Fig. 5.1 Vaccine-specific dose, zero-dose, and full immunization coverage in India among children (12–23 months), NFHS 1993–2021

Table S1 Vaccine-specific dose, zero-dose, and full immunization coverage in India among children (12–23 months), NFHS 1993–2021

All India (%)	1992–93	1998–99	2005–06	2015–16	2019–21
BCG	62.2	71.6	78.2	91.9	95.2
DPT 1	66.3	71.2	75.9	89.2	93.0
DPT 2	59.2	65.0	66.6	85.6	91.0
DPT 3	51.8	55.5	55.4	78.7	87.2
OPV 1	66.9	83.2	92.9	90.4	91.7
OPV 2	61.2	77.7	88.8	85.9	88.2
OPV 3	53.7	60.0	78.5	73.4	81.1
Measles	42.2	50.7	58.8	81.1	87.6
Full immunization	35.4	39.4	43.5	62.0	76.2
Partial immunization	34.6	46.2	51.1	32.0	20.2
Zero-dose (no vaccine)	30.0	14.4	5.3	6.0	3.6
Zero-dose (no DPT1)	33.7	28.8	24.1	10.8	7.0
Rural India (%)	1992–93	1998–99	2005–06	2015–16	2019–21
BCG	57.6	67.2	75.1	91.4	95.4
DPT 1	62.1	66.9	75.1	88.9	93.3
DPT 2	54.5	60.1	62.2	85.2	91.4
DPT 3	46.8	50.1	50.5	78.0	87.5
OPV 1	62.8	80.7	92.3	89.9	91.9
OPV 2	56.6	74.5	88.0	85.4	88.5
OPV 3	48.7	56.4	76.7	73.2	81.6
Measles	37.7	45.3	54.2	80.3	87.9
Full immunization	30.9	34.9	38.6	61.3	76.6
Partial immunization	35.1	48.4	55.5	32.3	20.0
Zero-dose (no vaccine)	34.0	16.8	6.0	6.4	3.4
Zero-dose (IA2030)	37.9	33.1	24.9	11.1	6.7
Urban India (%)	1992–93	1998–99	2005–06	2015–16	2019–21
BCG	77.6	86.8	86.9	93.2	94.8
DPT 1	80.5	85.9	84.3	90.0	92.2
DPT 2	75.2	81.9	78.0	86.7	89.9
DPT 3	68.8	73.8	69.3	80.5	86.3
OPV 1	80.8	91.9	94.7	91.7	91.1
OPV 2	76.9	88.6	91.0	87.0	87.5
OPV 3	70.4	72.2	83.3	73.4	79.7
Measles	57.5	69.2	71.8	83.2	86.9
Full immunization	50.7	54.8	57.6	63.9	75.2
Partial immunization	32.9	38.9	38.9	31.1	20.5

(continued)

Table S1 (continued)

All India (%)	1992–93	1998–99	2005–06	2015–16	2019–21
Zero-dose (no vaccine)	16.4	6.4	3.5	5.1	4.3
Zero-dose (IA2030)	19.5	14.1	15.7	10.0	7.8

form of pulse polio campaigns have played an instrumental role in increasing the OPV coverage. However, in recent years, coverage of OPV3 has been the lowest in both rural and urban areas and requires concerted engagements. It is also important to note that despite wide-ranging improvements and programmatic efforts, one-fifth of the children in India also remain partially immunized.

Progress Across States/UTs

Wide variations in immunization coverage across states and union territories (UTs) is a key feature of progress heterogeneity in India (Table S2). In 1992–93, the state of Goa had the highest level of full immunization coverage (74.9%) and the lowest was in Nagaland (3.8%). Whereas in 2019–21, the highest coverage is noted in Odisha (90.6%), but Nagaland (56.6%) continues to display the lowest coverage of full immunization. In general, the full immunization coverage in the northeastern states of India is the lowest. In 2019–21, seven states have full immunization coverage below 70% levels. Except for Uttar Pradesh (69.2%), all the other six states are from the northeast region of India *viz.* Nagaland (56.6%), Meghalaya (63.2%), Arunachal Pradesh (63.8%), Assam (65.9%), Tripura (68.4%), and Manipur (69.9%).

The progress in full immunization coverage across states/UTs has led to reductions in inter-state disparities. The inter-state coefficient of variation in full immunization coverage has declined from 0.517 in 1992–93 to 0.109 in 2019–21. The Gini coefficient also yields similar inferences whereby the magnitude of inter-state inequality has declined from 0.289 in 1992–93 to 0.061 in 2019–21. The full immunization coverage in rural and urban sectors shows the wide geographical heterogeneity of India (Table S3). In the early 1990s, the coverage varied from 0.9% in rural Nagaland to 75.2% in rural Goa. The rural sector variations continue to be substantial in 2019–21 (52.0% in rural Nagaland and 91.7% in rural Tamil Nadu). The rural-urban differentials were very high in 1992–93 and urban India was 19.8% point ahead of rural areas in full immunization coverage (Table S4). However, rural India has progress substantially in the last three decades and now has a lead of 1.3% point over urban India. The rural coverage across states was highly unequal in 1992–93 compared to the urban areas and had Gini coefficients of 0.318 and 0.195, respectively. In 2019–21, the inter-sectoral inequalities have reduced to 0.071 in rural and 0.063 in urban areas.

Table S2 Full immunization coverage (%) among children (12–23 months), States and UTs of India, NFHS 1993–2021

States/UTs	1992-93	1998-99	2005-06	2015-16	2019-21
Andaman & Nicobar Island	-	-	-	73.2	78.5
Andhra Pradesh	45.0	52.0	46.0	65.3	72.2
Arunachal Pradesh	22.5	18.5	28.4	38.2	63.8
Assam	19.4	16.1	31.4	47.1	65.9
Bihar	10.7	10.6	32.8	61.7	70.8
Chandigarh	-	-	-	79.5	80.2
Chhattisgarh	-	-	48.7	76.4	79.6
Dadra & Nagar Haveli	-	-	-	43.2	94.9
Daman & Diu				66.3	.
Delhi (NCT)	57.8	49.8	63.2	68.8	75.5
Goa	74.9	77.7	78.6	88.4	81.1
Gujarat	49.8	48.3	45.2	50.4	76.0
Haryana	53.5	60.3	65.3	62.2	77.2
Himachal Pradesh	62.9	81.2	74.2	69.5	88.9
Jammu & Kashmir	65.7	54.5	66.7	75.1	86.8
Jharkhand	-	-	34.2	61.9	73.4
Karnataka	52.2	56.0	55	62.6	84.1
Kerala	54.4	71.9	75.3	82.1	77.6
Ladakh	-	-	-	.	86.8
Lakshadweep	-	-	-	89.0	85.2
Madhya Pradesh	29.2	20.6	40.3	53.6	77.0
Maharashtra	64.1	72.7	58.8	56.2	73.6
Manipur	29.1	41.3	46.8	65.8	69.9
Meghalaya	9.7	12.2	32.9	61.4	63.2
Mizoram	56.4	59.6	46.5	50.7	72.6
Nagaland	3.8	12.1	21	35.4	56.6
Odisha	36.1	40.5	51.8	78.6	90.6
Puducherry	-	-	-	91.3	82.3
Punjab	61.9	71.5	60.1	89.1	75.5
Rajasthan	21.1	16.1	26.5	54.8	80.2
Sikkim	-	43.9	69.6	83.0	79.6
Tamil Nadu	64.9	88.1	80.9	69.7	88.6
Telangana	-	-	-	67.5	79.3
Tripura	19.0	39.5	49.7	54.5	68.4
Uttar Pradesh	19.8	20.1	23	51.1	69.2
Uttarakhand	-	-	60	57.6	82.0

(continued)

Table S2 (continued)

States/UTs	1992-93	1998-99	2005-06	2015-16	2019-21
West Bengal	34.2	43.7	64.3	84.4	88.1
All India	35.4	39.4	43.5	62.0	76.2

It is worth investigating whether the reduction in inter-state disparities in immunization coverage have occurred due to secular as well as programmatic improvements over the years or if these are also because of catching up phenomenon demonstrated by rural areas that had low coverage levels in the 1990s. The between-sector and within-sector decomposition of the state disparities in coverage levels is attempted using the generalized entropy (GE) indices with coverage difference sensitivity (disparity aversion) parameter set at 2. Technically, the GE(2) index is half of the squared coefficient of variation. In 1992–93 the decomposition of GE(2) index reveals that 88.9% of the inter-state disparities in full immunization coverage is attributable to within-sector differentials across states whereas only 10.1% was accounted by between-sector differentials. In 2019–21, the contribution of between-sector differentials in inter-state disparities is almost nil and all these disparities are emerging because of within-sector differentials across states.

Socioeconomic Disparities in Full Immunization

Table 5.1 presents the status of full immunization coverage by broad demographic and socioeconomic characteristics of the children. The coverage among females was discovered to be lower than males, and this pattern is consistent across the five rounds of NFHS (1992–93: Male 36.7% and Female 34.1%; 2019–21: Male 76.6% and Female 75.8%). In the 1990s, maternal age was a critical factor in determining full immunization coverage whereby children born to teenage mothers or those in their 40s were more disadvantaged. In recent years, the maternal age-related variations in full immunization are rather negligible though mothers above 40-years of age still demonstrate lower coverage. Maternal education, however, continues to be of high relevance for full immunization coverage. It is notable that throughout the five rounds of NFHS, the full immunization coverage among mothers with higher education (12+ years) was always about 70% or more. In contrast, in 1992–93, mothers with no formal schooling had full immunization coverage levels of 23.3% only. The education-related gradient persists even in 2019–21 though the slope is now much flatter than the previous decades.

In the 90s, the scheduled caste (SC, 26.5%) and scheduled tribe (ST, 24.8%) households had low levels of full immunization coverage compared to other social groups (38.2%). Nevertheless, it is worth highlighting that there are no social group disparities in full immunization coverage in 2019–21. The religion of the household is an important correlate as children from Muslim households (71.0% in 2019–21) display

Table S3 Full immunization coverage (%) among children (12–23 months) in rural and urban areas of States/UTs, India, NFHS 1993–2021

States / UTs	1992–93		1998–99		2005–06		2015–16		2019–21	
	Rural	Urban	Rural	Urban	Rural	Urban	Rural	Urban	Rural	Urban
A & N Island	–	–	–	–	–	–	82.5	61.8	86.1	72.1
Andhra Pradesh	39.7	58.3	48.9	61.0	42.9	51.2	67.2	60.4	73.3	69.9
Arunachal Pradesh	19.4	38.5	16.7	26.3	21.1	51.2	36.4	44.2	63.5	66.2
Assam	17.4	40.0	14.2	45.3	31.7	29.3	44.4	70.9	66.7	60.4
Bihar	9.1	21.5	9.4	22.4	31.2	45.6	61.9	59.7	71.5	65.8
Chandigarh	–	–	–	–	–	–	100.0	77.2	–	81.0
Chhattisgarh	–	–	–	–	43.1	74.7	74.3	84.9	80.4	76.6
D&N Haveli	–	–	–	–	–	–	35.1	53.7	100.0	89.5
Delhi (NCT)	55.8	58.0	57.7	48.9	63.2	63.2	33.0	41.6	72.1	75.7
Goa	75.2	74.6	82.2	70.3	40.1	83.5	62.4	67.8	87.7	77.1
Gujarat	46.2	57.0	45.0	54.3	73.0	54.7	80.6	68.6	75.8	76.5
Haryana	52.1	58.0	56.6	71.6	73.6	82.2	90.1	87.7	78.4	73.9
Himachal Pradesh	61.3	81.5	81.4	78.9	60.3	80.0	50.4	50.4	88.5	91.6
Jammu & Kashmir	62.8	84.9	51.0	71.7	29.5	73.0	65.1	57.0	87.4	84.8
Jharkhand	–	–	–	–	64.9	51.0	69.9	64.8	74.6	67.5
Karnataka	49.9	57.6	57.8	51.9	52.2	59.6	72.9	81.6	86.2	80.7
Kerala	54.0	55.7	71.2	74.7	69.4	87.5	60.7	67.0	77.5	77.8
Ladakh	–	–	–	–	–	–	64.8	59.8	90.1	76.0
Lakshadweep	–	–	–	–	–	–	82.0	82.2	83.4	86.1
Madhya Pradesh	25.6	43.0	15.3	38.8	32.6	68.7	100.0	86.1	77.0	76.9
Maharashtra	65.6	61.6	73.2	71.9	49.8	68.1	50.2	63.0	75.0	71.7
Manipur	21.2	45.2	41.7	40.3	42.8	59.7	56.6	55.8	66.1	77.9
Meghalaya	6.7	24.0	11.6	16.9	31.5	33.9	61.7	74.3	64.3	55.8
Mizoram	50.9	62.3	51.3	70.9	36.6	57.1	58.4	81.4	75.8	69.1
Nagaland	0.8	19.2	10.1	22.6	17.1	36.0	51.6	49.8	52.0	68.6
Odisha	34.7	43.8	38.8	55.3	51.6	52.8	79.2	75.0	90.5	91.6
Puducherry	–	–	–	–	–	–	85.4	93.9	70.0	85.5
Punjab	57.7	75.6	66.3	83.9	58.1	64.4	89.3	88.7	76.9	72.9
Rajasthan	16.1	45.9	13.1	26.4	22.1	44.3	53.1	60.9	79.4	83.2
Sikkim	–	–	43.1	50.0	66.7	85.4	83.7	81.4	83.1	68.8
Tamil Nadu	60.3	73.3	83.7	96.2	83.7	77.8	66.8	73.3	91.7	85.0
Telangana	–	–	–	–	–	–	68.3	66.7	81.5	75.6
Tripura	16.8	35.7	35.7	63.2	47.9	60.9	51.2	64.2	64.1	82.9
Uttar Pradesh	17.4	32.9	18.3	29.8	57.4	33.0	50.4	53.6	69.9	66.6
Uttarakhand	–	–	–	–	20.5	67.2	58.1	56.5	80.8	84.7

(continued)

Table S3 (continued)

States / UTs	1992–93		1998–99		2005–06		2015–16		2019–21	
	Rural	Urban	Rural	Urban	Rural	Urban	Rural	Urban	Rural	Urban
West Bengal	31.3	44.1	40.8	56.6	62.8	70.3	87.1	77.7	89.5	84.0
All India	30.9	50.7	34.9	54.8	38.6	57.6	61.3	63.9	76.6	75.2

lower levels of full immunization coverage compared to any of the other religion households. Economic status of the household was a key marker of full immunization. The coverage among children in the highest wealth quintile (18.4%) was more than three times that of the coverage level among the lowest wealth quintile (64.8%). The wealth-related gradient persists even in 2019–21 although the differentials between highest and lowest wealth quintiles have been bridged substantially.

Intersecting Prominent Axes of Inequalities

The recent literature on health and health care inequalities have demonstrated the importance and influence of multiple co-existing identities in determining the access to various services. In the Indian context, gender, caste, and place of residence have been a key aspect in determining access and utilization of publicly provided health care services such as immunization [17, 34]. Figure 5.2 shows the coverage of full immunization and the prevalence of zero-dose children across groups are cross-classified by gender (male and female), caste (SC/ST and others), and place of residence (rural and urban). This yields eight mutually exclusive subgroups as follows: (i) rural-SCST-female (RSCSTF), (ii) rural-SCST-male (RSCSTM), (iii) rural-others-female (ROF), (iv) rural-others-male (ROM), (v) urban-SCST-female (USCSTF), (vi) urban-SCST-male (USCSTM), (vii) urban-others-female (UOF), and (viii) urban-others-male (UOM).

In 1992–93, the full immunization coverage among the intersectional groups varied from 22.5% among RSCSTF to 53.0% among UOF. The disadvantageous status of RSCSTF is apparent and persisted throughout the last three decades. However, since 2015–16 the inter-group disparities in full immunization have reduced and further in 2019–21, the RSCST (75.6%) is no longer the most disadvantaged group in full immunization. In 2019–21, the lowest full immunization coverage is noted among USCSTF (74.2%) and the levels among USCSTM (74.3%) are similar. Reductions in the inter-group disparities in the last two rounds of NFHS are an important achievement of the immunization program in India. However, further efforts are warranted to increase the coverage and sustain the momentum.

Both the definitions of prevalence of zero-dose children show that RSCSTF were the most vulnerable group in non-receipt of vaccines. In 1992–93, 45.1% of RSCSTF had not received any of the basic vaccines whereas 49.4% had not received the DPT1 dose. The problem of zero-dose has been reducing since the 90s; and in 2019–21, the

Table S4 Urban–Rural Absolute Difference (%) and Rural/Urban Ratio Differentials in full immunization coverage among children (12-23 months), States/UTs of India, NFHS 1993–2021

States/UTs	1992–93		1998–99		2005–06		2015–16		2019–21	
	U–R	R/U	U–R	R/U	U–R	R/U	U–R	R/U	U–R	R/U
A & N Island	–	–	–	–	–	–	–20.7	0.7	–14.0	0.8
Andhra Pradesh	18.6	1.5	12.1	1.2	8.4	1.2	–6.8	0.9	–3.3	1.0
Arunachal Pradesh	19.1	2.0	9.6	1.6	30.1	2.4	7.8	1.2	2.7	1.0
Assam	22.6	2.3	31.1	3.2	–2.4	0.9	26.5	1.6	–6.3	0.9
Bihar	12.4	2.4	13.0	2.4	14.4	1.5	–2.2	1.0	–5.7	0.9
Chandigarh	–	–	–	–	–	–	–22.8	0.8	–	–
Chhattisgarh	–	–	–	–	31.6	1.7	10.6	1.1	–3.8	1.0
D & N Haveli	–	–	–	–	–	–	18.6	1.5	–10.6	0.9
Delhi (NCT)	2.2	1.0	–8.8	0.8	0.0	1.0	8.6	1.3	3.6	1.0
Goa	-0.5	1.0	–11.9	0.9	43.4	2.1	5.4	1.1	–10.6	0.9
Gujarat	10.8	1.2	9.3	1.2	-18.3	0.7	–12.0	0.9	0.7	1.0
Haryana	5.9	1.1	15.0	1.3	8.7	1.1	–2.4	1.0	–4.5	0.9
Himachal Pradesh	20.2	1.3	–2.4	1.0	19.7	1.3	0.0	1.0	3.1	1.0
Jammu & Kashmir	22.0	1.4	20.7	1.4	43.5	2.5	–8.0	0.9	–2.7	1.0
Jharkhand	–	–	–	–	–13.8	0.8	–5.1	0.9	–7.0	0.9
Karnataka	7.7	1.2	-5.9	0.9	7.4	1.1	8.7	1.1	–5.5	0.9
Kerala	1.6	1.0	3.5	1.0	18.1	1.3	6.3	1.1	0.3	1.0
Ladakh	–	–	–	–	–	–	-5.0	0.9	–14.1	0.8
Lakshadweep	–	–	–	–	–	–	0.2	1.0	2.7	1.0
Madhya Pradesh	17.5	1.7	23.4	2.5	36.0	2.1	–13.9	0.9	–0.1	1.0
Maharashtra	–4.0	0.9	–1.3	1.0	18.3	1.4	12.8	1.3	–3.3	1.0
Manipur	24.1	2.1	–1.5	1.0	16.9	1.4	–0.8	1.0	11.8	1.2
Meghalaya	17.3	3.6	5.3	1.5	2.4	1.1	12.6	1.2	–8.6	0.9
Mizoram	11.4	1.2	19.6	1.4	20.6	1.6	23.0	1.4	–6.8	0.9
Nagaland	18.5	25.6	12.5	2.2	18.9	2.1	–1.8	1.0	16.6	1.3
Odisha	9.1	1.3	16.5	1.4	1.1	1.0	-4.2	0.9	1.1	1.0
Puducherry	–	–	–	–	–	–	8.5	1.1	15.5	1.2
Punjab	17.9	1.3	17.5	1.3	6.3	1.1	-0.6	1.0	–4.0	0.9
Rajasthan	29.8	2.9	13.3	2.0	22.2	2.0	7.8	1.1	3.9	1.0
Sikkim	0.0	–	6.9	1.2	18.7	1.3	–2.3	1.0	–14.3	0.8
Tamil Nadu	13.0	1.2	12.5	1.1	-5.9	0.9	6.5	1.1	–6.7	0.9

(continued)

Table S4 (continued)

States/UTs	1992–93		1998–99		2005–06		2015–16		2019–21	
	U–R	R/U	U–R	R/U	U–R	R/U	U–R	R/U	U–R	R/U
Telangana	–	–	–	–	–	–	–1.6	1.0	–5.9	0.9
Tripura	18.9	2.1	27.4	1.8	13.0	1.3	12.9	1.3	18.9	1.3
Uttar Pradesh	15.5	1.9	11.5	1.6	–24.4	0.6	3.2	1.1	–3.2	1.0
Uttarakhand	–	–	–	–	46.7	3.3	–1.6	1.0	3.9	1.0
West Bengal	12.8	1.4	15.8	1.4	7.5	1.1	–9.4	0.9	–5.5	0.9
All India	19.8	1.6	19.9	1.6	19.0	1.5	2.6	1.0	–1.3	1.0

highest prevalence of zero-dose (no vaccine) and zero-dose (no DPT1) is observed among USCSTF (6.9% and 9.7%, respectively). The intersectional inequalities manifest along the various axes with a graded impact on the immunization coverage levels. In the 90s, bulk of the differentials were attributable to the rural-urban sectoral disparities followed by caste affiliations and gender disadvantages. However, in the recent years, the effect of these axes on inter-group differences in full immunization is offset by the broad-based coverage improvements. In fact, urban areas are now emerging as being at a disadvantage in terms of zero-dose prevalence.

Coverage Across Vulnerable Populations

The SDG commitment of leaving-no-one-behind has led to specific focus on the marginalized, vulnerable, and neglected population subgroups. Here we attempt to explore the status of immunization coverage among vulnerable populations identified based on slum residence status, wealth index as well as multidimensional poverty index (MPI) based economic status, health care deprivation status in terms of non-receipt of the mandated four ANC visits or iron and folic acid (IFA) supplements during pregnancy, and the migration status of the household. The migration status is further cross-classified by the economic status in terms of poorest migrant households if they belong to the lowest wealth quintile. Also, migration to rural or urban areas is also viewed as an important characteristic of the vulnerability among such poorest households.

Table 5.2 shows the immunization coverage status for the vulnerable population subgroups for the three rounds of NFHS (2005–06, 2015–16, and 2019–21). The NFHS rounds in the 90s had limited information on these indicators and hence were omitted from the analysis. In 2005–06, the slum area residents (census-based or observation-based) in selected urban areas had much higher full immunization coverage (65.4%) than the national average (43.5%). The urban advantage has since disappeared, and in 2015–16, slum areas exhibits lower coverage (54.8%) than all-India average (62.0%). The slum residency information is unavailable in NFHS 2019–21 resulting the trend cannot be further assessed but, nevertheless, the reversal

Table 5.1 Full immunization coverage (%) among children (12–23 months) by background characteristics, India, NFHS 1993-2021

Background characteristics	1992–93	1998–99	2005–06	2015–16	2019–21
Sex					
Male	36.7	40.4	45.3	62.1	76.6
Female	34.1	38.2	41.5	61.9	75.8
Maternal Age					
15–19	34.1	34.2	39.1	62.4	73.6
20–29	38.1	42.7	45.5	63.0	76.6
30–39	28.7	31.7	39.7	58.9	75.7
40–49	14.8	13.7	18.3	48.7	70.4
Maternal education					
No formal schooling	23.3	24.7	26.1	51.5	68.0
Primary	45.1	45.9	45.7	60.4	75.0
Secondary	62.6	58.5	61.7	66.5	78.7
Higher	76.2	69.0	79.9	70.5	78.3
Caste					
Scheduled caste	26.5	37.8	39.7	63.2	76.3
Scheduled tribe	24.8	24.8	31.3	55.8	76.3
Other backward classes	–	40.6	40.7	61.9	76.8
Others (+OBCs in 1992–93)	38.2	43.4	53.8	63.6	75.8
Religion					
Hindu	36.0	40.0	44.4	63.0	77.1
Muslim	26.3	29.8	36.3	55.4	71.0
Christian	42.4	56.0	56.3	61.7	77.2
Sikh	60.4	66.0	67.3	88.9	79.4
Others	57.7	59.9	41.7	61.4	80.5
Wealth Quintile					
Lowest	18.4	23.1	24.4	52.8	70.9
Second	24.4	29.0	33.2	60.6	75.0
Middle	31.0	38.3	46.9	64.2	79.5
Fourth	47.5	51.9	55.3	66.9	79.3
Highest	64.8	64.0	71.0	70.0	78.2
Place of Residence					
Urban	50.7	54.8	57.6	63.8	75.2
Rural	30.9	34.9	38.6	61.3	76.6
All India	35.4	39.4	43.5	62.0	76.2

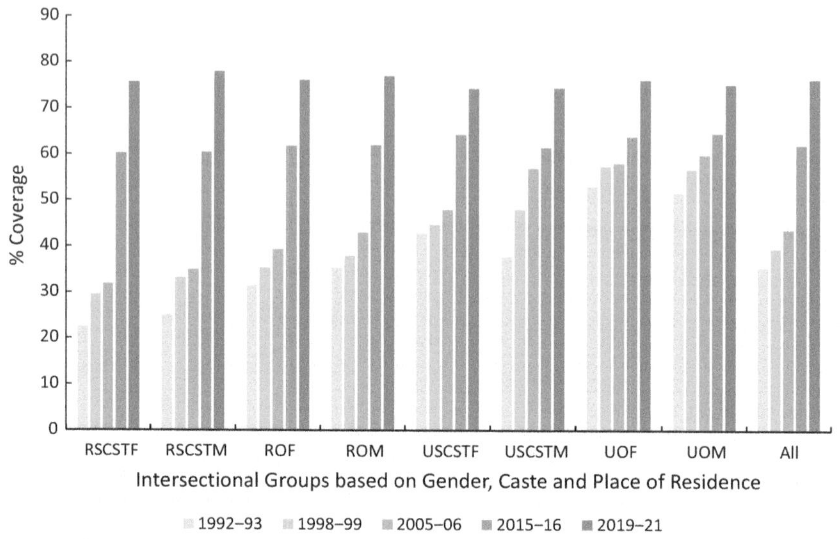

Fig. 5.2 Full immunization and zero-dose coverage (%) among children (12–23 months) by intersectional groups based on gender, caste, and place of residence, India, NFHS 1993–2021

in coverage trends is worrisome and this group emerges as a clear vulnerable section in immunization coverage. Poverty status of the household is also an important characteristic of vulnerability. In 2005–06, children from the poorest wealth quintile households in rural (24.2%) and urban (27.3%) areas had similar coverage but were much behind the national average. However, in 2019–21, the patterns have reversed as well as the gap between these groups has widened (urban lowest wealth quintile, 59.3% and rural lowest wealth quintile, 71.5%). Children categorized as MPI poor based on the NITI Aayog definition also have coverage levels (36.7% in 2005–06 and 72.2% in 2019–21) lower than the national average [1]. However, these children are not as disadvantaged as those from the poorest households, especially from the urban areas.

Non-receipt of basic antenatal care services such as mandated four ANC visits and provisioning of IFA supplements emerge as important markers of left-behind women and children. The immunization coverage among children with such deprivation in maternal health care is lower than the national average. The most vulnerable subgroups are those identified based on economic status of migrants into urban or rural areas. While migration per se is not particularly disadvantageous but the overall full immunization coverage among the migrant households is also not very different from the national average. The urban migrants used to have an edge over rural migrants in 2005–05 but this has disappeared in 2019–21. It may be largely attributed to the significant movement of populations from all economic sections whereby the influx in urban areas may be greater among the economically poor households. The poorest urban migrant households had a full immunization coverage of 25.3% in 2005–06 and this level continues to be the lowest (53.2% in 2019–21) among the

Table 5.2 Full immunization and zero-dose coverage (%) among children (12–23 months) by vulnerable groups and populations, India, NFHS 1993–2021

Vulnerable groups/populations	Full immunization (%)		
	2005–06	2015–16	2019–21
Slum area residents	65.4	54.8	–
Urban lowest WQ household	27.3	56.2	59.3
Rural lowest WQ household	24.2	52.6	71.5
MPI Poor (NITI Aayog definition)	36.7	56.2	72.2
0-3 ANC visits in last pregnancy	31.0	54.0	70.2
No IFA received in last pregnancy	28.9	50.0	68.5
Urban migrant (last 10 years reference)	59.0	66.8	70.2
Rural migrant (last 10 years reference)	47.6	69.9	75.7
Urban lowest WQ migrant household	25.3	48.9	53.2
Rural lowest WQ migrant household	31.1	54.4	64.5
Vulnerable groups/populations	Zero-dose (None vaccine)		
	2005–06	2015–16	2019–21
Slum area residents	3.8	8.1	–
Urban lowest WQ household	9.6	10.1	7.6
Rural lowest WQ household	9.4	10.0	4.5
MPI Poor (NITI Aayog definition)	6.0	8.5	4.5
0-3 ANC visits in last pregnancy	6.9	8.5	4.8
No IFA received in last pregnancy	8.2	11.8	6.5
Urban migrant (last 10 years reference)	2.6	2.3	4.1
Rural migrant (last 10 years reference)	5.7	4.1	2.4
Urban lowest WQ migrant household	1.6	19.3	25.3
Rural lowest WQ migrant household	7.5	12.1	5.0
Vulnerable groups/populations	Zero-dose (IA2030 DTP1)		
	2005–06	2015–16	2019–21
Slum area residents	9.7	16.7	–
Urban lowest WQ household	40.3	18.4	15.4
Rural lowest WQ household	40.0	16.0	9.0
MPI Poor (NITI Aayog definition)	28.6	14.5	8.8
0-3 ANC visits in last pregnancy	33.5	14.8	9.2
No IFA received in last pregnancy	38.8	19.2	11.3
Urban migrant (last 10 years reference)	13.9	7.9	7.7
Rural migrant (last 10 years reference)	19.5	7.2	5.4
Urban lowest WQ migrant household	38.9	20.1	26.0
Rural lowest WQ migrant household	34.5	15.7	8.8

identified vulnerable populations in Table 5.2. The status of lowest quintile rural migrants is relatively better than their urban counterparts.

The patterns in zero-dose prevalence also follows similar pattern of disadvantage among the identified vulnerable populations. In 2019–21 as per the zero-dose (DTP1) definition, the prevalence is found to be 26.0% among children from the poorest urban migrant households. In general, the prevalence among the urban poorest households (15.4%) is a major concern. Usually, the prevalence in terms of zero-dose (no vaccine) definition is lower than the other definition but, in this instance, it is worth noting that 25.3% of the children from the poorest urban migrant households have not received any vaccine. The SDG progress now critically depends on the performance of the immunization coverage program in urban areas with a particular emphasis on the poorest and the migrant households.

Econometric Associations with Correlates

Finally, the significance of the bivariate association of various demographic and socioeconomic correlates with immunization coverage is verified through logistic regression analysis (Table 5.3). The odds ratios (OR) and the 95% confidence interval (CI) for the mutually adjusted models are presented for the years 2005–06, 2015–16, and 2019–21. Females are less likely to receive full immunization. The likelihood was 24% lower in 2005–06 (OR 0.76: 95% CI [0.60; 0.96]) and continues to be significant in 2019–21 (OR 0.85: 95% CI [0.73; 0.98]). Since 2005–06, urban areas have displayed lower likelihood of full immunization, and this has further worsened with 40% lower chances of immunization in 2019–21 (OR 0.60: 95% CI [0.48; 0.77]). Wealth-related gradient in receipt of full immunization has disappeared in 2019–21 but this used to be significant in 2005–06. The change can be attributed to the free public provision of vaccines, which has made immunization a service accessible to all, particularly benefitting the poor.

Tables S6 and S7 present the logistic regression-based odds ratio for the two indicators defined here to understand zero-dose viz. no vaccine and no DPT1, respectively. The broad patterns of advantages and disadvantages are consistent in these models. Female child is found to be at greater risk of zero-dose than males. The risk is much higher in case of non-receipt of DPT1 dosage. Urban children are becoming increasingly disadvantaged in zero-dose irrespective of the employed definition of zero-dose. The risk of zero-dose shows a wealth gradient in case of the definition of zero-dose (no vaccine) whereas no significant gradient is noted for the definition of zero-dose (no DPT1). Maternal education continues to an influential factor in determining zero-dose status. There are no social group or caste-based advantages in zero-dose prevalence, but it is worth noting that Muslim households are at a greater risk of zero-dose than others. The odds of zero-dose (no vaccine) are higher in slum areas in 2015–16 whereas the patterns are consistent but not significant for the other definition. Health system factors again turn out to be a major deterrent in enabling access to vaccination services. Mothers who have not received four ANC visits or

Table 5.3 Logistic regression-based odds ratio (OR) for receipt of full immunization by children (12–23 months), India NFHS 2006–2021

Background characteristics	2005–06		2015–16		2019–21	
Sex of the child	OR	95% CI	OR	95% CI	OR	95% CI
Male	1.00		1.00		1.00	
Female	0.76**	[0.60; 0.96]	0.97	[0.87; 1.09]	0.85**	[0.73; 0.98]
Place of residence						
Rural	1.00		1.00		1.00	
Urban	0.78	[0.55; 1.09]	0.86*	[0.73; 1.01]	0.60***	[0.48; 0.77]
Wealth quintile (WQ)						
Lowest WQ	1.00		1.00		1.00	
Second WQ	1.28	[0.95; 1.73]	1.24***	[1.08; 1.41]	1.03	[0.86; 1.24]
Middle WQ	1.52**	[1.04; 2.20]	1.41***	[1.19; 1.66]	1.18	[0.93; 1.49]
Fourth WQ	2.15***	[1.38; 3.33]	1.72***	[1.38; 2.15]	1.46***	[1.12; 1.92]
Highest WQ	4.54***	[2.26; 9.13]	1.66***	[1.21; 2.27]	1.29	[0.92; 1.81]
Social group						
Scheduled caste	1.00		1.00		1.00	
Scheduled tribe	0.57***	[0.40; 0.83]	0.61***	[0.50; 0.74]	0.83	[0.65; 1.07]
Other backward classes	1.41**	[1.00; 1.98]	1.05	[0.90; 1.23]	0.96	[0.78; 1.18]
Others	1.14	[0.79; 1.66]	0.84*	[0.70; 1.02]	0.93	[0.72; 1.20]
Religion						
Hindu	1.00		1.00		1.00	
Muslim	0.53***	[0.39; 0.72]	0.58***	[0.50; 0.67]	0.69***	[0.57; 0.84]
Others	0.56***	[0.39; 0.80]	0.92	[0.66; 1.27]	0.66**	[0.47; 0.93]
Maternal age						
15–19 years	1.00		1.00		1.00	
20–29 years	1.24	[0.84; 1.84]	1.11	[0.86; 1.43]	1.08	[0.75; 1.55]
30–39 years	1.02	[0.65; 1.59]	0.91	[0.70; 1.19]	1.13	[0.78; 1.65]
40–49 years	0.96	[0.42; 2.20]	0.61***	[0.42; 0.90]	0.68	[0.36; 1.28]
Maternal education						
No formal schooling	1.00		1.00		1.00	
Primary	0.99	[0.72; 1.36]	1.34***	[1.15; 1.57]	1.65***	[1.32; 2.07]
Secondary	1.64***	[1.12; 2.38]	1.42***	[1.24; 1.63]	1.66***	[1.38; 1.99]
Higher	7.41***	[1.51; 36.4]	1.39**	[0.99; 1.96]	1.74***	[1.33; 2.30]
Slum Area household						
No	1.00		1.00		-	
Yes	0.76	[0.44; 1.32]	0.50	[0.20; 1.27]	-	
4+ ANC visits by mother						

(continued)

Table 5.3 (continued)

Background characteristics	2005–06		2015–16		2019–21	
Yes	1.00		1.00		1.00	
No	0.87	[0.61; 1.24]	0.60***	[0.52; 0.69]	0.67***	[0.57; 0.80]
IFA received by mother						
Yes	1.00		1.00		1.00	
No	0.45***	[0.35; 0.58]	0.41***	[0.37; 0.45]	0.54***	[0.45; 0.63]
Urban migrant x Lowest WQ						
No	1.00		1.00		1.00	
Yes	8.13**	[0.96; 69.1]	0.32	[0.04; 2.53]	0.19	[0.01; 3.22]
Rural migrant x Lowest WQ						
No	1.00		1.00		1.00	
Yes	1.30	[0.48; 3.51]	0.83	[0.46; 1.51]	0.93	[0.25; 3.51]

any IFA during pregnancy are also at greater risk of zero-dose. Despite sampling errors, poor urban migrant households also confront a higher risk of zero-dose.

ST children were 43% less likely to receive full immunization in 2005–06 (OR 0.57: 95% CI [0.40; 0.83]) compared to the SC children, the inter-group disparities are now not statistically significant. Muslim households, however, display much lower odds ratio for full immunization coverage with a continued pattern. Compared to Hindu households, children from other religion also show lower odds of full immunization. This suggests wide socioeconomic heterogeneity within the religious composition of the populations. While maternal age per se has no significant effect on full immunization coverage but maternal education plays a critical role. In 2019–21, maternal higher education provides a 1.74 times higher likelihood (OR 1.74: 95% CI [1.33; 2.30]) of full immunization than those without any formal schooling.

The adjusted models do not find any significant association between slum residency status and full immunization coverage. While the odds ratio is in the expected direction, the statistical significance may be affected because of low sample size. Similar effects are noted in case of poorest rural and urban migrant households whereby the coefficients are in the expected direction but are not statistically significant. However, the non-receipt of basic ANC care and IFA supplements during pregnancy period turns out to be the most significant factor in reducing the chances of full immunization. In 2019–21, women who had not completed four ANC visits had 33% less chances of having full immunization of the child (OR 0.67: 95% CI [0.57; 0.80]). Similarly, non-receipt of any IFA supplement during pregnancy reduces the chances of full immunization for children by 46% (OR 0.54: 95% CI [0.45; 0.63]). This indicates that barriers are much association with health system factors including availability and access rather than poverty and migration status of the households.

Discussion

Summary of Findings

The analysis yields certain novel insights on the trends and patterns in immunization coverage in India since the 90s. The five salient findings are listed as follows. First, there is acceleration in immunization coverage in India in recent years. The average annualized rate of progress (AARP) in immunization coverage between 1993 and 2006 was 1.6% per annum. The AARP has accelerated since the launch of the NRHM (3.5% per annum during 2006–2016) and has further accelerated in the IMI phase (4.1% per annum during 2016–21). Second, the remarkable feature of progress is the consistent bridging of the wide disparities in immunization coverage across gender, caste, and place of residence. The variations across income, education, and religious background have substantially shrunk in the last few years. Third, the high prevalence of zero-dose amidst such rapid improvements in immunization coverage is deplorable. The two alternative definitions of zero-dose put forth disconcerting evidence on the situation. Fourth, the geography of vulnerability in immunization coverage is gradually shifting toward the urban areas with greater concentration of the problem in the slum areas and among the urban poor. The migrants comprise of an increasing share of the urban poor, and they are now more vulnerable than their rural counterparts in the receipt of basic vaccines including DPT1. Finally, the econometric association signal the potential role of health system challenges that may be contributing to poor immunization coverage. While reaching out to women and children with health care services, it is likely that the system is still missing out on certain vulnerable sections and individuals. For instance, the magnitude of zero-dose is likely to be higher for mothers who have not received any IFA tablet during pregnancy or have not received four ANC visits. This correlation can stem from geographical inaccessibility or systemic barriers that discourage the migrants and the poor from seeking public health care services. The analysis, however, must be interpreted along with certain broad data limitations. The analysis is based on cross-sectional data and the observed associations may not be necessarily causal. The information on immunization coverage and vaccines received is partly based on recall by the mother/caregiver. Respondent bias and recall errors are plausible. The information on slums or migrants is not available consistently in all the five rounds of NFHS.

Disparities in Immunization Coverage

At the aggregate level, the gender disadvantage in full immunization coverage continues to persist with slightly lower coverage among female children. A major feature of the 1990s was the low immunization coverage among the SC and ST population. However, the primary health care services have performed well to eliminate the gap between SC, ST, and other social groups. This is a major accomplishment even though all the groups are yet to reach the target of universal coverage. With the focus on leaving no one behind, such achievements should nevertheless be skeptically viewed through alternative lens to examine equitable progress. Our analysis motivated by intersectionality lens with groups cross-classified by gender, caste, and place of residence suggests that the disadvantageous status of females from rural and SCST background (RSCSTF) that persisted throughout the 1990s are gradually eliminated. However, SC-ST population in urban areas are now at a position of relative disadvantage in full immunization, particularly zero-dose prevalence. The disparities in immunization coverage are now increasingly getting manifested alongside access and utilization of maternal health care services. This essentially includes the use of antenatal care services and provisions to ensure access to such services in urban areas. The migration status, poverty situation, and increasing urban proliferation of slums may pose additional challenges in managing the urban health services and ensure equity for all in-migrants. The patterns in zero-dose prevalence also follows similar pattern of disparities and disadvantage among the identified vulnerable populations. The inequities in immunization coverage can be further addressed through concerted with the urban poor households.

Corroboration of Findings

The global momentum in immunization coincides with the setting up of GAVI, The Vaccine Alliance in 2000 to support immunization programs and vaccine development across LMICs [24]. India also displays acceleration in immunization coverage in the post-NRHM phase and subsequently in the post-IMI phase [12, 37]. The success of MI and IMI can be attributed to improvements in governance and messaging (such as Jan Andolan campaigns) along with technical improvements in terms of expanding network of cold chain, improving microplanning, supervision and data systems, and dedicated attention to redress adverse event following immunization (AEFI) cases [10]. The pre-NRHM phase was marked with low coverage, huge prevalence of zero-dose, and wide inter-state, inter-group, and socioeconomic inequalities in immunization [17, 18, 20, 29]. Our findings confirm these patterns for the first few rounds of NFHS and unravel reductions in the disparities across these broad axes of inequities. Low likelihood of full immunization among the Muslim households is also an important and persistent feature in the Indian context [5, 20].

Rural to urban migrants are identified to be among the most vulnerable populations in receipt of immunization services [3]. Our findings are consistent with this widespread concern across LMICs. In fact, we reveal that poorest of the urban migrants also have the highest prevalence of zero-dose. The public health system in urban areas is dealing with a plethora of problems. These include huge influx of migrants that are not necessarily accommodated with corresponding expansion of infrastructure or human resources for health. Notwithstanding the gaps in knowledge and awareness among the poor urban migrants, systemic exclusion on account of non-recognition or delays in notification of slums further alienate the migrants from the health system [19, 25]. Studies have noted that often health worker insist upon beneficiary identification through vaccination card or Aadhar card [35]. These may be a major challenge for the urban migrants as they may lack papers or may be discouraged in revisiting the facility amidst their search for subsistence livelihoods. The list of concerns in urban health services delivery are manifold. For instance, observance of Urban Health and Nutrition Day (UHND) although focuses primarily on immunization services but it often neglects certain urban slum pockets and areas because of ill-defined location boundaries [4]. Inadequate training of frontline workers as well as indifference among community members and representatives further create disadvantages for women and children in receipt of these basic services.

Programmatic Implications

The trends and patterns although promising but also outline important areas for policy actions. First and foremost, the challenge of zero-dose and full immunization has gradually evolved as a major public health challenge in urban areas. The solution here lies in expansion of the urban health system services in areas that are underserved and are inhabited by vulnerable populations including urban poor and the low-income migrants. Scope for relaxations in documentation and identification evidence of beneficiary for universal basic services such as maternal and child health care should be reviewed, and specific budgetary norms and provisions should be put in place. The persistent challenge of low coverage should be addressed through greater stakeholder interactions in underserved and hard-to-reach areas. Vaccine hesitancy across communities has been a worldwide phenomenon. However, continued engagement and evidence on safety and efficacy helps to overcome reservations within communities.

The role of monetary and non-monetary incentives for frontline workers may also require timely review to meet the expectations while being consistent with their efforts in last mile delivery of these essential services in maternal and child health. Immunization programs should also aim to leverage alternative community-based platforms such as the POSHAN Abhiyaan, Ayushman Bharat—Health and Wellness Centres and Janani Suraksha Yojana (JSY). These platforms provide opportunity to address different facets of immunization. In addition, greater support in monitoring of the immunization programs can be instrumental in identifying priority areas and population subgroups. Various national and international developmental organizations that focus on urban health also offer such platforms for sustaining community engagement for primary health care services.

The immunization program must strengthen the gaps in supply chain. Geographic disparities are often driven by inadequate healthcare infrastructure. To improve access to vaccination services, it is essential to strengthen healthcare resources and planning for service delivery in remote areas. Individuals from lower socioeconomic backgrounds are disproportionately affected by lower immunization rates. Implementing outreach programs that educate these communities about the benefits of vaccination and make these services available is crucial. A significant barrier to immunization is a lack of awareness regarding its importance. By conducting educational campaigns within communities, we can encourage a greater number of people to get vaccinated. Integrating immunization efforts with broader health services and social welfare programs can increase access and uptake. For instance, linking immunization with nutrition programs can encourage greater participation in both initiatives.

Conclusion

In conclusion, it is worth reiterating the accelerated progress of India in full immunization coverage. The bridging of gap in immunization coverage across sectors and social groups stands out as a significant achievement of the three-decade journey. While vaccination remains an unfinished agenda, the biggest risk to further progress is the stagnancy in urban areas. The growing concentration of vulnerable populations in urban poor settlements is a major challenge in delivery of immunization services. The policy approach on urban immunization coverage will determine whether India is able to timely deliver on the SDG promise of leaving no one behind.

References

1. NITI Aayog. (2021). National Multidimensional Poverty Index: Baseline Report, .
2. Aayog, N. I. T. I. (2022). *The Indian Model of SDG Localization, United Nations High-Level Political Forum on Sustainable Development 2022.* NITI Aayog.
3. Awoh, A. B., & Plugge, E. (2016). Immunisation coverage in rural–urban migrant children in low and middle-income countries (LMICs): A systematic review and meta-analysis. *Journal of Epidemiology and Community Health, 70*(3), 305–311.
4. Banerjee, S., Selvaraj, K., Bandyopadhyay, K., Khan, M. F., Bisen, T., & Deshmukh, P. (2021). Urban health and nutrition day or only immunisation day? Barriers and bottlenecks in implementing urban health and nutrition day in an urban primary health centre of Nagpur, central India. *Journal of Mother and Child, 25*(1), 51–60.
5. Bellatin, A., Hyder, A., Rao, S., Zhang, P. C., & McGahan, A. M. (2021). Overcoming vaccine deployment challenges among the hardest to reach: Lessons from polio elimination in India. *BMJ Global Health, 6*(4), e005125.
6. Bettampadi, D., Lepkowski, J. M., Sen, A., Power, L. E., & Boulton, M. L. (2021). Vaccination inequality in India, 2002–2013. *American Journal of Preventive Medicine, 60*(1), S65–S76.
7. Bhadoria, A. S., Mishra, S., Singh, M., & Kishore, S. (2019). National immunization programme–mission Indradhanush programme: newer approaches and interventions. *The Indian Journal of Pediatrics, 86*, 633–638.
8. Bloom, D. E., Canning, D., & Weston, M. (2017). The Value of Vaccination. *World Economics, 6*(3), 15–39.

9. Cata-Preta, B. O., Santos, T. M., Mengistu, T., Hogan, D. R., Barros, A. J., & Victora, C. G. (2021). Zero-dose children and the immunisation cascade: Understanding immunisation pathways in low and middle-income countries. *Vaccine, 39*(32), 4564–4570.
10. Dhawan, V., Chakraborty, A. B., Dhandore, S., Dhalaria, P., Agarwal, D., & Singh, A. K. (2023). Mission Indradhanush and Intensified Mission Indradhanush—Success Story of India's Universal Immunization Program and the Role of Mann Ki Baat in Bridging the Immunization Gap. *Indian Journal of Community Medicine, 48*(6), 823–827.
11. Greenwood, B. (2014). *The contribution of vaccination to global health: past, present and future* (p. *369*). *Philosophical Transactions of the Royal Society B.*
12. Gurnani, V., et al. (2018). Improving vaccination coverage in India: lessons from Intensified Mission Indradhanush, a cross-sectoral systems strengthening strategy. *BMJ, 363*(K4782), 1–7.
13. Gurnani, V., et al. (2020). Programmatic assessment of electronic vaccine intelligence network (eVIN). *PLoS One, 15*(11), e0241369.
14. Gurnani, V., et al. (2021). Comprehensive review of the Universal Immunization Programme (UIP)–Identifying gaps and assist in formulating improvement plan for routine immunization in few states of India. *Clinical Epidemiology and Global Health, 12*, 100834.
15. Hogan, D., & Gupta, A. (2023). Why reaching zero-dose children holds the key to achieving the sustainable development goals. *Vaccines, 11*(4), 781.
16. IIPS and ICF. (2021). *National Family Health Survey (NFHS-5), 2019-21: India. International Institute for Population Sciences.*
17. Joe, W. (2015). Intersectional inequalities in immunization in India, 1992–93 to 2005–06: A progress assessment. *Health Policy and Planning, 30*(4), 407–422.
18. Johri, M., Rajpal, S., & Subramanian, S. V. (2021). Progress in reaching unvaccinated (zero-dose) children in India, 1992–2016: A multilevel, geospatial analysis of repeated cross-sectional surveys. *The Lancet Global Health, 9*(12), e1697–e1706.
19. Kulkarni, S., Thampi, V., Deshmukh, D., Gadhari, M., Chandrasekar, R., & Phadke, M. (2023). Trends in urban immunization coverage in India: a meta-analysis and meta-regression. *Indian Journal of Pediatrics, 90*, 38–48.
20. Mathew, J. L. (2012). Inequity in childhood immunization in India: A systematic review. *Indian Pediatrics, 49*, 203–223.
21. MoHFW. (2023a). *Brief Activities of Department of Health and Family Welfare.* Ministry of Health and Family Welfare.
22. MoHFW. (2023b). *G20 Health Ministers Meeting (18–19 August, 2023 at Gandhinagar, India).* Outcome Document and Chair's Summary.
23. MoSPI. (2024). *Sustainable Development Goals National Indicator Framework, Progress Report 2024.* Ministry of Statistics and Programme Implementation.
24. Muraskin, W. (2002). The last years of the CVI and the birth of the GAVI. In M. R. Reich (Ed.), *Public-private partnerships for public health* (pp. 115–168). Harvard University Press.
25. Nolan, L. B., Bloom, D. E., & Subbaraman, R. (2018). Legal status and deprivation in urban slums over two decades. *Economic and political weekly, 53*(15), 47.
26. Orenstein, W. A., & Ahmed, R. (2017). Simply put: Vaccination saves lives. *Proceedings of the National Academy of Sciences, 114*(16), 4031–4033.
27. Ozawa, S., *et al.* (2011). During the 'decade of vaccines,' the lives of 6.4 million children valued at $231 billion could be saved. *Health Affairs, 30*(6), 1010–1020.
28. Ozawa, S., et al. (2017). Estimated economic impact of vaccinations in 73 low-and middle-income countries, 2001–2020. *Bulletin of the World Health Organization, 95*(9), 629.
29. Pande, R. P., & Yazbeck, A. S. (2003). What's in a country average? Wealth, gender, and regional inequalities in immunization in India. *Social Science & Medicine, 57*(11), 2075–2088.
30. Patel, A. R., & Nowalk, M. P. (2010). Expanding immunization coverage in rural India: A review of evidence for the role of community health workers. *Vaccine, 28*(3), 604–613.
31. Piot, P., et al. (2019). Immunization: Vital progress, unfinished agenda. *Nature, 575*(7781), 119–129.
32. Pramanik, S., Muthusamy, N., Gera, R., & Laxminarayan, R. (2015). Vaccination coverage in India: a small area estimation approach. *Vaccine, 33*(14), 1731–1738.

33. Rajwar, E., et al. (2023). The utilization of systematic review evidence in formulating India's National Health Programme guidelines between 2007 and 2021. *Health Policy and Planning, 38*(4), 435–453.
34. Sen, G., Iyer, A., & Mukherjee, C. (2009). A methodology to analyse the intersections of social inequalities in health. *Journal of Human Development and Capabilities, 10*(3), 397–415.
35. Sharma, V., Singh, A., & Sharma, V. (2015). Provider's and user's perspective about immunization coverage among migratory and non-migratory population in slums and construction sites of Chandigarh. *Journal of Urban Health, 92*, 304–312.
36. Shattock, A. J., et al. (2024). Contribution of vaccination to improved survival and health: Modelling 50 years of the Expanded Programme on Immunization. *The Lancet, 403*(10441), 2307–2316.
37. Summan, A., Nandi, A., Deo, S., & Laxminarayan, R. (2021). Improving vaccination coverage and timeliness through periodic intensification of routine immunization: evidence from Mission Indradhanush. *Annals of the New York Academy of Sciences, 1502*(1), 110–120.
38. United Nations. (2015). *Transforming our World: The 2030 Agenda for Sustainable Development, A/RES/70/1*. United Nations General Assembly.
39. United Nations. (2017). *Work of the Statistical Commission pertaining to the 2030 Agenda for Sustainable Development, A/RES/71/313*. United Nations General Assembly.
40. WHO; UNICEF (2024). Progress and Challenges with Achieving Universal Immunization Coverage. 2023 WHO/UNICEF Estimates of National Immunization Coverage (WUENIC); World Health Organization: .
41. WHO, UNICEF and Gavi, the Vaccine Alliance. (2023). *The big catch-up: An essential immunization recovery plan for 2023 and beyond*. WHO, UNICEF and Gavi, The Vaccine Alliance.

Chapter 6
Impact on Long-Term Health: Nutritional Challenges and Interventions

Subhasree Ray

Introduction

Food is essential for survival, as it provides the necessary fuel for the body to function. According to the World Health Organization (WHO, 2019), establishing healthy dietary habits from an early age, starting with breastfeeding, is not only essential for physical growth but also for cognitive development [1]. This early foundation of nutrition is vital for ensuring well-being as individuals grow. A nutritious diet during childhood plays a crucial role in promoting long-term health, reducing the risk of metabolic disorders, weight-related issues, and the development of non-communicable diseases later in life. On the other hand, unhealthy eating habits combined with a sedentary lifestyle and little physical activity are major contributors to health risks [2]. When individuals consume food that lacks essential nutrients, they are at risk of developing malnutrition, which poses a serious threat to human health especially for children.

Malnutrition can manifest in different forms including undernutrition (wasting, stunting, and underweight), deficiencies in vitamins or minerals, overweight, obesity, and the associated diet-related non-communicable diseases [3]. Globally, in 2022, an estimated 149 million children under the age of five were stunted (too short for their age), 45 million were wasted (too thin for their height), and 37 million were either overweight or living with obesity [4]. Almost half of the deaths among children under five years are related to undernutrition, with the majority occurring in low- and middle-income countries [3]. The impact of malnutrition on individuals, families, communities, and locations is significant and enduring, with implications for development, economy, society, and health. Figure 6.1 demonstrates the global trends from 2020 to 2022 in the prevalence of various spectra of malnutrition among children under five years [5].

S. Ray (✉)
Section Head - Wellness at TVS Motor Company, Hosur, Tamil Nadu, India
e-mail: roysubhoshree@gmail.com

S. Suri (ed.), *Child Health and Nutrition from Conception to Age Two*,
https://doi.org/10.1007/978-981-95-7868-9_6

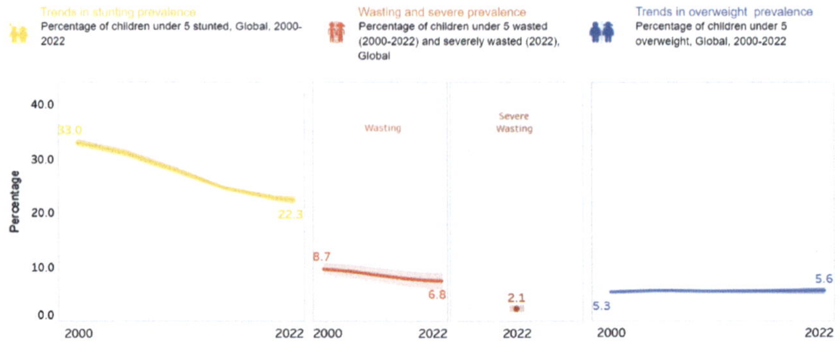

Fig 6.1 Global Overview of Child Nutrition: World Health Organization

The nutritional foundation established during the early childhood has a lasting impact on the long-term health of a child. Nutrition is essential for the physical growth, cognitive development, and overall well-being of children. The first 1000 days of life, from conception to a child's second birthday, are a critical window for shaping lifelong health [6]. Nutritional status during this period impacts physical growth, brain development, and immune function. Inadequate nutrition can lead to stunted growth, cognitive impairment, and an increased risk of chronic diseases, while optimal nutrition enhances development and educational outcomes, promoting healthier adulthood. However, challenges persist, and issues like poverty, food insecurity, and limited access to nutrient-rich foods hinder adequate nutrition [7, 8], while cultural practices, misconceptions, and lack of knowledge contribute to suboptimal feeding [9, 10]. In high-income countries, processed foods and sedentary lifestyles have led to rising childhood obesity rates, posing long-term health risks.

Nutritional Challenges: The Critical Determinants

Malnutrition in children under the age of five years is caused by a combination of factors related to food and healthcare accessibility and their utilization [3]. Specific issues include inadequate food intake, poor caregiving and parenting, improper feeding methods, and infectious diseases. Additionally, broader factors such as food insecurity, limited economic resources, and poor access to education, healthcare, and hygiene also contribute to malnutrition in this age group.

Individual risk factors for malnutrition include age, gender, birthweight, breastfeeding practices, childhood comorbidities, teenage pregnancy, low maternal education, lack of breastfeeding, and personal food preferences. Low birthweight is an individual factor but is strongly influenced by maternal health, nutritional status, and household food security. The influence of gender and a mother's literacy on malnutrition in children under five is well-established. Protein-energy malnutrition (PEM) is most common during the third year of life and lowest in the second [11]. Undernutrition primarily affects children aged 24–59 months, while those under one year are less vulnerable [12], with wasting most prevalent among younger children [13, 14]. Gender differences in undernutrition vary with age. Boys are more vulnerable to wasting and stunting up until 30 months, after which the gap between boys and girls reduces [15]. However, the lower risk of undernutrition typically observed in girls is less noticeable in South Asia compared to other regions [16]. In some African cultures, gender bias against female children places them at a greater nutritional risk [17]. Additionally, PEM weakens immunity, increasing susceptibility to infections like tuberculosis, diarrhea, and measles, further deteriorating the nutritional status of affected children [18].

The level of a mother's education is an important determinant of the nutritional status of children under five years. Educated mothers, due to their awareness of health practices and nutrition literacy, tend to provide better primary care, delay childbearing, and reduce infant mortality [18]. Mothers who completed elementary school were found to be 1.167 times more likely to perform exclusive breastfeeding compared to mothers who never attended school [19]. Children born to older mothers were found to be at a lower risk of malnutrition than younger mothers [17]. On the other hand, children of uneducated mothers are more likely to experience stunting, and maternal education also influences the prevalence of underweight and wasting [20]. The literacy rate of females is further dependent on a country's income and other social factors [21]. The socioeconomic benefits of education, such as higher income and better living conditions, further contribute to child health [22]. However, working mothers, particularly in informal or slum settings, may face challenges in balancing childcare, potentially increasing the risk of malnutrition [23].

Household, environmental, and socioeconomic factors, such as geographic location, family income, household size, food security, and healthcare access, play a vital role in child malnutrition. Cultural beliefs, community practices, and feeding habits also contribute to malnutrition in children under five. Factors like poverty, large family sizes, and neglect of children's health worsen malnutrition, as fewer resources are available for food per child. Higher family income provides better food security, dietary adequacy, and improved child nutrition [24]. In rural areas, especially in South Africa, poor infrastructure and limited access to services increase the risk of childhood malnutrition [25].

In recent times, conflicts, climate, and pandemics such as COVID-19 are critical determinants of global food security and poverty that directly link to the economic condition of a country. The National Income Dynamics Study–Coronavirus Rapid Mobile Survey (NIDS–CRAM) revealed a significant increase in household and food insecurity during the COVID-19 pandemic, emphasizing the economic roots of malnutrition [25]. The climatic change on the other hand significantly impacts agriculture, food production, availability, and security—all of which affect child nutrition and health outcomes [26]. Climate change coupled with COVID-19 worsened critical determinants for child nutritional status such as dietary diversity, nutrient quality, and maternal nutrition status. Child malnutrition and children's living conditions are significantly affected by social instability. The combined effects of inequality, unrest, and poverty result in 1 in 4 children worldwide facing severe food insecurity. The magnitude of child malnutrition and children's living experience is heavily impacted by the armed conflicts. The combined impact of inequity, conflict, and poverty leaving 1 in 4 children globally live with severe child food poverty [27].

Forms of Early Childhood Malnutrition and Their Long-Term Health Impacts

The spectrum of malnutrition in children under the age of five can take various forms, such as underweight, stunting, wasting, and severe acute malnutrition (SAM), all of which can have serious consequences [28]. These conditions are the consequences of severe food insecurity, nutrition inadequacy, and other social determinants. Figure 6.2 illustrates various forms of malnutrition according to the WHO classification, adopted from Obasohan *et al.*, 2020 [29].

Figure 6.2 presents the schematic classification of the various forms of malnutrition, delineated through standardized anthropometric indicators and their respective Z-scores. The figure employs three primary indices: height-for-age Z-score (HAZ), weight-for-height Z-score (WHZ), and weight-for-age Z-score (WAZ), each serving as a proxy for distinct manifestations of nutritional deficiency or excess.

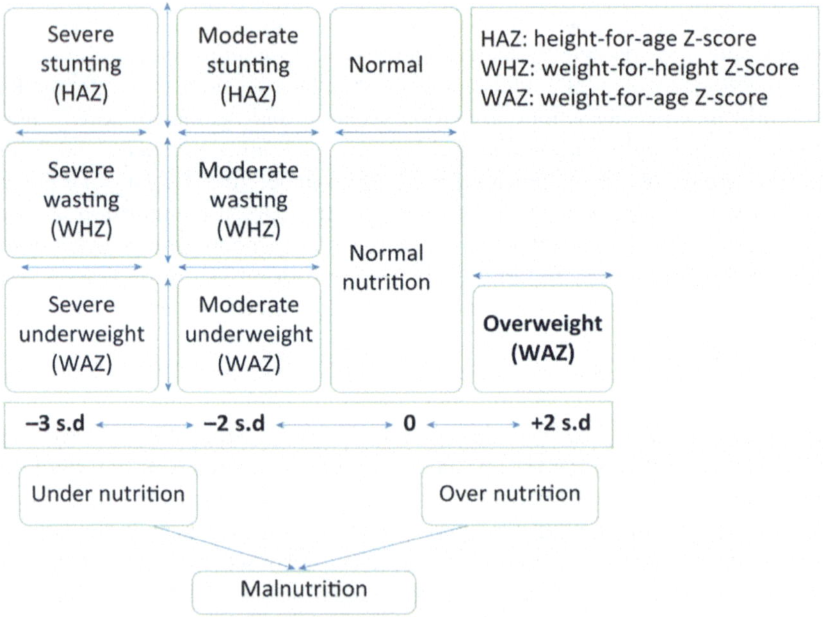

Fig 6.2 Various Forms of Malnutrition

HAZ is used to assess stunting, which reflects chronic undernutrition often resulting from prolonged dietary inadequacies or repeated infections. WHZ captures wasting, indicative of acute undernutrition and rapid weight loss typically associated with recent episodes of food deprivation or illness. WAZ, a composite measure, is applied to identify underweight status, encapsulating both acute and chronic undernutrition. The classification system is aligned with World Health Organization standards, using standard deviation (s.d.) thresholds to categorize severity: values below –2 s.d. denote moderate malnutrition, while values below –3 s.d. indicate severe forms. Individuals with Z-scores between –2 s.d. and +2 s.d. are considered to have normal nutritional status. Conversely, Z-scores exceeding +2 s.d. reflect overnutrition, typically manifesting as overweight. This bidirectional framework underscores malnutrition as a spectrum encompassing both undernutrition and overnutrition, thereby informing public health strategies and interventions aimed at achieving optimal growth and nutritional well-being across populations.

Stunting is defined as height-for-age Z-score that is more than 2 standard deviations below the median [30]. It indicates chronic malnutrition in children and results in slow growth and overall growth deficits. Stunting has significant and often irreversible effects on a child's physical and cognitive development, especially within the first 1,000 days from conception. According to a 2020 report by UNICEF, WHO, and the World Bank, approximately 144 million or 21.9% of children under five globally suffer from stunting [31]. Although stunting rates are decreasing worldwide, the African and Asian regions have seen an alarming increase. Stunting is the most frequent form of child malnutrition [32]. All forms of malnutrition in early life of a child are associated with significant physiological changes, inflammation, protein deficiency, micronutrient deficiency, altered leptin levels, and elevated glucocorticoids, which can lead to epigenetic modifications [33]. These alterations are linked to neurodevelopmental disorders, disruptions in neurogenesis, increased cell apoptosis, and synaptic dysfunction, all contributing to developmental delays. The association between stunting and impaired cognitive function has been well-documented [34]. Children with long-term stunting demonstrated significantly lower cognitive abilities compared to their non-stunted peers. The neurocognitive effects of stunting are severe, resulting in 'stunted brains' and 'stunted lives', which impede the development of entire communities. Growth faltering typically begins in utero and can continue through the first two years of life, resulting in irreversible physical and neurocognitive damage. Stunted children are at an increased risk of delays in both motor and gross development resulting in inadequate muscle functions, poor physical development, and delay of striated muscles, which regulate involuntary actions [35]. Co-ordinated voluntary movements are also impaired in stunted children due to inadequate muscle development. These findings align with research showing that acute malnutrition in children around the age of one year is linked to delays in gross motor skills, fine motor skills, social interactions, and language development [36]. The impact of child stunting has been exacerbated by the COVID-19 pandemic as the economic downturn has further limited parents' ability to meet their children's nutritional needs, leading to a rise in stunting cases. The high incidence of stunting poses a significant burden for the country, highlighting the need for further research into its impact on child development.

Acute malnutrition, characterized by wasting, can lead to increased morbidity, mortality, and disability, as well as impaired cognitive and physical development, making affected children more susceptible to infections. Wasting, which is defined as a low weight-for-height *Z*-score of less than –2 standard deviations from the median of the reference population, indicates acute undernutrition and often reflects recent and severe weight loss due to food scarcity or infectious diseases like diarrhea [27]. Children experiencing moderate to severe wasting episodes face an increased risk of death, particularly in regions with poor access to healthcare, inadequate food security, and insufficient sanitation and hygiene services. SAM represents the most extreme form of malnutrition, defined by a weight-for-height *Z*-score of less than –3 standard deviations, along with a mid-upper-arm circumference of less than 115 mm and the presence of bilateral nutritional edema [37]. Acute malnutrition is divided into moderate acute malnutrition (MAM) and SAM, depending on the severity. SAM is complex and goes beyond wasting with a detrimental effect on the gut, liver, skin, brain as well as the immune, metabolic, and hormonal systems [38]. In sub-Saharan Africa, the mortality rate goes up to 40% in children hospitalized with complicated SAM (CSAM), which is characterized by severe edema, cognitive dysfunctions like loss of appetite, and apathy or severe infections [39]. The risk of death from Severe Acute Malnutrition (SAM) is not fully eliminated in children during the initial stabilization phase, even when they receive therapeutic feeding in the hospital. The mortality rate, one year post discharge, was found to be 9.4% among children in Zimbabwe and Zambia that is similar to the mortality rate noted during hospitalization [40]. Research across nine sites in Africa and South Asia also found that children aged 2–23 months with severe wasting or Kwashiorkor had a mortality rate of 11.2% within 180 days after discharge, a rate seven times higher than that of well-nourished children [41].

SAM in children under five significantly elevates both short- and long-term health risks [42]. In the short term, SAM increases mortality risk with affected children up to nine times more likely to die than their well-nourished counterparts. In many developing countries, case fatality rates for SAM in hospitals range from 20 to 30% [10]. SAM also weakens the immune system, leading to frequent, severe infections and a detrimental cycle of malnutrition and illness due to impaired mucosal barriers and altered gut microbiota [38]. In the long term, SAM can cause irreversible damage, especially if it occurs during the critical first 1,000 days of life [43]. It is closely associated with stunting, cognitive deficits, and reduced academic and work performance, limiting future earning potential [44]. Women who experienced SAM as children may face complications during childbirth, including delivering infants with low birthweight. Additionally, SAM increases the risk of chronic diseases such as cardiovascular disease, diabetes, and obesity in adulthood, illustrating the impact of early-life malnutrition [44].

Underweight, another form of malnutrition, is defined by a low weight-for-age *Z*-score of less than –2 standard deviations from the median [45]. This condition is a composite measure resulting from either stunting, wasting, or both. In contrast, overweight, an emerging concern in childhood malnutrition, is defined by a weight-for-height Z-score above +2 standard deviations from the median [37]. The global prevalence of overweight children has risen to 38.3 million driven by greater access to processed foods and lower levels of physical activity.

Interventions—Current Status and Challenges

Addressing malnutrition is a multifaceted challenge that requires interventions extending beyond healthcare settings. A comprehensive, multisectoral approach is essential for effectively managing malnutrition in children under five. Primary healthcare workers, often the first point of contact for health concerns outside the home, play a crucial role of managing and preventing malnutrition in this vulnerable age group.

Optimum Maternal Nutrition

Prevention of malnutrition in children starts intra-utero, emphasizing the importance of optimum maternal nutrition. Pregnancy and lactation cause major changes in a mother's metabolism and physiology, which are important for supporting the developing fetus and preparing the body for childbirth and breastfeeding. A woman's age and overall health significantly influence her experience during pregnancy. Proper nutritional intake, before and during pregnancy, as well as during lactation, is crucial for maintaining maternal health and promoting optimal fetal growth and development. Nutritional imbalance can lead to negative outcomes such as low birth weight and fetal malformations. Additionally, poor maternal nutrition increases the risk of chronic health conditions like obesity and heart disease in offspring later in life. Nutritional needs during pregnancy are significantly different from those of non-pregnant women, and despite available guidelines, these needs are often not met due to socioeconomic, dietary, and food accessibility challenges.

The current approach to improving maternal nutrition focuses on a 'one-size-fits-all' strategy and often ignores individual factors that affect a mother's overall nutritional status [46]. Optimal nutrition during pregnancy is highly personalized and influenced by physiological, socioeconomic, and cultural factors. Dietary habits, influenced by geographic location and personal preferences, significantly impact nutritional status. The Global Dietary Database, designed to assess worldwide dietary trends, shows that various regions face unique challenges in meeting nutritional needs, directly impacting pregnant and lactating women. Pre-existing conditions such as Type 2 diabetes and obesity can have negative effects on maternal health. Specialized diets like veganism, vegetarianism, and gluten-free diets are becoming more popular, making it complex to ensure adequate nutrient intake. With veganism's increasing popularity, these diets can lead to imbalances in key nutrients like iron, vitamins B-12 and D, protein, and omega-3 fatty acids, which are particularly important for pregnant women as their nutritional demands increase to support fetal development. Fast-evolving dietary trends often outpace scientific recommendations, leaving gaps in formalized nutritional guidelines. As these consumer-driven shifts continue, the scientific community must investigate their effects, particularly during critical life stages like pregnancy, to better understand their long-term impacts on both maternal and fetal health. Effective nutrition strategies must take individual needs into account to promote positive pregnancy outcomes.

Exclusive Breastfeeding and Complementary Feeding

Adequate nutrition during infancy and early childhood is crucial for ensuring optimal growth, health, and cognitive development. Globally, breastfeeding is considered the best form of nutrition for infants, offering significant health benefits to both the mother and the child. It also provides economic and social advantages for families, healthcare systems, and employers. The World Health Organization (WHO) recommends exclusive breastfeeding during the first six months of life, followed by continued breastfeeding alongside complementary foods until two years of age or beyond [47]. Exclusive breastfeeding is associated with numerous health benefits, such as reducing the incidence of gastrointestinal infections, pneumonia, otitis media, and urinary tract infections in infants [48]. For mothers, it helps with postpartum weight loss and lowers the risk of Type 2 diabetes. However, many women struggle in following breastfeeding recommendations [49]. Factors such as nipple pain, perceived insufficient milk production, and societal obstacles—such as employment and short maternity leave—pose significant barriers to sustained exclusive breastfeeding. Additionally, limited breastfeeding knowledge, insufficient familial and societal support, and inadequate guidance from healthcare providers often lead to early cessation. The promotion and use of infant formula, pacifiers, and bottles further add to the reduction in breastfeeding duration [50]. Although infant formula is formulated to meet the dietary needs of infants, it may lead to nutritional imbalances, such as deficiencies in water-soluble vitamins, and increase the risk of exposure to pathogens due to improper handling and preparation. Breastfeeding should be sustained alongside the introduction of complementary foods until at least two years of age or beyond, and it should be provided on demand, responding to the child's needs. Between the ages of 6 and 12 months, breast milk continues to meet at least half of a child's energy requirements, while between 12 and 24 months, it supplies approximately one-third of the child's energy and essential nutrients [51]. In comparison to complementary foods, breast milk remains a superior source of high-quality nutrients and contains protective components that support the child's immune system. During illness, breast milk becomes especially important, providing essential energy and nutrients and significantly reducing mortality among malnourished children [52]. As the introduction of complementary foods often leads to a decrease in breastfeeding frequency, it is essential to actively promote and encourage continued breastfeeding to ensure adequate intake of breast milk alongside complementary feeding.

As infants develop, breast milk or formula alone no longer satisfies their nutritional requirements, necessitating the introduction of complementary foods [53]. The WHO recommends introducing solid foods at around six months, as the gastrointestinal and renal systems of infants are not mature enough for earlier weaning [54]. Optimal complementary feeding not only involves the type of food offered but also the way it is provided. Responsive feeding, a concept rooted in psycho-social care, encourages caregivers to feed infants directly and assist older children, ensuring a patient and attentive approach without forcing food intake [55]. It is important to use individual utensils for each child to monitor adequate food consumption. Cultural practices dictate whether feeding is done with a spoon or clean hands, with the utensil being age appropriate. Since microbial contamination of complementary foods is a significant cause of diarrheal diseases in children aged 6–12 months, ensuring proper hygiene and food safety is critical [56]. Safe food preparation and storage, such as washing hands and utensils thoroughly, can prevent contamination. The introduction of complementary foods should occur at six months, starting with small amounts and gradually increasing as the child grows. Complementary foods should be rich in nutrition to meet the child's growing needs and avoid malnutrition [55]. A child's appetite generally dictates the quantity of food consumed, although caregivers should provide extra assistance during illness to ensure adequate intake for recovery. During this period, many mothers face challenges such as feeding refusal, colic, and vomiting, which often impact feeding practices and consequently infant's nutritional intake [50]. In addition, issues such as perceived insufficient breast milk, early introduction of complementary foods, heavy maternal workloads, poverty, and lack of partner support can hinder optimal feeding. Some mothers may give water or cow milk if breast milk is delayed, or they may continue exclusive breastfeeding beyond six months if the child refuses solid foods.

Community-Based Nutritional Interventions

Community-based nutrition programs are crucial in addressing malnutrition because they offer customized interventions directly within affected communities. These programs improve access to essential nutrients by distributing fortified foods and supplements locally, cater to specific dietary needs, and encourage healthy eating habits. By involving community members, these initiatives promote better comprehension and adherence to nutrition recommendations. Additionally, they make use of local resources and knowledge, which enhances sustainability and effectiveness. Such programs play an important role in promptly addressing emerging nutritional issues and reaching underserved populations, thereby enhancing overall health and reducing malnutrition rates.

Supplementary foods are specially designed, energy-dense, and nutrient-rich products formulated to address the specific nutritional needs of vulnerable populations, particularly infants and young children [57]. These foods, which include fortified blended foods and lipid-based nutrient supplements, help transition infants aged six months and older to family meals gradually. They are essential in managing acute malnutrition by addressing deficiencies in protein, fat, and micronutrients. Conversely, therapeutic foods are designed to treat SAM. These include therapeutic milk formulas like F-75 and F-100, used in inpatient stabilization and rehabilitation phases, while ready-to-use therapeutic foods (RUTF) are employed in outpatient settings [58]. RUTF or ready-to-use supplementary foods (RUSF) have shown promising results in managing severe and moderate acute malnutrition in children. Recent advances have seen the incorporation of locally sourced ingredients in RUTF and RUSF formulations, further enhancing their nutritional recovery impact.

In India, supplementary nutrition is provided under the Integrated Child Development Services (ICDS) Scheme to children aged 6 months to 6 years, as well as to pregnant and lactating mothers, to bridge the gap between the Recommended Dietary Allowance (RDA) and the Average Daily Intake (ADI) [59]. The provision of supplementary nutrition varies by category under the ICDS Scheme. For children aged 6–36 months, Take Home Rations (THR) provide 500 calories and 12–15 grams of protein daily in the form of micronutrient-fortified or energy-dense foods. Children aged 3–6 years receive similar nutritional support, including snacks such as milk, bananas, or seasonal fruits along with a hot cooked meal. Severely underweight children receive 800 calories and 20–25 grams of protein per day. Pregnant and lactating mothers are provided with 600 calories and 18–20 grams of protein daily through micronutrient-fortified foods as THR. However, key challenges include inconsistent quality of services across regions due to varying levels of implementation and supervision [60]. There is a shortage of adequately trained staff and resources, impacting the effectiveness of nutrition and health interventions. Additionally, inadequate monitoring and evaluation mechanisms hinder the program's ability to address gaps and inefficiencies. The program also struggles with coordination issues among multiple stakeholders, including government departments and non-governmental organizations. These limitations contribute to suboptimal outcomes in combating malnutrition and improving child health in India. In South Africa, the Integrated Nutrition Programme (INP), introduced in 1994, involves multiple sectors such as health, social development, and agriculture to combat malnutrition [61]. In Latin America, Brazil's Programa Bolsa Família provides conditional cash transfers as financial aid to low-income families for health and nutritional needs in order to encourage these families to seek regular health check-ups, vaccinations, and dietary counseling [62]. Covering over 13.2 million households, it aims to reduce impact of poverty on maternal and child health. However, evidence on the effectiveness in improving health outcomes, particularly through large-scale, long-term studies, remains limited for this program. In Bangladesh, the Bangladesh Rehabilitation Assistance Committee (BRAC) has utilized female volunteer Community Health Workers (CHWs) known as Shasthya Shebika (SS) to carry out health and nutrition programs [63]. To reduce anemia, these volunteers are trained to deliver essential healthcare services, such as selling packets of micronutrient powder (MNP) and providing nutrition counseling as part of the Maternal, Infant, and Young Child Nutrition (MIYCN) Phase II program. Volunteer CHWs encounter challenges like high dropout rates, irregular visits, and inadequate home contact. This study aims to investigate the factors, including individual characteristics, organizational dynamics, and socio-cultural influences, that impact the performance of the SS in delivering community health services.

Facility-Based Interventions to Manage Severe Malnutrition

Health facility-based management programs for SAM are essential for addressing the medical and nutritional needs of children facing life-threatening complications related to malnutrition [64]. These programs are globally implemented and focus on providing therapeutic feeding and comprehensive medical care in inpatient settings. During stabilization and rehabilitation phases in sub-Saharan Africa, countries like Ethiopia and Kenya have established health facility-based programs where children with SAM receive specialized therapeutic foods such as F-75 and F-100 formulas [65]. These interventions, guided by international organizations such as UNICEF and WHO, not only include therapeutic feeding but also the administration of antibiotics, deworming, and treatment for dehydration and infections that frequently co-occur with SAM. The integration of inpatient care has been crucial in reducing mortality among severely malnourished children in these regions. In India, the management of SAM with medical complications is conducted through Nutrition Rehabilitation Centers (NRCs) [66]. These centers, supported by government initiatives like the Integrated Child Development Services (ICDS) and the National Health Mission (NHM), provide a multidisciplinary approach involving medical treatment, therapeutic feeding, and nutritional counseling. The caregivers in these centers are well trained on feeding practices, hygiene and focus on reducing the recurrence of malnutrition in inpatient children. The Bal Poshan Yojana is being implemented in Dwarka, Gujarat, India under a public-private partnership (PPP) model to manage SAM in children [67]. Private practitioners and centers have been trained and high-risk SAM cases are referred to approved Bal Poshan Centers for a 14-day treatment. The program includes anthropometric measurements, medical evaluations, and a structured follow-up process. Similarly, in Bangladesh, facility-based management of SAM is integrated into the healthcare system through programs run by organizations such as BRAC. Hospitals and health centers offer medical stabilization, therapeutic nutrition, and ongoing support to families. These programs are further strengthened by community health workers to ensure follow-up care and provide education on nutritional practices at home, fostering long-term behavioral changes to prevent malnutrition. In South Asia, countries such as Pakistan, Afghanistan, and Nepal adopt blended inpatient and outpatient care models for SAM management [68–70].

The facility-based management of SAM continues to face several significant gaps that undermine its effectiveness [71]. One critical issue is the limited access to adequately equipped healthcare facilities, particularly in rural and remote areas of low- and middle-income countries, which restricts vulnerable populations' access to essential life-saving interventions. Additionally, many healthcare workers lack comprehensive training in SAM management, leading to inconsistent care provision. This is further exacerbated by shortages of therapeutic foods, medicines, and other essential resources in many health centers. Weak referral systems between community health workers and facility-based care also create delays in the identification and timely treatment of SAM cases. Moreover, post-discharge follow-up is frequently insufficient, increasing the risk of relapse and compromising the long-term success of SAM interventions. The absence of robust monitoring and evaluation mechanisms further limits the ability to track treatment outcomes effectively. Financial and logistical barriers, such as transportation difficulties and costs associated with seeking care, present additional challenges for families, making it difficult for them to access and sustain treatment. Furthermore, the integration of SAM management with broader health services, such as immunization, antenatal care, and maternal health programs, remains inadequate, limiting the scope of comprehensive care. Addressing these gaps is essential to enhancing the overall effectiveness of facility-based SAM management strategies.

Future-Forward Recommendations

Childhood malnutrition is a significant global health challenge, especially in low- and middle-income countries. Inadequate nutrition not only impacts physical growth but also hinders cognitive development, leading to long-term health, educational, and economic problems. While global efforts have reduced malnutrition rates, new challenges such as climate change and armed conflict have deteriorated the situation. These crises disrupt food systems, displace populations, and impact access to essential healthcare and nutritional services. Maternal nutrition also plays a crucial role in child health outcomes as malnourished mothers are more likely to give birth to undernourished infants, continuing the cycle of malnutrition.

In the context of conflict and climate change, addressing childhood malnutrition through nutrition interventions requires adaptable, resilient, and comprehensive strategies. Effective interventions must prioritize access, sustainability, and context-specific solutions that recognize the multifaceted challenges presented by these global crises.

First, it is important to include nutrition interventions in emergency preparedness plans in conflict zones and areas heavily affected by climate change. This involves ensuring access to nutrition support, such as RUTF and fortified products, through mobile clinics, local health centers, and community-based distribution networks. Strengthening local food systems by empowering communities to grow nutrient-rich crops using climate-resilient agricultural practices is also crucial, as it reduces reliance on external aid and promotes long-term food security. In conflict zones, partnerships with humanitarian organizations and local authorities are essential for establishing nutrition programs in refugee camps and conflict-affected areas, ensuring that vulnerable populations, especially children, receive essential nutritional support.

Second, it is necessary to enhance the role of community health workers (CHWs) and local volunteers. These frontline workers, when properly trained to screen, treat, and monitor malnutrition in crisis settings, can ensure timely intervention and expand the reach of nutrition programs. Additionally, the use of technology, such as mobile health platforms, can facilitate real-time data collection, monitoring, and nutritional counseling, improving service delivery in remote or conflict-affected regions.

Third, addressing childhood malnutrition in the context of climate change and conflict requires a comprehensive approach that integrates nutrition with water, sanitation, and hygiene (WASH), maternal and child healthcare, and social protection systems. Maternal nutrition plays a crucial role in preventing childhood malnutrition. Improving maternal health and nutritional status, particularly during pregnancy and lactation, ensures optimal fetal and early childhood development, enhancing resilience to malnutrition. Policies should focus on mitigating the impact of climate change on food security through sustainable agricultural practices, efficient water management, and the promotion of climate-resilient crops.

Finally, collaboration between global and local stakeholders is essential for ensuring sustainable funding, policy frameworks, and innovative partnerships. This will enable nutrition interventions to be adaptable, scalable, and responsive to the evolving challenges due to conflict and climate change, while safeguarding maternal and child health.

References

1. World Health Organization. (2019). *Healthy Diet* (Vol. No. WHO-EM/NUT/282/E). World Health Organization. Regional Office for the Eastern Mediterranean.
2. Ssewanyana, D., Abubakar, A., Van Baar, A., Mwangala, P. N., & Newton, C. R. (2018). Perspectives on underlying factors for unhealthy diet and sedentary lifestyle of adolescents at a Kenyan coastal setting. *Frontiers in Public Health, 6*, 11.
3. World Health Organization. (2016). *The Double Burden of Malnutrition: Policy Brief* (Vol. No. WHO/NMH/NHD/17.3). World Health Organization.
4. World Health Organization. (2023). *The State of Food Security and Nutrition in the World 2023: Urbanization, Agrifood Systems Transformation and Healthy Diets Across the Rural–Urban Continuum*. Food & Agriculture Org.
5. World Health Organization. (2023). *Levels and Trends in Child Malnutrition Child Malnutrition: UNICEF/WHO/World Bank Group Joint Child Malnutrition Estimates: Key findings of the* (2023rd ed.). World Health Organization.
6. Cusick, S. E., & Georgieff, M. K. (2016). The role of nutrition in brain development: the golden opportunity of the "first 1000 days". *The Journal of Pediatrics, 175*, 16–21.
7. Black, M. M., Trude, A. C., & Lutter, C. K. (2020). All children thrive: integration of nutrition and early childhood development. *Annual Review of Nutrition, 40*(1), 375–406.

8. Vilar-Compte, M., et al. (2021). Urban poverty and nutrition challenges associated with accessibility to a healthy diet: a global systematic literature review. *International Journal for Equity in Health, 20*, 1–19.
9. Chakona, G. (2020). Social circumstances and cultural beliefs influence maternal nutrition, breastfeeding and child feeding practices in South Africa. *Nutrition Journal, 19*, 1–15.
10. Lenters, L., Wazny, K., & Bhutta, Z. A. (2016). Management of severe and moderate acute malnutrition in children. *Reproductive, Maternal, Newborn, and Child Health: Disease Control Priorities, 3rd Edition,* Washington, DC: World Bank, 205–223.
11. Baranwal, K., Gupta, V. M., Mishra, R. N., Prakash, S., & Pandey, O. N. (2010). Factors influencing the nutritional status of under five (1–5 years) children in urban-slum area of Varanasi. *Indian Journal of Community Health, 22*(1), 13–17.
12. Sinha, R. K., Dua, R., Bijalwan, V., Rohatgi, S., & Kumar, P. (2018). Determinants of stunting, wasting, and underweight in five high-burden pockets of four Indian states. *Indian Journal of Community Medicine, 43*(4), 279–283.
13. Olack, B., et al. (2011). Nutritional status of under-five children living in an informal urban settlement in Nairobi, Kenya. *Journal of Health, Population, and Nutrition, 29*(4), 357.
14. Myatt, M., et al. (2018). Children who are both wasted and stunted are also underweight and have a high risk of death: a descriptive epidemiology of multiple anthropometric deficits using data from 51 countries. *Archives of Public Health, 76*, 1–11.
15. Garenne, M., et al. (2022). Changing sex differences in undernutrition of African children: findings from Demographic and Health Surveys. *Journal of biosocial science, 54*(5), 847–857.
16. Thurstans, S., et al. (2020). Boys are more likely to be undernourished than girls: a systematic review and meta-analysis of sex differences in undernutrition. *BMJ global health, 5*(12), e004030.
17. Nyaruhucha, C. N., Msuya, J. M., Mamiro, P. S., & Kerengi, A. J. (2006). Nutritional status and feeding practices of under-five children in Simanjiro District. *Tanzania. Tanzania Journal of Health Research, 8*(3), 162–167.
18. Gwela, A., Mupere, E., Berkley, J. A., & Lancioni, C. (2019). Undernutrition, host immunity and vulnerability to infection among young children. *The Pediatric Infectious Disease Journal, 38*(8), e175–e177.
19. Laksono, A. D., Wulandari, R. D., Ibad, M., & Kusrini, I. (2021). The effects of mother's education on achieving exclusive breastfeeding in Indonesia. *BMC Public Health, 21*, 1–6.
20. Lawal, S. A., Okunlola, D. A., Adegboye, O. A., & Adedeji, I. A. (2023). Mother's education and nutritional status as correlates of child stunting, wasting, underweight, and overweight in Nigeria: Evidence from 2018 Demographic and Health Survey. *Nutrition and Health, 02601060221146320.*
21. Rezaeizadeh, G., et al. (2024). Maternal education and its influence on child growth and nutritional status during the first two years of life: a systematic review and meta-analysis. *eClinicalmedicine, 71*, 102574.
22. Zajacova, A., & Lawrence, E. M. (2018). The relationship between education and health: reducing disparities through a contextual approach. *Annual Review of Public Health, 39*(1), 273–289.
23. Win, H., Shafique, S., Mizan, S., Wallenborn, J., Probst-Hensch, N., & Fink, G. (2022). Association between mother's work status and child stunting in urban slums: A cross-sectional assessment of 346 child-mother dyads in Dhaka, Bangladesh (2020). *Archives of Public Health, 80*(1), 192.
24. Chaudhury, R. H. (1984). Determinants of dietary intake and dietary adequacy for pre-school children in Bangladesh. *Food and Nutrition Bulletin, 6*(4), 1–10.
25. Govender, I., Rangiah, S., Kaswa, R., & Nzaumvila, D. (2021). Malnutrition in children under the age of 5 years in a primary health care setting. *South African Family Practice, 63*(1), e1–e6.
26. Agostoni, C., Baglioni, M., La Vecchia, A., Molari, G., & Berti, C. (2023). Interlinkages between climate change and food systems: the impact on child malnutrition—Narrative review. *Nutrients, 15*(2), 416.

27. Clark, H., et al. (2020). A future for the world's children? A WHO–UNICEF–Lancet Commission. *The Lancet, 395*(10224), 605–658.
28. Wali, N., Agho, K., & Renzaho, A. M. (2019). Past drivers of and priorities for child undernutrition in South Asia: a mixed methods systematic review protocol. *Systematic Reviews, 8*, 1–8.
29. Obasohan, P. E., Walters, S. J., Jacques, R., & Khatab, K. (2020). A scoping review of the risk factors associated with anaemia among children under five years in sub-Saharan African countries. *International Journal of Environmental Research and Public Health, 17*(23), 8829.
30. Vollmer, S., Harttgen, K., Kupka, R., & Subramanian, S. V. (2017). Levels and trends of childhood undernutrition by wealth and education according to a composite index of anthropometric failure: evidence from 146 demographic and health surveys from 39 countries. *BMJ Global Health, 2*(2), e000206.
31. Unicef, & WHO, W. (2020). *Levels and trends in child malnutrition: key findings of the 2019 Edition of the Joint Child Malnutrition Estimates. World Health Organization.*
32. De Onis, M., & Branca, F. (2016). Childhood stunting: a global perspective. *Maternal & Child Nutrition, 12*, 12–16.
33. Martins, V. J., et al. (2011). Long-lasting effects of undernutrition. *International Journal of Environmental Research and Public Health, 8*(6), 1817–1846.
34. Ocansey, M. E., et al. (2019). The association of early linear growth and haemoglobin concentration with later cognitive, motor, and social–emotional development at preschool age in Ghana. *Maternal & Child Nutrition, 15*(4), e12834.
35. Mustakim, M. R., Irawan, R., Irmawati, M., & Setyoboedi, B. (2022). Impact of Stunting on Development of Children between 1–3 Years of Age. *Ethiopian Journal of Health Sciences, 32*(3), 569–578.
36. Abessa, T. G., Bruckers, L., Kolsteren, P., & Granitzer, M. (2017). Developmental performance of hospitalized severely acutely malnourished under-six children in low-income setting. *BMC Pediatrics, 17*, 1–10.
37. World Health Organization. (2017). Guideline: assessing and managing children at primary health-care facilities to prevent overweight and obesity in the context of the double burden of malnutrition.
38. Sturgeon, J. P., et al. (2023). Inflammation: the driver of poor outcomes among children with severe acute malnutrition? *Nutrition reviews, 81*(12), 1636–1652.
39. Tickell, K. D., & Denno, D. M. (2016). Inpatient management of children with severe acute malnutrition: a review of WHO guidelines. *Bulletin of the World Health Organization, 94*(9), 642.
40. Bwakura-Dangarembizi, M., *et al.* & HOPE-SAM study team. (2021). Risk factors for post-discharge mortality following hospitalization for severe acute malnutrition in Zimbabwe and Zambia. *The American Journal of Clinical Nutrition, 113*(3), 665–674.
41. Diallo, A. H., et al. (2022). Childhood mortality during and after acute illness in Africa and south Asia: a prospective cohort study. *The Lancet Global Health, 10*(5), e673–e684.
42. Alflah, Y. M., & Alrashidi, M. A. (2023). Severe acute malnutrition and its consequences among malnourished children. *Journal of Clinical Pediatrics Research, 2*(1), 1–5.
43. Lelijveld, N. J. M. (2016). *Long-term effects of severe acute malnutrition on growth, body composition, and function; a prospective cohort study in Malawi.* (Doctoral dissertation,. UCL (University College London)).
44. Mwene-Batu, P., et al. (2020). Long-term effects of severe acute malnutrition during childhood on adult cognitive, academic and behavioural development in African fragile countries: The Lwiro cohort study in Democratic Republic of the Congo. *PLoS One, 15*(12), e0244486.
45. Desyibelew, H. D., Bayih, M. T., Baraki, A. G., & Dadi, A. F. (2020). The recovery rate from severe acute malnutrition among under-five years of children remains low in sub-Saharan Africa. A systematic review and meta-analysis of observational studies. *PloS One, 15*(3), e0229698.
46. Brink, L. R., Bender, T. M., Davies, R., Luo, H., Miketinas, D., Shah, N., et al. (2022). Optimizing maternal Nutrition: the importance of a tailored Approach. *Current Developments. Nutrition, 6(9), nzac118.*

47. Ribeiro, J. R. & Antunes, H. (2018). World Health Organization (WHO) recommends exclusive breastfeeding in the first six months of life.
48. Gupta, A., Holla, R., Dadhich, J. P., Suri, S., Trejos, M., & Chanetsa, J. (2013). The status of policy and programmes on infant and young child feeding in 40 countries. *Health Policy and planning, 28*(3), 279–298.
49. Whalen, B., & Cramton, R. (2010). Overcoming barriers to breastfeeding continuation and exclusivity. *Current Opinion in Pediatrics, 22*(5), 655–663.
50. Motee, A., & Jeewon, R. (2014). Importance of exclusive breastfeeding and complementary feeding among infants. *Current Research in Nutrition and Food Science Journal, 2*(2), 56–72.
51. Dewey, K. G., & Brown, K. H. (2003). Update on technical issues concerning complementary feeding of young children in developing countries and implications for intervention programs. *Food and Nutrition Bulletin, 24*(1), 5–28.
52. Brown, K. H., Stallings, R. Y., de Kanashiro, H. C., de Romana, G. L., & Black, R. E. (1990). Effects of common illnesses on infants' energy intakes from breast milk and other foods during longitudinal community-based studies in Huascar (Lima), Peru. *The American Journal of Clinical Nutrition, 52*(6), 1005–1013.
53. Golley, R. K., et al. (2012). An index measuring adherence to complementary feeding guidelines has convergent validity as a measure of infant diet quality. *The Journal of Nutrition, 142*(5), 901–908.
54. World Health Organization. (2023). *WHO Guideline for complementary feeding of infants and young children 6-23 months of age. World Health.* Organization.
55. World Health Organization. (2009). Infant and Young Child Feeding: Model Chapter for Textbooks for Medical Students and Allied Health Professionals. *World Health Organization, 3.*
56. Bern, C., Martines, J., De Zoysa, I., & Glass, R. I. (1992). The magnitude of the global problem of diarrhoeal disease: a ten-year update. *Bulletin of the World Health Organization, 70*(6), 705.
57. Visser, J., McLachlan, M. H., Maayan, N., & Garner, P. (2018). Community-based supplementary feeding for food insecure, vulnerable and malnourished populations–an overview of systematic reviews. *Cochrane Database of Systematic Reviews, 11*(11), CD010578. (11).
58. Fetriyuna, F., et al. (2023). *Ready-to-use therapeutic/supplementary foods from local food resources: Technology accessibility, program effectiveness, and sustainability, a review. Heliyon.*
59. Antier, C., Kumar, S., Bhagwat, S., & Sankar, R. (2014). Production of fortified food for a public supplementary nutrition program: performance and viability of a decentralised production model for the Integrated Child Development Services Program, India. *Asia Pacific Journal of Clinical Nutrition, 23.*
60. Sahoo, J., Mahajan, P. B., Paul, S., Bhatia, V., Patra, A. K., & Hembram, D. K. (2016). Operational assessment of ICDS scheme at grass root level in a rural area of Eastern India: Time to introspect. *Journal of Clinical and Diagnostic Research: JCDR, 10*(12), LC28.
61. Brits, H., Joubert, G., Eyman, K., De Vink, R., Lesaoana, K., & Moeketsi, K. (2017). An assessment of the integrated nutrition programme for malnourished children aged six months to five years at primary healthcare facilities in Mangaung, Free State. *South Africa. South African Family Practice, 59*(6), 214–218.
62. Falcão, I. R., et al. (2022). Evaluating the effect of Bolsa Familia, Brazil's conditional cash transfer programme, on maternal and child health: a study protocol. *Plos One, 17*(5), e0268500.
63. Sarma, H., et al. (2020). Performance of volunteer community health workers in implementing home-fortification interventions in Bangladesh: A qualitative investigation. *PLoS One, 15*(4), e0230709.
64. Modjadji, P., & Madiba, S. (2019). Childhood undernutrition and its predictors in a rural health and demographic surveillance system site in South Africa. *International Journal of Environmental Research and Public Health, 16*(17), 3021.
65. Abebe, A., Simachew, Y., & Delbiso, T. D. (2023). Effect of ready-to-use therapeutic foods on time to recovery among children with severe acute malnutrition in Ethiopia: a prospective cohort study. *BMC Pediatrics, 23*(1), 340.

66. Dasgupta, R., Ahuja, S., & Yumnam, V. (2014). Can nutrition rehabilitation centers address severe malnutrition in India? *Indian Pediatrics, 51*, 95–99.
67. Soni, J., et al. (2022). Bal Poshan Yojana: A Novel Approach to Facility-Based Severe Acute Malnutrition Management. *Cureus, 14*(8).
68. Ahmed, N., Umar, F., Saleem, F., Iqbal, Q., Haider, S., & Bashaar, M. (2023). Treatment Outcomes of Severe Acute Malnutrition and Its Determinants Among Paediatric Patients in Quetta City. *Pakistan. Journal of Multidisciplinary Healthcare*, 2809–2821.
69. Levitt, E., Kostermans, K., Laviolette, L., & Mbuya, N. (2010). *Malnutrition in Afghanistan: Scale, scope, causes, and potential response. World Bank*. Publications.
70. Haag, K. C., Sharma, A., Parajuli, K., & Adhikari, A. (2020). Experiences of the integrated management of acute malnutrition (IMAM) programme in Nepal: From pilot to scale up.
71. Fahim, S. M., et al. (2022). A qualitative assessment of facility readiness and barriers to the facility-based management of childhood severe acute malnutrition in the public healthcare settings in Bangladesh. *Public Health Nutrition, 25*(11), 2971–2982.

Part III
Child Nutrition and Development

Chapter 7
The Influence of Maternal Health and Nutrition on Fetal Development

Shweta Khandelwal and Aamir Siddiqui

Introduction

Maternal health and nutrition are not only essential for the immediate well-being of both mother and fetus but also for shaping the child's future health trajectory. The period from conception to the first 1000 days of life, often referred to as the "window of opportunity", is when the mother's health and nutrition exert the greatest influence on fetal growth, development, and long-term health outcomes [1–3]. Key nutrients, such as iron, folic acid, calcium, and essential fatty acids, play a critical role during this period, supporting fetal brain development, skeletal growth, and overall cellular function. Optimal maternal health is essential for placenta to function properly, which is key to ensuring the exchange of nutrients and oxygen between mother and baby. However, various factors that can compromise maternal health are pre-existing medical conditions, poor diet, infections, and inadequate access to healthcare. For instance, maternal anemia is a widespread issue in low- and middle-income countries, contributing to adverse pregnancy outcomes such as preterm birth, low birthweight (LBW), and increased maternal mortality rates. Conversely, conditions such as gestational diabetes and preeclampsia, common in cases of maternal overnutrition, can also affect pregnancy outcomes by increasing the risk of macrosomia and complications during childbirth. Likewise, maternal nutrition is critical in supplying the nutrients needed for fetus development. Nutrient imbalances, whether deficiencies or excesses, can lead to adverse pregnancy outcomes, affecting both the mother and the fetus [4].

Malnutrition in women—whether in the form of underweight, short stature, anemia, or overweight—remains a major global concern with direct implications

S. Khandelwal (✉) · A. Siddiqui
Social and Economic Empowerment, IPE Global Limited, New Delhi, India
e-mail: skhandelwal@ipeglobal.com

A. Siddiqui
e-mail: asiddiqui@ipeglobal.com

S. Suri (ed.), *Child Health and Nutrition from Conception to Age Two*,
https://doi.org/10.1007/978-981-95-7868-9_7

for pregnancy outcomes and fetal development. Current estimates suggest that 170 million women (9.1%) worldwide are underweight, while 610 million (32.5%) are overweight, and 7% have short stature. Anemia affects 30.7% of women globally, with a higher burden among pregnant women (35.5%) [5]. In India, the challenge is even more pronounced: according to NFHS-5 (2019–21), 57% of women of reproductive age and 52% of pregnant women are anemic. These conditions heighten the risk of intrauterine growth restriction, low birthweight, preterm birth, and other adverse outcomes. Simultaneously, the rise in overweight and obesity—affecting 1.11 billion women globally, including 180 million in India—has contributed to the growing incidence of gestational diabetes, hypertensive disorders of pregnancy, and birth complications such as macrosomia. Micronutrient deficiencies—including iron, folate, vitamins B12 and D, iodine, and zinc—are prevalent across all body types, further compromising maternal and fetal health. These patterns highlight the need for integrated strategies across the continuum of care. India's flagship initiatives, such as Anemia Mukt Bharat and Poshan Abhiyaan, offer vital platforms to strengthen antenatal nutrition services, improve dietary intake, and deliver targeted supplementation. Furthermore, evidence shows that every $1 invested in maternal and child nutrition yields up to $20 in economic returns, underscoring not only the health imperative but also the developmental and financial rationale for prioritizing maternal nutrition [6].

The objective of this chapter is to examine how maternal health and nutrition directly influence fetal growth and long-term outcomes. By understanding these critical relationships, the chapter will explore public health strategies and interventions aimed at improving maternal care.

This includes a focus on global and regional disparities, particularly in South Asia, where the burden of maternal and child malnutrition is significant. The chapter will also highlight evidence-based policies and programs that can enhance maternal nutrition and health services, ensuring better pregnancy outcomes and healthier long-term development for children.

Maternal Health & Nutrition: A Life-Course 360 Approach

Evidence affirms that maternal health and nutrition should be approached as a continuum, starting from preconception period, continuing through pregnancy, childbirth, and beyond. This life-course 360-degree approach emphasizes the importance of addressing health and nutritional needs at all stages to ensure optimal outcomes for both mother and child. The preconception period is critical, yet often neglected both in India and across the world.

Several well-known trials have demonstrated the importance of investing even before the conception period. The Pune Rural Intervention in Young Adolescents (PRIYA) is a pre-conceptional trial involving vitamin B12 and multi-micronutrient supplementation in adolescent participants from the Pune Maternal Nutrition Study.

This trial noted an improved maternal B12 status and better offspring neurodevelopment at 2 years of age in the supplemented group [7]. The Mumbai Maternal Nutrition Project (SARAS) demonstrated the benefits of micronutrient-rich food supplements during preconception period on birthweight of their offspring and reduced prevalence of gestational diabetes [8]. The Women and Infants Integrated Interventions for Growth Study (WINGS) showed that a package of health, nutrition, psychosocial care, water, sanitation, and hygiene interventions delivered during preconception, pregnancy, and early childhood reduces the risk of low birthweight and stunting at 24 months of age. Preconception interventions deliver impact on birth outcomes but not on outcomes at 24 months of age. Preconception and pregnancy interventions improved several maternal outcomes—higher hemoglobin concentration and gestational weight gain, and reduced risk of reproductive tract infections, moderate to severe anemia, and pregnancy induced hypertension [9].

Given the growing recognition of preconception care (PCC) as a critical intervention for improving maternal and child health outcomes, there is a clear opportunity to develop national guidelines and a comprehensive care package tailored specifically for the Indian context. While India currently lacks a dedicated and integrated PCC framework within its health system, several existing guidelines offer a foundational starting point. For instance, the **India Newborn Action Plan (INAP)** incorporates elements of PCC by advocating for screening of anemia and hypertensive disorders, alongside balanced energy-protein supplementation. The **Indian Academy of Pediatrics (IAP)** guidelines highlight the importance of promoting healthy lifestyles and mental well-being before conception, whereas the **World Health Organization (WHO)** Preconception Care Package outlines a broader set of interventions, including nutritional support, tobacco cessation, and infectious disease screening. These frameworks present valuable components that can be adapted and unified into a national strategy, ensuring more comprehensive and equitable coverage of preconception health across India.

Using the Lives Saved Tool, Hofmeyr et al. (2023) estimated that eight proven preventive interventions, i.e., (1) multiple micronutrient supplementation, (2) balanced protein and energy supplementation, (3) low-dose aspirin, (4) progesterone provided vaginally, (5) education for smoking cessation, (6) malaria prevention, (7) treatment of asymptomatic bacteriuria, and (8) treatment of syphilis), if fully implemented in 81 low-income and middle-income countries, could prevent 5.202 million SVN births (sensitivity bounds 2.398–7.903) and 0.566 million stillbirths (0.208–0.754) per year. These interventions, combined with two measures aimed at reducing complications from preterm births (<37 weeks' gestation) births antenatal corticosteroids and delayed cord clamping have the potential to prevent 0.476 million neonatal deaths (range: 0.181–0.676) per year [10].

Poor maternal health increases the risk of obesity, insulin resistance, and related disorders, perpetuating a cycle of intergenerational health problems such as cardiometabolic diseases (See Fig. 7.1). This concept is well captured in the Developmental Origins of Health and Disease (DOHaD) hypothesis, which highlights the critical importance of early embryonic and fetal life in determining future risk of metabolic disturbances. Maternal lifestyle—both before conception and during

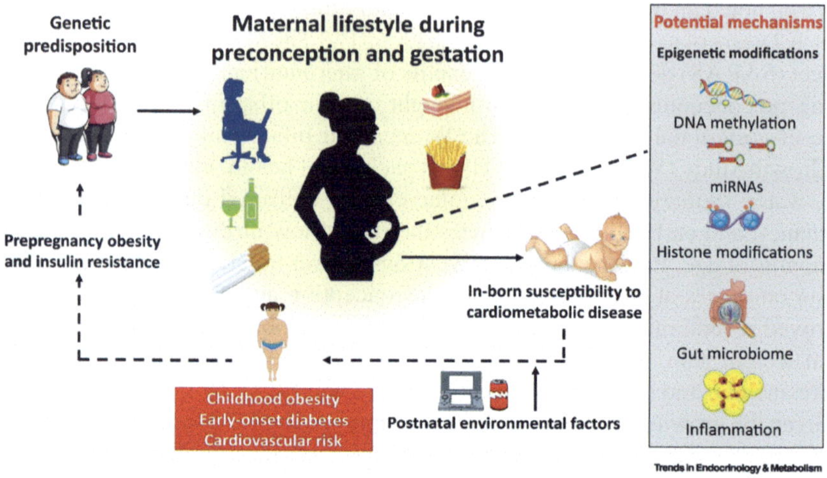

Fig. 7.1 The intergenerational cycle of chronic cardiometabolic disorders [10]

pregnancy—plays a key role in shaping the epigenetic programming of the offspring. Poor preconception and gestational behaviors can thus predispose both mother and child to adverse outcomes, contributing to a cycle of obesity, insulin resistance, and associated disorders across generations. Promoting healthy behaviors during these critical periods is essential to break this cycle and improve both maternal and child health outcomes [11].

Pregnancy-Related Diseases and Nutritional Interventions

Pregnancy-Induced Hypertension (PIH)

Pregnancy-induced hypertension, including preeclampsia, is a leading cause of maternal and perinatal morbidity and mortality. It is associated with increased risks of intrauterine growth restriction (IUGR), preterm birth, and long-term health complications for both mother and child. PIH is linked to poor dietary habits and rising rates of maternal obesity, which have become more prevalent due to a dietary transition marked by increased consumption of high fat, sugar, and salt (HFSS) foods. The increase in hypertension among pregnant women in India is also reflective of this shift in dietary patterns [12, 13].

As unhealthy diets account for 56.4% of the total disease burden in India, addressing these dietary patterns can lead to a significant reduction in hypertension, and other related conditions [14]. Nutritional interventions to manage PIH include supplementation with calcium and magnesium, which has been shown to reduce the incidence of hypertensive disorders. In addition to supplementation, nutrition counseling during antenatal care (ANC) is crucial in guiding pregnant women toward healthier dietary patterns. Evidence supports that counseling can help women reduce their consumption of HFSS foods and adopt diets rich in fruits, vegetables, and whole grains, thus reducing PIH risk. The World Health Organization (WHO) recommends integrating nutrition counseling into routine ANC, combining it with other nutritional support like food or micronutrient supplements for optimal maternal and fetal health outcomes [15, 16].

Gestational Diabetes Mellitus

Gestational diabetes mellitus (GDM) is another prevalent condition in India, ranging from 3–35%. GDM increases the risk of adverse pregnancy outcomes such as macrosomia (large birthweight), preterm birth, and neonatal hypoglycaemia. It also predisposes both mother and child to long-term metabolic conditions such as Type 2 diabetes and cardiovascular disease [17].

Proper management of GDM through maternal nutrition therapy (MNT) is critical for minimizing these risks. Dietary interventions for GDM focus on controlling caloric intake to manage gestational weight gain (GWG), particularly in overweight or obese women. Nutritional recommendations include a balanced diet rich in fiber, low in refined carbohydrates, and supplemented with iron and folic acid. Regular physical activity is also advised to improve insulin sensitivity and support overall glucose management. Addressing the rising rates of maternal obesity through dietary changes can significantly reduce the incidence of GDM [18]. Incorporating nutrition counseling into this management strategy has been shown to significantly improve maternal glycemic control and gestational weight gain (GWG). Counseling helps women to better understand and implement dietary practices that are rich in fiber and low in refined carbohydrates, further supporting insulin sensitivity and overall glucose management. Research has shown that counseling improves adherence to dietary recommendations, thus lowering the incidence of excessive GWG and reducing complications associated with GDM [19, 20].

Maternal Undernutrition and Overnutrition

Maternal undernutrition or overweight/obesity represent two forms of malnutrition that contribute significantly to adverse pregnancy outcomes in India. This often is perpetuated in their offspring and adversely impacts height, cognition, and productivity across a lifetime. Undernutrition is usually the result of inadequate intake of key macronutrients like proteins, carbohydrates, and fats that are also inextricably linked with deficiency of several key micronutrients such as iron, folic acid, calcium, and iodine. Proteins are critical for fetal tissue growth, particularly the brain, while carbohydrates are the primary energy source. Fats are crucial for the development of the fetal brain and nervous system. The pathway of maternal undernutrition begins with inadequate nutrient intake during preconception and pregnancy, impairing placental development and reduces placental blood flow and nutrient transfer. This leads to intrauterine growth restriction (IUGR) and developmental adaptations known as fetal programming, which predispose the child to long-term metabolic diseases such as type 2 diabetes and cardiovascular disorders [21].

On the other hand, overnutrition, driven by the increasing consumption of HFSS foods and the resultant rise in obesity rates, is associated with complications such as GDM, PIH, and macrosomia. Overnutrition also contributes to poor maternal and fetal outcomes, as excessive gestational weight gain increases the risk of cesarean delivery and long-term metabolic diseases in both mother and child. The pathway of maternal overnutrition involves an excess intake of calories, fats, and sugars, which overstimulates placental nutrient transfer, leading to fetal overgrowth (macrosomia) and altered metabolic programming. This excess nutrient supply increases the risk of developing obesity, insulin resistance, and related metabolic disorders later in the child's life. Additionally, maternal inflammation caused by overnutrition can further impair placental function, compounding the risks of adverse outcomes [22–24].

To address these challenges, nutritional interventions for undernourished women should focus on increasing the intake of micronutrient-rich foods, including fruits, vegetables, whole grains, and fortified foods, to meet the heightened nutritional demands of pregnancy. For women experiencing overnutrition, interventions should prioritize limiting the consumption of HFSS foods and encouraging a balanced diet rich in essential nutrients, combined with regular physical activity. The dietary transition in India, marked by increased consumption of HFSS foods, has led to an increase in the prevalence of hypertension, obesity, and related metabolic disorders among pregnant women. Controlling these dietary shifts is crucial, as up to 80% cases of type 2 diabetes and other non-communicable diseases (NCDs) could be prevented through lifestyle modifications, including improved diet and regular physical activity [14]. Nutrition counseling is effective in addressing both undernutrition and overnutrition. For undernourished women, counseling combined with food supplementation helps ensure an adequate intake of key nutrients like proteins, carbohydrates, fats, and essential micronutrients such as iron and folic acid, which are vital for fetal development. For overweight or obese women, counseling helps in controlling excessive calorie intake and in promoting a healthier dietary balance, thus preventing excessive gestational weight gain and reducing the risk of complications such as GDM and preeclampsia. Counseling empowers women to make informed food choices based on their specific nutritional needs during pregnancy, leading to better pregnancy outcomes [17].

Perinatal Mental Disorders

Mental health is a critical, yet often overlooked aspect of maternal health. Perinatal mental disorders, including depression, anxiety, and stress, affect a significant proportion of women during pregnancy and the postpartum period. These mental health conditions can have serious implications for both maternal and fetal outcomes. For instance, depression during pregnancy is associated with preterm birth, low birthweight, and developmental delays in children. Prenatal stress has been linked to adverse neurodevelopmental outcomes in children, with research showing that children born to mothers who experienced significant stress during pregnancy are at a higher risk for cognitive, motor, and social-emotional developmental delays [25].

The compounded effects of perinatal mental disorders can extend beyond infancy, influencing the child's health trajectory into adolescence. Children exposed to maternal mental health issues in utero are at an increased risk of developing psychiatric disorders, including anxiety and depression, later in life [26].

To mitigate these risks, access to mental health services is essential during the perinatal period. Early screening and intervention for mental health conditions can improve both maternal and child health outcomes. Psychological counseling, support networks, and, when necessary, pharmacological treatment should be available to all women during pregnancy and the postpartum period. Nutritional counseling has also been found to have a positive effect on maternal mental health. By promoting adequate nutrient intake and helping women feel more in control of their health, counseling can reduce stress and anxiety during pregnancy, contributing to improved mental well-being and better fetal outcomes. This holistic approach not just positively impacts the physical health of the mother and baby, but also supports emotional and psychological resilience [27].

Effects of Micronutrient Deficiencies During Pregnancy

Micronutrient deficiencies or hidden hunger during pregnancy can have severe consequences for both the mother and the developing fetus. Micronutrients like iron, folic acid, calcium, and vitamin D play vital roles in ensuring a healthy pregnancy, from supporting hemoglobin production to preventing neural tube defects (NTDs) and ensuring proper bone development. Deficiencies in these key nutrients can lead to adverse pregnancy outcomes such as preterm birth, low birthweight, and congenital anomalies [28, 29]. Evidence indicates that deficiencies in iron, folate, calcium, vitamin D, zinc, iodine, and vitamin A are widespread during pregnancy, especially in low-resource settings where dietary diversity is limited and physiological demands are elevated. Iron deficiency, the most prevalent micronutrient deficiency, not only contributes to maternal anemia but is also associated with a heightened risk of preterm delivery and intrauterine growth restriction. Folic acid deficiency is a leading cause of NTDs and is also linked to preeclampsia and fetal growth impairment. Calcium and vitamin D insufficiencies are associated with gestational hypertension, reduced fetal bone mass, and adverse skeletal outcomes. Inadequate intake of zinc and iodine has been associated with compromised immune function, prolonged labor, and impaired neurodevelopment. These deficiencies often coexist, making targeted single-nutrient interventions insufficient in many cases. Supplementation strategies that address multiple micronutrient needs during pregnancy have shown greater benefits in reducing the risk of low birthweight, stillbirths, and neonatal mortality compared to iron and folic acid alone. Ensuring adequate and balanced micronutrient intake throughout pregnancy is therefore crucial for safeguarding maternal health, supporting fetal development, and improving perinatal survival and long-term outcomes [30].

Nutrient Requirements for Pregnant and Lactating Women

(Adapted from ICMR NIN 2024)

Pregnancy and lactation are the periods of heightened nutritional demand. Ensuring proper nutrition during pregnancy and lactation involves meeting these nutritional requirements to support maternal and infant health. Macronutrients like carbohydrates, proteins, and fats provide the energy needed for fetal growth, while micronutrients like iron, calcium, and folic acid are vital for preventing complications such as anemia, neural tube defects, and impaired bone development [31].

The daily nutrient requirements for pregnant and lactating women, as outlined by the Indian Council of Medical Research–National Institute of Nutrition (ICMR-NIN), 2024, provide detailed and evidence-based guidance to meet these heightened needs. These recommendations include an additional 350 kcal/day during pregnancy and up to 600 kcal/day during lactation to support increased metabolic activity. Protein intake is advised at approximately 78–90 g per day, varying by trimester, to support the rapid growth of maternal and fetal tissues. Iron requirements increase to 27 mg/day during pregnancy to account for expanded maternal blood volume and fetal iron stores. Folic acid intake of 600 μg/day is recommended to reduce the risk of neural tube defects, while 1200 mg/day of calcium is essential for fetal bone mineralization and to preserve maternal bone health. Similarly, the inclusion of iodine (250 μg/day), zinc (12 mg/day), vitamin A (900 μg/day), and vitamin D (10 μg/day) is necessary for optimal thyroid function, immune competence, organ development, and calcium absorption.

These nutrient targets are foundational not only for individual clinical practice but also for shaping public health nutrition strategies aimed at improving maternal and child health outcomes. By incorporating the ICMR-NIN 2024 guidelines into antenatal and postnatal care, India's public health programs—such as Poshan Abhiyaan, Anemia Mukt Bharat, and the Janani Shishu Suraksha Karyakram (JSSK)—can better align service delivery with physiological requirements. Such alignment is critical for preventing nutrient deficiencies, supporting healthy pregnancies, and enhancing infant survival, growth, and development through improved maternal nutrition.

Impact of Maternal Lifestyle and Behavior on Fetal Development

Maternal lifestyle and behavior during pregnancy play a critical role in shaping fetal development, with far-reaching implications for both immediate and long-term health outcomes. As suggested by the Barker hypothesis, adverse maternal conditions during pregnancy can predispose offspring to a range of diseases in adulthood, emphasizing the need for a healthy maternal lifestyle throughout pregnancy. Diet, physical activity, smoking, alcohol consumption, and mental health are among the most significant maternal factors that interact to influence the intrauterine environment, directly affecting fetal growth and development [32].

Physical activity is an influential factor, with regular, moderate exercise during pregnancy being linked to improved maternal metabolic health and enhanced fetal growth patterns. However, both excessive physical activity and a sedentary lifestyle can result in adverse outcomes such as preterm birth or impaired fetal growth. Maternal mental health also significantly affects fetal development, with conditions like depression and anxiety potentially leading to long-term cognitive and behavioral issues in offspring [33].

Behavioral factors such as smoking and alcohol consumption are particularly detrimental to fetal health. Maternal smoking increases the risk of low birthweight, preterm birth, and neurodevelopmental disorders, while alcohol consumption can cause fetal alcohol spectrum disorders (FASD), resulting in physical, cognitive, and behavioral impairments. Even moderate alcohol intake has been shown to disrupt fetal brain development, reinforcing the recommendation for complete abstinence during pregnancy [34, 35].

Socioeconomic and cultural influences further shape maternal behaviors and access to resources, often exacerbating health disparities in fetal outcomes. Women from lower socioeconomic backgrounds face barriers in accessing healthcare, nutrition, and mental health services, contributing to poor maternal and fetal health outcomes. Stressors related to financial insecurity and lack of social support can adversely affect maternal mental health, creating additional risks for fetal development [36].

Maternal lifestyle and behavior during pregnancy significantly influence fetal development, with implications for both immediate and long-term health outcomes. One critical aspect of this is nutritional counseling, which plays a vital role in guiding expectant mothers toward healthier dietary choices. Nutritional counseling can help pregnant women understand the importance of a balanced diet rich in essential nutrients, such as folic acid, iodine, and iron, which are crucial for fetal growth and development. Evidence suggests that tailored nutritional interventions can improve maternal health outcomes and reduce the risk of complications such as gestational diabetes and hypertension. Additionally, education on avoiding harmful substances like alcohol and tobacco is vital, as these can lead to severe developmental issues in the fetus. By fostering a supportive environment, that encourages healthy eating habits and lifestyle changes, healthcare providers can empower women to make informed decisions that benefit both their health and that of their unborn child [37].

In conclusion, maternal health and nutrition should be addressed holistically, starting from the preconception period, and continuing through pregnancy and lactation. Ensuring nutritional requirements, particularly micronutrients, is essential for preventing adverse maternal and fetal outcomes in women. Comprehensive nutritional interventions, combined with lifestyle modifications, can significantly reduce the health risks associated with poor dietary habits and improve outcomes for both mothers and their children. By embracing this holistic, life-course approach, we can disrupt the cycle of poor maternal and child health across generations.

Case Studies

Understanding how maternal nutrition interventions can translate into measurable improvements requires engagement with on-the-ground implementation experiences. While global frameworks provide strategic direction, it is the contextual adaptation, delivery mechanisms, and behavioral engagement strategies that often determine effectiveness. This section presents a series of case studies that exemplify varied approaches to improving maternal and newborn nutrition—ranging from large-scale social and behavior change programs and conditional cash transfers to community-based trials and participatory group models. Together, these cases reflect both the diversity of delivery platforms and the consistent emphasis on early intervention, systems strengthening, and community engagement.

Case Study 1

The Alive & Thrive (A&T) initiative represents one of the most systematically implemented and evaluated large-scale social and behavior change (SBC) efforts aimed at improving maternal, infant, and young child nutrition (MIYCN) across six countries—Bangladesh, Burkina Faso, Ethiopia, India, Nigeria, and Vietnam. Drawing on a unified implementation model anchored in interpersonal communication, community mobilization, and mass media, A&T sought to shift normative practices around breastfeeding, complementary feeding, and maternal nutrition. Interpersonal counseling, primarily delivered through government and community-based health workers, was the cornerstone of the approach and demonstrated strong associations with improved exclusive breastfeeding rates, dietary adequacy for children, and antenatal consumption of iron–folic acid supplements. Community mobilization activities were targeted at influential actors—particularly husbands, mothers-in-law, and religious leaders—through mechanisms such as community meetings, religious forums, and peer groups. Mass media strategies were designed based on formative research and media habit assessments, and included localized, memorable campaigns that were adapted for low-access settings via "media-dark" strategies. A&T's India model was notably distinct in its focus on technical support to integrate SBC within existing government platforms, prioritizing sustainability over intervention intensity. Impact evaluations revealed substantial improvements in exclusive breastfeeding in most countries, modest but significant gains in minimum dietary diversity in specific geographies (e.g., Bangladesh and Ethiopia), and an increase in IFA tablet consumption. However, the intervention's impact on early initiation of breastfeeding and maternal dietary diversity was inconsistent across settings. The initiative underscores critical lessons for program design: the value of tailoring counseling to life-stage needs, the importance of involving key household decision-makers, and the necessity of using real-time data for course correction. A&T's experience demonstrates that SBC, when implemented across multiple channels and institutionalized within public health systems, can effect measurable changes in nutrition behaviors at scale—though contextual challenges and programmatic fidelity remain central determinants of success [38].

Case Study 2

The **RajPusht** initiative in Rajasthan, India, is a large-scale program that operationalizes a life-course nutrition approach through strengthened government cash transfer schemes and sustained behavior change communication (SBCC). Aligned with India's Poshan Abhiyaan and PMMVY efforts, RajPusht focuses on maternal nutrition, capacity building of community workers, data-driven monitoring, and technology-based solutions, targeting districts with high malnutrition prevalence, especially among Adivasi communities.

RajPusht, in collaboration with the Government of Rajasthan, has been instrumental in addressing maternal and child malnutrition by focusing on reducing the prevalence of low birthweight and wasting in five tribal-dominated districts: Udaipur, Dungarpur, Pratapgarh, Banswara, and Baran. These areas suffer from high rates of underweight children and anemia, with over half of children under five being underweight and nearly two-thirds of women anemic. RajPusht has shown success in strengthening two key cash transfer schemes—Pradhan Mantri Matru Vandana Yojana (PMMVY) and Indira Gandhi Matritva Poshan Yojana (IGMPY)—enabling approximately 379,000 pregnant and lactating women to receive cash benefits, which has helped improve their dietary diversity and access to antenatal care (ANC). The project has reached 336,967 households with nutrition counseling, promoting diverse and adequate meals for mothers. Accurate birth weight recording for over 331,465 newborns has been ensured using digital weighing machines, vital for tracking and preventing wasting. Through its multi-tiered social and behavior change communication (SBCC) strategy, RajPusht has engaged Poshan Champions to deliver tailored counseling, improving maternal diet diversity and empowering mothers to make informed nutrition choices. The project's holistic approach, including the training of 21,419 frontline workers, real-time data monitoring, and sustained engagement with stakeholders, has been instrumental in addressing systemic gaps, thereby contributing to reducing low birthweight and wasting among children in Rajasthan [39].

Case Study 3

The **Projahnmo study in Sylhet, Bangladesh**, aimed to reduce neonatal mortality through a community-based newborn care intervention delivered via two models: home-care and community-care. Conducted across 24 clusters with ~120,000 people, the home-care arm involved trained female CHWs who identified pregnant women, provided two antenatal visits for birth and newborn preparedness, postnatal visits on days 1, 3, and 7, and treatment for neonatal illnesses—including injectable antibiotics when facility access was limited. In the community-care arm, male and female mobilizers led group sessions on birth preparedness and care-seeking but did not provide direct postnatal care. Over 30 months, neonatal mortality was reduced by 34% in the home-care arm compared to the control, with significant improvements in maternal practices like antenatal visits, clean cord-cutting, delayed bathing, and early breastfeeding. No mortality reduction occurred in the community-care arm. The cost per neonatal death averted was USD 2,995, indicating high cost-effectiveness. Despite success, challenges such as CHW workload and delayed birth notifications were noted. The study highlights that integrating home-based newborn care with existing systems can significantly improve maternal and neonatal outcomes in low-resource settings [40].

Case Study 4

In rural Nepal, the **Makwanpur trial** assessed the impact of participatory women's groups on maternal and neonatal health. Across 24 village development committees, local female facilitators led monthly meetings where women identified key health issues and implemented community-driven solutions such as emergency transport schemes, clean delivery kits, and maternal care funds. Although only 8% of women attended regularly, the intervention influenced 37% of newly pregnant women. Results showed a 30% reduction in neonatal mortality and an 80% drop in maternal mortality. Women in intervention areas were more likely to access antenatal care, deliver in facilities, and adopt safer practices. The low-cost, scalable model demonstrated that participatory groups can significantly improve outcomes in resource-limited settings [41].

Together, these cases demonstrate that measurable improvements in maternal and newborn health are achievable through well-designed and contextually adapted interventions. Whether through national platforms, community-based trials, or subnational initiatives, these experiences highlight the critical role of timely counseling, social norm change, and system integration in enabling sustained improvements in health and nutrition outcomes. Importantly, they also reinforce the need for multisectoral collaboration, tailored messaging, and continuous monitoring to ensure program effectiveness and equity across diverse settings.

Public Health Policies and Programs

Public health policies and programs play a pivotal role in improving maternal health and nutrition by providing a comprehensive framework to address healthcare gaps, enhance access to services, and ensure better health outcomes for women and children. Globally, initiatives like the WHO's maternal health guidelines, preconception Care (PCC) strategies, and the Sustainable Development Goals (SDGs) have significantly contributed to reducing maternal and child mortality. These initiatives have helped shape national efforts by emphasizing the need for universal health coverage, quality healthcare services, and reducing health inequalities. Particularly, SDG 3, which focuses on ensuring healthy lives and promoting well-being, has been crucial in guiding countries to strengthen maternal and child healthcare systems.

India has made considerable progress in maternal and child health through a series of focused national programs. Key initiatives such as *Anemia Mukt Bharat* (AMB), *Poshan Abhiyaan*, and *Pradhan Mantri Surakshit Matritva Abhiyan* (PMSMA) have played a crucial role in tackling major health challenges like anemia, malnutrition, and lack of antenatal care. Alongside these, initiatives like the *Janani Suraksha Yojana* (JSY), *Rashtriya Kishor Swasthya Karyakram* (RKSK), and *Surakshit Matritva Aashwasan* (SUMAN) are geared toward improving safe childbirth practices, adolescent health, and ensuring respectful, quality maternal care. Programs such as the *Public Distribution System* (PDS), which provides subsidized food grains, and the *National Iodine Deficiency Disorders Control Program* (NIDDCP), which aims to eliminate iodine deficiency, have further strengthened India's public health interventions by addressing nutritional gaps.

In addition, guidelines for managing *Gestational Diabetes Mellitus* (GDM), the *Janani Shishu Suraksha Karyakram* (JSSK), and *Facility-based Severe Acute Malnutrition management* (FSAM) provide critical care for at-risk mothers and children, emphasizing the importance of early detection and treatment. The interventions and beneficiaries of these initiatives, including targeted efforts like iron and folic acid supplementation, fortified food distribution, and comprehensive maternal healthcare, are outlined in Table 7.1. While India has made notable progress, sustained efforts are necessary to achieve the long-term goals of equitable healthcare access and improved maternal and child health outcomes.

Evidence-Based Recommendations

The intersection of maternal nutrition and child health is pivotal in ensuring favorable long-term health outcomes. Evidence-based interventions are crucial in guiding maternal healthcare practices, particularly in low- and middle-income countries where malnutrition, both undernutrition and rising obesity, coexist. Addressing maternal nutrition requires a life-course approach, with emphasis on preconception care, appropriate gestational weight gain (GWG), combating hidden hunger, promoting diet diversity, and ensuring sustainable interventions that can be integrated into public health systems.

Overcoming these complex challenges require a comprehensive bouquet of interventions that spans the entire reproductive cycle. The recommendations can be condensed in the form of an **N-O-U-R-I-S-H** framework, which provides a multi-sectoral strategy that incorporates nutrition education, community engagement, technology integration, and supportive environments to improve maternal, fetal, and newborn health outcomes. This framework was conceptualized by the authors through a comprehensive literature review of published interventions, review papers, government policy documents, and policy briefs available in the public domain, ensuring that it is grounded in evidence-based practices. Under each recommendation area, examples of activities are provided from a triple lens, i.e., government, research/academia and development partners, and NGOs, to ensure that it is scalable, sustainable, and adaptable within diverse public health frameworks. The framework can be tailored by users to suit their specific needs and context. NOURISH: An evidence-based recommendation framework to improve maternal, fetal, and newborn, health and nutrition outcomes in India.

N: Nutrition Education and Support

- Government-led efforts should focus on creating preconception care programs that are integrated within existing maternal health services. These programs must ensure early nutritional interventions, including micronutrient supplementation, to address deficiencies and reduce the risk of poor pregnancy outcomes.
- Empirical research is needed to evaluate the impacts of appropriate gestational weight gain (GWG) across different population groups, providing data-driven

Table 7.1 Indian initiatives to improve maternal and child health

Program/Policy	Main Interventions	Beneficiaries	Ministry
AMB (Anemia Mukt Bharat)	- Iron and folic acid supplementation - Deworming - Behavior Change Communication campaigns on iron-rich diet, breastfeeding, delayed cord clamping, and anemia screening - Use of digital tools for anemia testing and treatment - Iron and folic acid fortified foods - Address non-nutritional causes of anemia like malaria, hemoglobinopathies, and fluorosis	Pregnant and lactating women, children, adolescents, and women in reproductive age (15–49 years)	Ministry of Health and Family Welfare
POSHAN Abhiyaan	- Focus on reduction in stunting, wasting, and anemia through convergence, use of technology, and behavior change via Jan Andolan - Poshan Vatikas (Nutri-gardens) set up across the country for access to nutritious food - Now integrated with Mission Saksham Anganwadi and Poshan 2.0, emphasizing millets, diet diversity, and food fortification - Real-time monitoring through Poshan Tracker for better service delivery	Children under 6, adolescent girls, pregnant and lactating women	Ministry of Women & Child Development

(continued)

Table 7.1 (continued)

Program/Policy	Main Interventions	Beneficiaries	Ministry
ICDS (Integrated Child Development Services)	- Supplementary Nutrition - Immunization - Health Check-up and Referral Services - Pre-school non-formal education - Nutrition and Health Education for women (15–45 years) - Special feeding programs for malnourished children - Growth monitoring and breastfeeding awareness	Children below 6, pregnant and lactating mothers, and women (15–45 years)	Ministry of Women & Child Development
PMSMA (Pradhan Mantri Surakshit Matritva Abhiyan)	- Free, quality antenatal care - Tracking and management of high-risk pregnancies - Referral services to First Referral Units (FRUs)	Pregnant women, especially those in rural and underserved areas	Ministry of Health and Family Welfare
GDM Guidelines (Gestational Diabetes Mellitus)	- Routine blood glucose screening for all pregnant women - Medical Nutrition Therapy (MNT) for those diagnosed with GDM - Lifestyle modifications and timely interventions to prevent complications	Pregnant women at risk of or diagnosed with gestational diabetes	Ministry of Health and Family Welfare
PDS (Public Distribution System)	- Subsidized food grains for low-income households - Distribution of fortified rice under Mission Poshan 2.0	Low-income families, pregnant and lactating women	Ministry of Consumer Affairs, Food & Public Distribution

(continued)

Table 7.1 (continued)

Program/Policy	Main Interventions	Beneficiaries	Ministry
FSAM (Facility-based Severe Acute Malnutrition management)	- Therapeutic feeding for severely malnourished children - Growth monitoring and health check-ups - Nutrition surveillance and care for malnourished children	Severely malnourished children	Ministry of Health and Family Welfare
PMMVY (Pradhan Mantri Matru Vandana Yojana)	- Cash benefit of ₹5000 for the first child - ₹6000 for the second child if it's a girl - Maternity benefits and support for socially and economically disadvantaged women	Pregnant and lactating women, particularly for first live birth and second child (if a girl)	Ministry of Women & Child Development
JSSK (Janani Shishu Suraksha Karyakram)	- Free maternal care, medicines, diagnostics, and transportation - Free care for newborns until 30 days after birth - Reduction of out-of-pocket expenses for maternal care in public hospitals	Pregnant women and newborns	Ministry of Health and Family Welfare
JSY (Janani Suraksha Yojana)	- Cash incentives to promote institutional deliveries - Focus on safe delivery practices in rural and underserved areas	Pregnant women, particularly those below the poverty line (BPL)	Ministry of Health and Family Welfare
NIDDCP (National Iodine Deficiency Disorders Control Programme)	- Universal salt iodization - Awareness campaigns to prevent iodine deficiency disorders	General population, pregnant women, children	Ministry of Health and Family Welfare

(continued)

Table 7.1 (continued)

Program/Policy	Main Interventions	Beneficiaries	Ministry
SUMAN (Surakshit Matritva Aashwasan)	- Free services for maternal and newborn healthcare - Assured delivery of quality healthcare services - Focus on dignified, respectful care with zero tolerance for denial of services	Pregnant women, mothers, and newborns	Ministry of Health and Family Welfare
RBSK (Rashtriya Bal Swasthya Karyakram)	- Screening for Defects at birth, Diseases, Deficiencies, and Development delays (4Ds) - Free treatment for 32 common health conditions, including surgeries - Early intervention services and follow-up care at district level	Children from birth to 18 years (0–6 years at Anganwadis, 6–18 years in schools)	Ministry of Health and Family Welfare

guidelines that minimize risks associated with both underweight and obesity during pregnancy.

- o Collaborations with international organizations are necessary to implement large-scale awareness campaigns targeting hidden hunger, ensuring women receive education on nutrient-rich diets and the importance of iron, folic acid, and other key micronutrients.

O: Optimize Community Understanding and Engagement

- o Public health systems must leverage local governance structures to integrate nutrition-focused community health worker (CHW) programs into maternal care. This would ensure sustained delivery of nutrition education and regular monitoring of pregnant women in underserved regions.
- o Studies on community-based nutrition interventions should be prioritized to understand local food security dynamics and optimize the design of culturally appropriate solutions, with a specific focus on promoting diet diversity.
- o NGOs should play a critical role in community engagement by organizing grassroots initiatives that address life-course nutritional needs, emphasizing the importance of nutrition across all stages of life, from adolescence to pregnancy and beyond.

U: Utilize Technology and Tracking Systems

- Governments should integrate digital tracking systems into maternal health services to monitor essential data, such as nutritional intake and gestational weight gain (GWG), enabling timely interventions for women at risk.
- Research on the application of mHealth technologies for delivering personalized nutrition advice and reminders on micronutrient supplementation should be expanded, focusing on cost-effectiveness and scalability in low-resource settings.
- Development partners can support the deployment of digital tools that enable real-time monitoring of maternal and child health indicators, ensuring that healthcare providers have up-to-date information on the prevalence of hidden hunger and nutritional deficiencies.

R: Reinforce Healthy and Diverse Diets

- National policies must prioritize diet diversity by ensuring equitable access to nutrient-dense foods through public distribution systems, particularly in regions prone to food insecurity. These efforts should be coupled with education on balanced diets to prevent both undernutrition and the rising tide of obesity.
- Research into the effectiveness of dietary diversity in improving pregnancy outcomes should be expanded, with findings directly informing government nutrition guidelines to ensure that maternal diets are aligned with optimal fetal development.
- International development organizations should collaborate with local agricultural sectors to enhance food availability and diversity, addressing regional vulnerabilities to hidden hunger by promoting the cultivation and consumption of micronutrient-rich foods.

I: Integrate Information Technology for Capacity Building

- Governments should incorporate digital capacity-building initiatives for healthcare workers, equipping them with tools and training to deliver education on nutrition and monitor the nutritional status of pregnant women.
- Researchers should investigate the potential of telemedicine and digital platforms to enhance maternal nutrition services, focusing on improving access to information on preconception care and gestational nutrition.
- Development partners can fund the expansion of digital health platforms, ensuring that technology is accessible to marginalized populations for real-time guidance on nutrition and health during pregnancy and lactation.

S: Support, Sustain, and Nurture a Supportive Environment

- Government policies must focus on creating environments that support maternal and child health by ensuring access to quality healthcare services, including preconception counseling and continuous nutritional support during pregnancy and beyond. Family's engagement (especially the male counterparts) in providing nurturing care and positive environment for women goes a long way in ensuring optimal mental health during pregnancy.

- o Research should focus on the long-term impacts of integrated maternal health interventions, assessing how combining nutrition, psychosocial support, and mental health services enhances outcomes for both mother and child.
- o Collaborations with global development partners can help create sustainable community-based maternal health initiatives, which not only address nutrition but also foster mental and physical well-being throughout the reproductive cycle.

H: Holistic Health Interventions

- o Governments should develop integrated public health programs that provide a continuum of care, addressing not only nutrition but also mental health, sanitation, and immunization to ensure comprehensive support for maternal and child health.
- o Research into holistic maternal care models should be prioritized to evaluate the combined effects of multi-sectoral interventions on reducing maternal mortality and improving fetal health outcomes.
- o International agencies should work with local governments to implement holistic health interventions covering all determinants of maternal and child health, ensuring that even the most vulnerable populations benefit from integrated healthcare services.

The *NOURISH* package provides a comprehensive, evidence-based framework designed to address the multifaceted challenges in maternal and child nutrition. By implementing these recommendations, we can move toward a future where good health is not a privilege but a standard—ensuring that every mother and child could thrive.

Conclusion

Maternal health and nutrition play a vital role in fetal development and the long-term health outcomes of both the mother and child. As explained throughout this chapter, the critical window from conception through the first 1000 days is a pivotal period during which the foundation for lifelong health is laid. Adequate maternal nutrition is essential not only to prevent adverse outcomes such as low birthweight, preterm birth, and congenital anomalies but also for ensuring optimal placental function and fetal growth.

Over time, the landscape of nutritional challenges has shifted dramatically. Initially, the focus was on combating undernutrition, which was prevalent and led to significant public health issues. However, as economic and social conditions improved, there has been a rise in obesity and non-communicable diseases (NCDs), creating a new set of challenges. This telescoping of nutrition issues—from undernutrition to obesity—reflects the complex dual burden of malnutrition that many populations, especially in low- and middle-income countries, now face.

To address these challenges effectively, it is important to promote the need for appropriate nutrition throughout the life-course. The focus should not be limited to pregnancy alone; instead, a holistic approach that encompasses all stages of life—from preconception through pregnancy, infancy, childhood, and beyond—is necessary. Without consistent and comprehensive nutritional interventions, the benefits of good maternal nutrition during pregnancy can quickly diminish, failing to support long-term health and well-being.

Furthermore, promoting a healthy, affordable diet and ensuring dietary diversity are key strategies for combating both undernutrition and obesity. It is essential to make nutrient-rich foods accessible to all, ensuring that individuals from all socioeconomic backgrounds can benefit from a balanced diet. Achieving this requires a concerted effort to address food security, improve nutritional literacy, and support sustainable agricultural practices that prioritize health.

Emerging research areas, such as advancements in understanding maternal gut health and the microbiome's impact on fetal development, the effects of climate change and global warming on birth outcomes, and improvements in compliance with government-provided schemes, supplements, and services, are urgently needed.

Finally, good nutrition alone is not enough; it must be supported by a nourishing and nurturing environment. This includes ensuring access to quality healthcare, fostering supportive family and community networks, and addressing the social determinants of health that influence nutritional status. By creating an environment that supports both physical and emotional well-being, he effectiveness of nutritional interventions can be enhanced that will contribute to better health outcomes across generations.

In conclusion, the interplay between maternal nutrition, fetal development, and long-term health is profound and multifaceted. Addressing the evolving nutritional challenges through a life-course approach, promoting dietary diversity and equity, and fostering supportive environments are essential steps in ensuring that both current and future generations can thrive.

References

1. Black, R. E., et al. (2013). Maternal and Child Undernutrition and Overweight in Low-income and Middle-Income Countries. *The Lancet, 382*(9890), 427–51. Retrieved from https://doi.org/10.1016/s0140-6736(13)60937-x
2. Likhar, A., & Patil, M. S. (2022). Importance of Maternal Nutrition in the First 1000 Days of Life and Its Effects on Child Development: A Narrative Review. *Cureus, 14*(10), e30083. Retrieved from https://doi.org/10.7759/cureus.30083. PMID: 36381799; PMCID: PMC9640361.
3. Apostolopoulou, A., Tranidou, A., Tsakiridis, I., Magriplis, E., Dagklis, T., & Chourdakis, M. (2024). Effects of Nutrition on Maternal Health, Fetal Development, and Perinatal Outcomes. *Nutrients, 16*(3), 375. Retrieved from https://doi.org/10.3390/nu16030375. PMID: 38337660; PMCID: PMC10857165. Retrieved from https://archive.org/details/mothersbabieshea0000bark/mode/2up
4. Cetin, I., Berti, C., & Calabrese, S. (2023). Maternal Nutrition and Fetal Development. *Current Opinion in Clinical Nutrition & Metabolic Care, 26*(3), 231–238.
5. *Anaemia in women and children.* (n.d.). Retrieved June 26, 2025, from https://www.who.int/data/gho/data/themes/topics/anaemia_in_women_and_children

6. *Why we should invest in maternal and child health | World Economic Forum.* (n.d.). Retrieved June 26, 2025, from https://www.weforum.org/stories/2024/09/how-investing-in-maternal-and-child-health-fuels-prosperity-for-women-young-people-and-children-in-africa/
7. D'souza, N., et al. (2021). Pre-conceptional Maternal Vitamin B12 Supplementation Improves Offspring Neurodevelopment at 2 Years of Age: PRIYA Trial. *Front Pediatric, 7*(9), 755977. Retrieved from https://doi.org/10.3389/fped.2021.755977. Erratum in: Front Pediatr. 2022 February 21; 10:860732. Retrieved from https://doi.org/10.3389/fped.2022.860732. PMID: 34956975; PMCID: PMC8697851.
8. *Mumbai Maternal Nutrition Project (SARAS)–MRC Lifecourse Epidemiology Centre.* (n.d.). Retrieved from https://generic.wordpress.soton.ac.uk/mrclec/cohorts/mrclec-collaborations-in-india/mumbai-maternal-nutrition-project-saras/
9. Taneja, S., et al. (2020). Impact of An Integrated Nutrition, Health, Water Sanitation and Hygiene, Psychosocial Care and Support Intervention Package Delivered During the Pre- and Peri-Conception Period and/or During Pregnancy and Early Childhood on Linear Growth of Infants in the First Two Years of Life, Birth Outcomes and Nutritional Status of Mothers: Study Protocol of a Factorial, Individually Randomized Controlled Trial in India. *Trials, 21*(1), 127 Retrieved from https://doi.org/10.1186/s13063-020-4059-z
10. Hofmeyr, G., et al. (n.d.). Evidence-Based Antenatal Interventions to Reduce the Incidence of Small Vulnerable Newborns and Their Associated Poor Outcomes. *The Lancet, 401*(10389), 1733–1744.
11. Moholdt, T., & Hawley, J. A. (2020). Maternal Lifestyle Interventions: Targeting Preconception Health. *Trends in Endocrinology & Metabolism, 31*(8), 561–569. Retrieved from https://doi.org/10.1016/j.tem.2020.03.002
12. Roberts, J. M., & Hubel, C. A. (2009). The Two Stage Model of Preeclampsia: Variations on the Theme. *Placenta, 30*(Suppl A), S32–37. Retrieved from https://doi.org/10.1016/j.placenta.2008.11.009. Epub 2008 December 13. PMID: 19070896; PMCID: PMC2680383.
13. Reynolds, L. P., Borowicz, P. P, Caton, J. S., Crouse, M. S., Dahlen, C. R., & Ward A. K. (2019). Developmental Programming of Fetal Growth and Development. *Veterinary Clinics of North America: Food Animal Practice, 35*(2), 229–247. Retrieved from https://doi.org/10.1016/j.cvfa.2019.02.006. PMID: 31103178.
14. Indian Council of Medical Research. (2024). *Dietary Guidelines for Indians* https://main.icmr.nic.in/sites/default/files/upload_documents/DGI_07th_May_2024_fin.pdf
15. *Interventions* (n.d.). Retrieved from https://www.who.int/tools/elena/interventions/nutrition-counselling-pregnancy
16. Muktabhant, B., Lawrie, T. A., Lumbiganon, P., & Laopaiboon, M. (2015). Diet or Exercise, or Both, for Preventing Excessive Weight Gain in Pregnancy. *Cochrane Database of Systematic Reviews* (6). Art No.: CD007145. Retrieved from https://doi.org/10.1002/14651858.cd007145.pub3
17. Mantri, N., et al. (2024). National and Regional Prevalence of Gestational Diabetes Mellitus in India: A Systematic Review and Meta-analysis. *BMC Public Health, 24*, 527. Retrieved from https://doi.org/10.1186/s12889-024-18024-9
18. Diagnosis & Management of Gestational Diabetes Mellitus Technical and Operational Guidelines. Retrieved from https://nhm.gov.in/New_Updates_2018/NHM_Components/RMNCH_MH_Guidelines/Gestational-Diabetes-Mellitus.pdf
19. Girard, A. W., & Olude, O. (2012). Nutrition Education and Counselling Provided During Pregnancy: Effects on Maternal, Neonatal and Child Health Outcomes. *Paediatric Perinatal Epidemiol, 26*(1), 191–204. Retrieved from https://doi.org/10.1111/j.1365-3016.2012.01278.x. PMID: 22742611.
20. Tuncalp, Ö., et al. (2020). WHO Recommendations on Antenatal Nutrition: An Update on Multiple Micronutrient Supplements. *BMJ Global Health, 5*(7), e003375. Retrieved from https://doi.org/10.1136/bmjgh-2020-003375. PMID: 32732247; PMCID: PMC7394017.
21. Wu, G., Bazer, F. W., Cudd, T. A., Meininger, C. J., & Spencer T. E. (2004). Maternal Nutrition and Fetal Development. *Journal of Nutrition, 134*(9), 2169–2172. Retrieved from https://doi.org/10.1093/jn/134.9.2169. PMID: 15333699.

22. King, J. C. (2016). A Summary of Pathways or Mechanisms Linking Preconception Maternal Nutrition with Birth Outcomes. *Journal of Nutrition, 146*(7), 1437S–44S. Retrieved from https://doi.org/10.3945/jn.115.223479. PMID: 27281808; PMCID: PMC4926847.
23. Guelinckx, I., Devlieger, R., Beckers, K., & Vansant, G. (n.d.). Maternal Obesity: Pregnancy Complications, Gestational Weight Gain and Nutrition. *Obesity Review, 9*, 140–50. Retrieved from https://doi.org/10.1111/j.1467-789X.2007.00464.x
24. Li, C., Liu, Y., Zhang, W., & Obukhov, A. G. (2015). Joint and Independent Associations of Gestational Weight Gain and Pre-pregnancy Body Mass Index with Outcomes of Pregnancy in Chinese Women: A Retrospective Cohort Study. *PLoS ONE, 10*(8), e0136850. Retrieved from https://doi.org/10.1371/journal.pone.0136850
25. Chauhan, A., & Potdar, J. (2022). Maternal Mental Health During Pregnancy: A Critical Review. *Cureus, 14*(10), e30656. Retrieved from https://doi.org/10.7759/cureus.30656. PMID: 36426343; PMCID: PMC9681705.
26. Stein, A., et al. (2014). Effects of Perinatal Mental Disorders on the Fetus and Child. *The Lancet, 384*(9956), 1800–1819. Retrieved from https://doi.org/10.1016/s0140-6736(14)61277-0
27. Dewidar, O., et al. (2023). Effectiveness of Nutrition Counseling for Pregnant Women in Low- and Middle-income Countries to Improve Maternal and Infant Behavioral, Nutritional, and Health Outcomes: A Systematic Review. *Campbell Systematic Review, 19*(4), e1361. Retrieved from https://doi.org/10.1002/cl2.1361. PMID: 38034903; PMCID: PMC10687348.
28. Allen, L. H. (2000). Anemia and Iron Deficiency: Effects on Pregnancy Outcome. *American Journal of Clinical Nutrition, 71*(5), 1280S-S1284.
29. Berry, R. J., et al. (1999). Prevention of Neural-tube Defects with Folic Acid in China. *New England Journal of Medicine, 341*(20), 1485–1490.
30. Walle, B. M., Adekunle, A. O., Arowojolu, A. O., Muluken Walle, B., Dugul, T. T., & Mebiratie, A. L. (2020). <p>Micronutrients Deficiency and Their Associations with Pregnancy Outcomes: A Review</p>. *Nutrition and Dietary Supplements, 12*, 237–254. https://doi.org/10.2147/NDS.S274646
31. Mousa, A., Naqash, A., & Lim, S. (2019). Macronutrient and Micronutrient Intake During Pregnancy: An Overview of Recent Evidence. *Nutrients, 11*(2), 443. Retrieved from https://doi.org/10.3390/nu11020443. PMID: 30791647; PMCID: PMC6413112.
32. Muglia, L. J., et al. (2022). Maternal Factors During Pregnancy Influencing Maternal, Fetal, and Childhood Outcomes. *BMC Med, 20*, 418. Retrieved from https://doi.org/10.1186/s12916-022-02632-6
33. Bauer, I., et al. (2020). Spotlight on the Fetus: How Physical Activity During Pregnancy Influences Fetal Health: A Narrative Review. *BMJ Open Sports Exercise Medicine, 6*(1), e000658. Retrieved from https://doi.org/10.1136/bmjsem-2019-000658. PMID: 32206341; PMCID: PMC7078670
34. Lee, Y. J., et al. (2020). Alcohol Consumption Before Pregnancy Causes Detrimental Fetal Development and Maternal Metabolic Disorders. *Scientific Reports, 10*, 10054. Retrieved from https://doi.org/10.1038/s41598-020-66971-1.
35. Murawski, N. J., Moore, E. M., Thomas, J. D., & Riley, E. P. (2015). Advances in Diagnosis and Treatment of Fetal Alcohol Spectrum Disorders: From Animal Models to Human Studies. *Alcohol Research, 37*(1), 97–108.
36. S, Janaki., & Prabhakar S. (2024). Examining Socioeconomic Factors Influencing Maternal Health in Pregnancy. *Journal of Human Behavior in the Social Environment, 34*, 1–19. https://doi.org/10.1080/10911359.2024.2310272
37. Bagherzadeh, R., et al. (2021). Pregnancy: An Opportunity to Return to a Healthy Lifestyle: A Qualitative Study. *BMC Pregnancy Childbirth, 21*, 751. Retrieved from https://doi.org/10.1186/s12884-021-04213-6
38. Flax, V. L., Bose, S., Escobar-DeMarco, J., & Frongillo, E. A. (2023). Changing Maternal, Infant and Young Child Nutrition Practices Through Social and Behaviour Change Interventions Implemented at Scale: Lessons Learned from Alive & Thrive. *Maternal & Child Nutrition, 21*(2), Article e13559. https://doi.org/10.1111/MCN.13559

39. *About* (n.d.). Rajpusht. Retrieved from https://rajpusht.in/about/
40. Baqui, A. H., et al. (2008). Projahnmo Study Group. Effect of Community-based Newborn-Care Intervention Package Implemented Through Two Service-Delivery Strategies in Sylhet District, Bangladesh: A Cluster-Randomised Controlled Trial. *Lancet, 371*(9628), 1936–1944. Retrieved from https://doi.org/10.1016/S0140-6736(08)60835-1. PMID: 18539225.
41. Manandhar, D. S., et al. (2004). Members of the MIRA Makwanpur Trial Team. Effect of a Participatory Intervention with Women's Groups on Birth Outcomes in Nepal: Cluster-Randomised Controlled Trial. *Lancet, 364*(9438), 970–979. Retrieved from https://doi.org/10.1016/S0140-6736(04)17021-9. PMID: 15364188.

Chapter 8
Programmes and Policies Promoting Maternal Well-Being During Pregnancy

Seema Puri and Anshu Sharma

Introduction

A healthy pregnancy is essential not only for healthy growth and development of the foetus, but also substantially reduces the life-threatening complications during childbirth, such as haemorrhage, infection, and difficult labour as well as infant mortality and morbidity. Nutrition during this time can impact a child's health and productivity throughout life.

Ensuring good maternal health also has economic and social benefits. It helps to reduce poverty and promote gender equality. Healthy women can contribute to the workforce, support their families, and improve their economic status.

India has made significant progress in reducing maternal and infant mortality; still annually 97 women per lakh live births die due to pregnancy-related causes and the infant mortality rate stands at 35.2 per thousand live births, according to NFHS 5 data [1]. Many of these deaths are preventable if quality health care is provided to pregnant women during their antenatal period and timely detection and management of high-risk factors such as severe anaemia, pregnancy-induced hypertension, etc., is carried out.

Optimum nutrition is important for women throughout life, due to their special nutritional needs associated with physiological changes such as menstruation, growth spurt, pregnancy, lactation, and menopause. During pregnancy and lactation, the nutritional requirements increase tremendously as the mother has to cater to the additional needs of the growing foetus or the infant being breastfed.

S. Puri (✉) · A. Sharma
Institute of Home Economics, Department of Food and Nutrition, University of Delhi, Delhi, India
e-mail: dr.seemapuri@gmail.com

S. Suri (ed.), *Child Health and Nutrition from Conception to Age Two*,
https://doi.org/10.1007/978-981-95-7868-9_8

The First 1000 Days: Window of Opportunity

The first 1000 days of a child's life, from conception to age two, are a critical period for nutrition and development of their body, brain, metabolism, and immune system. The growth and development of the child during this period is significantly impacted by the nourishment and care received by the mothers and the infants.

The health of the mother and her child are intertwined during the first 1000 days. During this period, numerous factors contribute to growth, including diet, genetic and epigenetic factors, and hormonal regulation. Pregnancy complications caused by both inadequate and excessive nutrition and weight may influence pregnancy outcomes for the mother and child. The foetus is dependent on the mother's body for his/her nourishment. If the woman is malnourished, foetal development will be affected, with lifelong impact on the child's health.

A healthy, balanced maternal diet before conception and during pregnancy ensures that the growing foetus is well nourished and helps build adequate stores in the mother for breastfeeding. Several nutrients play specific roles throughout the first 1000 days, namely, carotenoids (lutein + zeaxanthin), choline, folate, iodine, iron, omega-3 fatty acids, and vitamin D. Other nutrients for maternal, newborn, and toddler health include magnesium, vitamin A, vitamin B complex, and other trace elements. Folic acid and iodine, essential for foetal neurodevelopment, are often deficient in pregnant women's diets. Moreover, this period provides a window of opportunity for modulating the gut microbiota through interventions such as diet, use of probiotics, prebiotics, or faecal microbiota transplantation so as to promote healthy growth and development [2, 3].

Preconception Care

Research has shown that individuals' health and lifestyle choices before conception can significantly influence the health outcomes of their offspring. Preconception care can reduce the incidence of various neonatal and birth disorders, leading to healthier pregnancies and improved long-term health outcomes for both mothers and their offspring.

Potential risk factors may be addressed during this phase to optimize health before pregnancy. This creates a favourable environment for conception, implantation, and embryonic development. Various physiological processes crucial for the embryo's development, such as organ formation, occur early in pregnancy even before a woman realizes that she is pregnant. Therefore, it becomes crucial to intervene during the preconception period to mitigate risks and promote healthy development right from the earliest stages. Some aspects of preconception care which need to be addressed include health promotion and education about healthy lifestyle, screening and management of medical conditions, genetic counselling and testing, immunization, family planning and contraception and psychosocial well-being and mental health.

Disseminating information and guidance about healthy lifestyle, such as maintaining a balanced diet, exercising regularly, managing stress, and avoiding addictions like tobacco, alcohol, and drugs empowers them to adopt health supporting behaviours and increase their chances of a healthy pregnancy. Screening and counselling for existing medical conditions, risk of inherited genetic disorders, effective contraceptive options allow them to make informed decisions about their reproductive choices. Preconception care also includes the prevention and management of infections that may pose risks during pregnancy. It is also imperative to address emotional well-being, support stress management, screen for mental health conditions, and provide appropriate referrals for counselling or treatment so as to help women achieve optimal mental health before conception [4].

Maternal Health Challenges

In spite of a large number of health initiatives over the last few decades, India continues to be plagued with high maternal mortality rates, inadequate access to healthcare, nutritional inadequacies, and mental health issues. These are further compounded by caste and economic status concerns. While the Government has been focusing on bringing about improvements in maternal health indicators and reducing preventable maternal deaths in the past two decades, coverage of life-saving health interventions and practices remains low due to gaps in knowledge, policies, and availability of resources [5].

Other concerns affecting maternal and child health include rise in c-section deliveries, commercialization of medical services, lack of timely detection of complications, inadequate training facilities, barriers to maternal education and lack of awareness about existing government initiatives [5].

Maternal Mortality: India has a high maternal mortality rate, with significant differences in utilization of maternal healthcare services and maternal health outcomes across different states. Maternal Mortality Ratio (MMR) stands at 97/100,000 live births, lower by 33 points, from 130/100,000 live births in 2014–16 [6].

Nearly two-thirds of all maternal deaths are due to complications during delivery, severe bleeding (mostly after childbirth), postnatal infections, pre-eclampsia and eclampsia, and unsafe abortions. Pregnancy-related complications are the primary cause of death among 15–19-year-old girls.

Access to Healthcare: Although the utilization of Maternal, Newborn and Child Health (MNCH) services has increased, it still varies widely between and within states, between the rich and poor, and urban and rural areas.

In India, even though there has been a significant increase in institutional births over the last several years, there has also been a disturbing increase in C-section deliveries, often performed without medical indications, leading to long-term adverse effects on both women's and children's health.

Maternal Nutrition: Poor maternal malnutrition is associated with a higher risk of maternal morbidity, preterm deliveries, and intrauterine growth retardation. Many women in India enter pregnancy with anaemia or a low Body Mass Index (BMI), which increases the risk of adverse pregnancy outcomes. Furthermore, nutritional inadequacy during the first 1000 days of life is highly detrimental to foetal and child growth.

Nguyen et al. [7] has reported that diets of pregnant women in India were characterized by low energy intakes, macronutrient imbalance, and inadequate micronutrient content. Constraints to consuming healthy diets included poor food availability, poor economic status, ignorance and gaps in knowledge due to inadequate nutrition counselling, food restrictions and taboos, adverse family influences, gender norms.

Mental Well-being: Post-partum depression is emerging as a growing health concern in India, affecting both rural and urban women. Beyond hormonal and psychological factors, sociocultural determinants, most often, relating to women's position within families and society, influence the development of post-partum depression. These factors must be recognized and targeted while developing interventions and policies concerning women's maternal health and mental well-being.

Sociocultural Influences: Various reports reiterate the association of increasing household income and higher women's education with increasing use of maternal health services, both in rural and urban areas. Religious and cultural practices also influence the utilization of maternal health services, nutrition care, and childcare practices. Early marriages were linked to low ANC usage and institutional deliveries. Studies also reported that if the husband was educated, it increased the likelihood of the wife's use of maternal health services. Gender, particularly the low status of women (in terms of autonomy and decision making) and son preference are strong influences on maternal health. Women with greater autonomy were more likely to use maternal health services in India [8].

Studies from Indian states reported a very high percentage of maternal deaths (50–80%) among the socially backward castes like scheduled tribes (ST), scheduled castes (SC), and other backward castes or socially and economically backward castes (OBC/SEBC). This factor was also associated with lower use of MNCH services such as ANCs and institutional deliveries [8].

The Government of India, under the umbrella of different ministries, has launched many programmes and framed various policies for improving the health and nutritional status of vulnerable sections of our population like adolescent girls, pregnant and lactating women, infants, and children. All these groups have to be targeted simultaneously to break the vicious cycle of malnutrition and reduce morbidity and mortality. These programmes aim to provide approachable, affordable, and need-based quality health services.

National Health Policy

The National Health Policy (NHP) was released in 2017 to achieve universal health coverage and improved health outcomes for all individuals in India. It emphasizes a preventive and promotive healthcare approach, ensuring access to quality health services without financial hardship. The policy focuses on strengthening primary healthcare through Health and Wellness Centres.

Key objectives include reducing infant mortality rates, enhancing maternal health, and addressing non-communicable diseases. The policy also prioritizes equity, aiming to minimize disparities related to gender, poverty, and social exclusion. It advocates for community participation and inter-sectoral collaboration to tackle the social determinants of health. The NHP seeks to ensure that vulnerable groups receive adequate support and services.

The NHP has various components like Reproductive, Maternal, Newborn, Child, Adolescent Health and Nutrition (RMNCAH + N), communicable and non-communicable diseases, health strengthening systems, and infrastructure maintenance. The RMNCAH + N component has strategies encompassing health throughout the lifecycle including newborn, child, adolescent and maternal health, and nutrition. The nutrition component is very critical for vulnerable groups including pregnant women. Many interventions have been initiated by Ministry of Health and Family Welfare (MoHFW) under the National Health Mission [9].

Programmes Addressing Preconception Health

Preconceptional maternal status plays a very crucial role in the growth and development of the newborn during pregnancy and post-partum too. In India, while the official age of marriage is 18 years, in rural areas many girls get married earlier and conceive at a very young age, often in early adolescence. Proper nutrition is of utmost importance during adolescence (10–19 years) to ensure their development as healthy women, minimize complications during pregnancy, and ensure the birth of a healthy infant.

Weekly Iron Folic Acid Supplementation (WIFS)

MoHFW launched the Weekly Iron and Folic Acid Supplementation (WIFS) Program to meet the challenge of high prevalence and prevalence of anaemia among adolescent girls and boys aged 10 to 19 years, enrolled in government/government-aided schools/ municipal schools, and outside school adolescents, both in rural and urban areas. Under this programme, a weekly iron folic acid supplement (100 mg elemental iron and 500 ug folic acid) is given to students on a fixed day. Biannual deworming

(Albendazole 400 mg), six months apart, and haemoglobin screening of the target groups are also a part of WIFS. Moderately/severely anaemic adolescents are referred to a health facility. Behaviour change communication (BCC) along with health talks and counselling sessions has also been integrated into WIFS to make the adolescents aware about anaemia [9, 10]

Weekly IFA tablet distribution is carried out by the teachers in schools. They are responsible for procurement, distribution, recording, and compliance tracking whereas Anganwadi workers do this for out-of-school adolescents. BCC is mostly done during assembly time and parent-teacher meetings and individual counselling, if required to address barriers such as fear of side-effects is carried out [10].

Implementation Gaps

While millions of adolescents have been enrolled under WIFS, its effective impact still remains a challenge. Reports indicate that only 9.4% of in-school girls and 7.1% of in-school boys received the intended four tablets in a month [11]. This low adherence is attributed to inadequate provision of tablets and poor consumption rates. Ignorance about and resistance to the WIFS Program is another issue. Both adolescents and their parents are often unaware of the importance of IFA supplementation for health [11, 12]. Some communities exhibit resistance to the programme, which stems from cultural beliefs or misinformation [11]. Lack of sufficient training of health workers and educators along with lack of supervision and follow-up, results in inconsistent messaging and delivery of services [13]. Due to absence of sound monitoring and evaluation, it is difficult to assess programme effectiveness and identify areas for improvement [14].

Rashtriya Kishor Swasthya Karyakram (RKSK)

To ensure the holistic development of adolescents, MoHFW launched Rashtriya Kishor Swasthya Karyakram (RKSK) in 2014 to reach out to 253 million adolescents—boys and girls, rural and urban, married and unmarried, in and out-of-school adolescents with special focus on marginalized and underserved groups. The programme addresses their diverse needs including nutrition, sexual and reproductive health, prevention of injuries, and violence, non-communicable diseases, mental health, and substance misuse. The community-based interventions include peer education, adolescent health and wellness days and outreach by counsellors [15, 16].

The strength of the programme is it's health promotion approach using a multi-pronged delivery strategy through community, facility, and school-based interventions with active participation of teachers and frontline workers. It attempts to reach adolescents in their own environment, such as in schools, families, and communities; and is different from clinic-based services. The facility-based services are delivered through Adolescent Friendly Health Clinics (AFHCs) wherein the core package includes preventive, promotive, curative, and counselling services, routine checkups at primary, secondary, and tertiary levels of care. At the school level, programmes like WIFS and School Health and Wellness Programme help in extending the RKSK's outreach [15, 16].

RKSK has expanded adolescent access to health information and services. The setting up of thousands of AFHCs, implementing peer education, and school-based programmes have boosted the utilization of services. Operational data indicate better knowledge, attitudes, and health-seeking behaviours among adolescents in the intervention areas. There is also greater uptake of IFA supplements, menstrual hygiene products, and early detection of high-risk behaviours, leading to improved adolescent health outcomes [15–17].

Implementation Gaps

Despite having a strong framework, the RKSK continues to have some shortfalls in its implementation. Reaching out to out-of-school, rural, and marginalized adolescents is difficult [16, 17]. Many AFHCs lack the necessary infrastructure, particularly at higher care facilities. Issues such as insufficient privacy and absence of dedicated spaces for counselling sessions have been reported. Further, there is a lack of trained counsellors and healthcare providers to effectively deliver RKSK services, as many are overburdened with multiple responsibilities [12, 16]. A study by Barua et al. [17] has reported the peer educator model struggles with issues of recruitment, retention, and capacity building.

Erratic supply of items like sanitary pads and other essentials has been a significant barrier to implement menstrual hygiene initiatives and also led to decreased utilization of services aimed at improving adolescent health. Additionally, many adolescents and their families are ignorant about the services available to them, which limits their engagement with the programme. Factors such as the COVID-19 pandemic have reduced participation rates which has further impacted the programme's outreach and effectiveness. Apart from this, inefficient monitoring and evaluation mechanisms has made it difficult to assess the programme's impact effectively [12, 16].

School Health and Wellness Programme

Schools are critical platforms for health promotion, disease prevention, and holistic development of students. Recognizing this importance, school-based health promotion activities, through knowledge upgradation, teaching life skills and positive attitudes to make informed health choices, have been incorporated as a part of the Health and Wellness component of the Ayushman Bharat Program [18]. SHWP, a joint venture of MoHFW and Ministry of Human Resource Development, is being implemented in government and government-aided schools in all districts, including aspirational districts, since 2020.

Under SHWP, two teachers, one male and one female, in every school, designated as "Health and Wellness Ambassadors" are trained to transact with school children on eleven thematic areas regarding health promotion and disease prevention. These areas include nutrition, mental health, gender equality, reproductive health, substance abuse prevention, and digital safety and are transacted to the students for one hour weekly using interactive methods, activity kits and digital resources. SHWP also includes student volunteers designated as "Health and Wellness Messengers"—to reinforce the key messages among peers, community, and families. Monitoring and supervision of the programme is done through electronic health records, reporting and intermittent review meetings at different levels [18–21].

Since its inception, SHWP has reached more than 15 million learners across various age groups showing improvement in taking preventive services, life skills, and improving health awareness. Students have become more open in discussing mental health and gender issues and have been reported to have responsible behaviour, specifically among adolescents [18–20].

Implementation Gaps

Several implementation gaps have been highlighted. Insufficient training of teachers designated as "Health and Wellness Ambassadors" and lack of time to implement the programme effectively are such gaps. Schools may lack the necessary infrastructure, materials, and financial resources to support comprehensive health and wellness initiatives. Many programmes focus on basic health screening rather than promoting holistic well-being, including mental health and healthy lifestyle. Trained healthcare providers are needed to counsel students, particularly for sensitive issues like mental health. Robust monitoring and evaluation mechanisms are needed to track progress, identify challenges, and ensure accountability. There was a need for better coordination between health and education departments, as well as with other relevant stakeholders like parents, community health workers, and NGOs [22].

Programmes for Adult Women, Pregnant, and Lactating Women

Anaemia Mukt Bharat (AMB)

Pregnancy anaemia has been a major public health problem in India for more than 5 decades now. Since 1971, numerous anaemia control programmes have been introduced, but they have failed to achieve a significant impact. Launched in 2018, the Anemia Mukt Bharat under the Intensified National Iron Plus Initiative (I-NIPI), is a flagship programme under POSHAN Abhiyaan by the MoHFW. The programme aims to reduce anaemia prevalence by 3% points every year in all target groups. It uses the $6 \times 6 \times 6$ strategy and aims to reduce the prevalence of anaemia among 6 stakeholder groups including children (6 months–9 years), adolescents (10–19 years), pregnant women, lactating women, and women in reproductive age (15–49 years) using 6 interventions and 6 institutional mechanisms [23]. The interventions include:

1. *Prophylactic Iron and Folic Acid Supplementation*: Pregnant women are advised to take one iron and folic acid tablet daily (second trimester onwards) and continue it till delivery (minimum 180 days during pregnancy) and even after delivery (for 180 days). Each tablet contains 60 mg elemental Iron +500 mcg Folic Acid.
2. *Deworming:* All pregnant women are advised deworming during their antenatal checkups in the second trimester.
3. *Intensified Year-Round Behaviour Change Communication Campaign* focusing on four key behaviours:
   - Improving compliance to iron folic acid supplementation and deworming
   - Appropriate infant and young child feeding practices
   - Increase in intake of iron-rich food through diet diversity/quantity/frequency and/or fortified foods with a focus on harnessing locally available resources
   - Ensuring delayed cord clamping after delivery (by 3 min) in health facilities.
4. *Testing and Treatment of Anaemia*, using digital methods and point-of-care treatment, with special focus on pregnant women and school-going adolescents.
5. *Mandatory provision of iron and folic acid fortified foods* in government-funded public health programmes.
6. *Intensifying awareness, screening, and treatment of non-nutritional causes of anaemia* in endemic pockets with focus on malaria, haemoglobinopathies, and fluorosis [23].

AMB is implemented with the convergence of ministries—MoHFW, Ministry of Women and Child Development and Ministry of Human Resource Development and Ministry of Rural Development. The community-based platforms for implementing AMB include Anganwadi centres, schools, village Health Sanitation and Nutrition Days and Health and Wellness Centres (HWCs) under Ayushman Bharat, for screening and counselling. The digital monitoring tools of the programme are AMB Dashboard on the HMIS portal tracks programme indicators and use of Anaemia Tracker App and PMSMA for service delivery tracking [23].

However, periodic national level surveys show that inspite of a robust framework, the prevalence of anaemia has increased in NFHS-5 as compared to NFHS-4, across all vulnerable groups [1, 24]. After the launch of the AMB strategy, the IFA supplementation coverage between 2017–2018 and 2019–2020 increased for all beneficiary groups including pregnant women (78%–90%); lactating mothers (34%–49%); school-going adolescent girls (23%–40%) and out-of-school adolescent girls (6%–23%). Increase in coverage alone does not necessarily have the desired impact if the quality aspect of coverage, including frequency of IFA distribution and consumption adherence is not adequately focused upon [25].

Implementation Gaps

The AMB programme faces several implementation gaps including low coverage and consumption of IFA supplements, weak supply chains for IFA tablets, challenges in procuring point-of-care devices and lack of effective strategies for addressing causes of non-nutritional anaemia like genetic disorders. Additionally, variations in coverage exist between states and departments, and knowledge gaps persist among beneficiaries and health workers. Training and orientation of health workers needs to be strengthened. Addressing these gaps through targeted interventions, improved training, robust supply chains, and enhanced monitoring and evaluation is crucial for achieving the goals of the Anemia Mukt Bharat programme [25, 26].

Mission Indradhanush

Mission Indradhanush was launched in 2014 by MoHFW. This scheme ensures that all pregnant women and children in India receive full immunization coverage, especially in areas where immunization rates are dismally low. The programme focuses on providing vaccines to protect against serious diseases and helps prevent outbreaks of diseases like polio, measles, and tetanus [33].

The objective of the Intensified MI (IMI) programme, launched in 2017, is to achieve more than 90% immunization coverage, targeting under-2 children and pregnant women. MI began with 201 high-focussed districts, later expanding to cover more districts and urban areas with low immunization rates [27–29]. Reports indicate that a total of 5.46 crore children and 1.32 crore pregnant women have been vaccinated in all phases of MI conducted so far [29].

This programme is implemented through collaboration of MoHFW, MWCD, Panchayati Raj, Urban Development, etc. Detailed mapping is done so that all target groups are covered. The state and district task forces co-ordinate, plan, implement, monitor, and report so that corrective measures may be taken. Local workers and leaders are approached for social mobilization. All health workers are trained to carry out MI successfully [28, 29].

Implementation Gaps

Logistic issues in implementation include difficulty in reaching remote and hard-to-access populations, including those living in tribal areas, urban slums, and construction sites. These groups often experience higher rates of missed vaccinations due to logistical challenges [29, 30]. Other challenges are inadequate vaccination infrastructure, limited awareness, and resistance to vaccination among some communities. Inadequate infrastructure and insufficient trained healthcare personnel, ASHA and Anganwadi workers, as well as poor coordination among various stakeholders can compromise the quality of immunization services. Many health facilities are ill-equipped to handle the demands of vaccination campaigns, leading to inefficiencies. Strengthening of the system and practice changes could make it more effective. Better communication and counselling skills tailored to local beliefs are needed to deal with barriers to seeking vaccinations [30].

Maternal Health Component of rMNCH + A

This programme addresses the major causes of mortality and morbidity among women and children and those specifically for maternal well-being are discussed here.

Surakshit Matritva Aashwasan (SUMAN)

The SUMAN programme is a national initiative by MoHFW, aimed at ensuring free, quality healthcare services for pregnant women and newborn babies, with focus on eliminating preventable maternal and newborn deaths. It provides comprehensive antenatal care, promotes institutional deliveries, and nutritional support, maternal health education and ensures timely access to healthcare services for pregnant women, end denial of services to pregnant women and children, and provide a positive birthing experience. By integrating services and utilizing technology for monitoring, SUMAN seeks to reduce maternal mortality rates and improve health outcomes for mothers and newborns. The initiative also fosters community participation to empower women to make informed health decisions [31].

The programme works with the existing schemes like Janani Suraksha Yojna (JSY) and Janani Shishu Suraksha Karyakram (JSSK). Some of the benefits of SUMAN include free access to healthcare to pregnant women, newborns, and mothers up to six months after delivery at public health facilities, free transportation from home to the health facility and back after discharge, respectful care with privacy and support for breastfeeding and grievance redressal [31].

The SUMAN initiative employs multi-level committees at national, state, district, and block levels for oversight, monitoring, and review. All public health facilities, including medical colleges and district hospitals, assessed and notified for SUMAN service packages, must achieve LaQshya certification within set timeframe to ensure quality. Community engagement under SUMAN is carried out by volunteers, self-help groups (SHGs), and village health sanitation and nutrition committees (VHSNCs). A robust grievance redressal system is operated through call centres, web portals, and facility-level help desks [31, 32]. As of early 2025, the SUMAN initiative has expanded significantly, with over 10,000 health facilities across India notified as SUMAN-compliant. Studies indicate high utilization rates for free diagnostic tests, IFA supplements, and delivery services among the beneficiaries [33].

Implementation Gaps

Lack of awareness among pregnant women, particularly in rural and marginalized communities, regarding the SUMAN scheme and its benefits, was leading to underutilization of available services and preventing women from accessing essential maternal care. Inadequate infrastructure, insufficient medical supplies, and trained personnel in many healthcare facilities compromise service delivery. While SUMAN encourages community participation through volunteers, actual engagement at the grassroots level remains inconsistent. Lack of adequate training on the specific protocols of SUMAN affects many healthcare providers especially in rural areas. This gap can lead to variations in service quality and adherence to best practices [33].

The scheme promises free transport for pregnant women to health facilities; however, timely availability of ambulances is often lacking critically affecting maternal and newborn health outcomes during emergencies. Despite the intent to provide zero-cost services, many beneficiaries report incurring significant out-of-pocket expenses for medications, diagnostics, and other necessary care not covered under the scheme. A study conducted in Lucknow showed that only 7% of the eligible women reported utilization of SUMAN services, only 54% received free drugs and 80% did not receive free transportation [33].

Janani Suraksha Yojana (JSY)

Janani Suraksha Yojana (JSY) is a safe motherhood intervention under the National Rural Health Mission (NRHM) being implemented to reduce maternal and neonatal mortality by promoting safe institutional delivery among poor pregnant women, especially those in rural and low-income areas. The programme provides financial support to encourage women to give birth in healthcare centres rather than at home. A cornerstone of the JSY programme is the provision of financial assistance to pregnant women, as an incentive for institutional deliveries. In rural areas, women receive Rs. 1400, while in urban areas, the amount is Rs. 1000. The programme has identified ASHA workers as the key facilitators to mobilize beneficiaries and ensure uptake of services by them [34, 35].

Under JSY scheme, ASHAs are incentivized to identify the pregnant woman as a beneficiary, counsel her for institutional delivery and facilitate registration for ANC; assist in obtaining necessary certifications; provide and/or help the women receive at least three ANC checkups including TT injections, IFA tablets; identify a functional Government health centre or an accredited private health institution for referral and delivery; escort the beneficiary woman to the pre-determined health centre and stay with her till discharge; arrange to immunize the newborn till the age of 14 weeks; inform about the birth or death of the child or mother to the ANM/MO; conduct postnatal visit within 7 days of delivery to track mother's health after delivery and facilitate in obtaining care, wherever necessary; counsel for initiation of breastfeeding to the newborn within one hour of delivery and its continuance till 3 to 6 months and promote family planning [34].

JSY has been successful in promoting institutional deliveries with NFHS–5 data reporting that the institutional deliveries in India have risen to 89% [1]. The payments under JSY have been associated with a decline in perinatal and neonatal deaths. Trained personnel assisted deliveries and postnatal checkups have increased. Studies show that almost 70% beneficiaries know about the scheme with 88% utilization rate [35].

JSY coverage is highly variable across different regions with an overall utilization rate of only 36.4% in India. States like Jharkhand, Chhattisgarh, Bihar, and Uttar Pradesh exhibit very low coverage, highlighting socio-economic inequalities in access to services [36].

Implementation Gaps

Besides a general lack of awareness among women in rural areas, there are reports of delays in payment disbursement, discrepancies in eligibility criteria, and insufficient health facilities in remote areas. The conditional nature of the cash transfer can exclude certain vulnerable groups, such as younger mothers or those with more than two children [37].

Facilities lack essential resources such as emergency obstetric care and trained staff, leads to complications being referred to private facilities, which deters women from utilizing JSY services. High out-of-pocket costs continue to burden families despite the cash transfer scheme. Many beneficiaries report incurring additional expenses for drugs, diagnostics, and user charges that exceed the cash incentive provided by JSY. Poor programme management has been highlighted, including inadequate monitoring of fund allocation and irregular payments to ASHA workers which affects their motivation and performance [37, 38].

Janani Shishu Suraksha Karyakram (JSSK)

JSSK is a scheme launched by MoHFW, designed to eliminate out-of-pocket expenditure for pregnant women and sick infants who access public health facilities. This scheme entitles all pregnant women delivering in public health institutions to completely free and costless delivery including Caesarean section. It stipulates free drugs, diagnostics, blood, and diet, besides free transport from home to institution, between facilities in case of a referral and drop back home. All antenatal and postnatal complications are carefully addressed. The scheme includes all unwell newborns up to one year of age [39].

JSSK is operationalized through all public health facilities and is closely integrated with other maternal and child health services in both urban and rural areas. The scheme aims at benefitting almost 12 million pregnant women annually [39]. The data show a significant decline in maternal and infant mortality rates, especially among the low socio-economic communities. Utilizing JSSK facilities enhanced the uptake of free diagnostics, drugs, and transport services which have improved timely care-seeking behaviour and reduced financial hardship for families [40].

Implementation Gaps

The implementation of JSSK varies significantly across states with some regions facing more challenges than others in delivering the benefits effectively [40, 41]. Implementation challenges include financial constraints, inconsistent service quality, limited outreach in remote regions, understaffed hospitals, and lack of proper tracking of services provided. Due to inadequate access or awareness of JSSK benefits, a notable percentage of women still deliver at home or in private facilities though there has been an overall increase in institutional deliveries. For example, only 67% of deliveries occurred in government institutions in some areas as reported by Chaudhary et al., 2017 [39–41].

Significant out-of-pocket expenses are incurred by many beneficiaries, related to drugs, diagnostics, and user charges despite the scheme's intent to provide cashless services. A study indicated that 83.5% participants reported out-of-pocket expenditures during childbirth [41, 42]. Issues such as overcrowding in hospitals, lack of trained staff, and insufficient facilities like delays in emergency referrals, inconsistent quality of care, unreliable transport services, can deter women from utilizing JSSK services. Numerous beneficiaries have proposed enhancements in hospital management, and staff cooperation as well as more efficient grievance redressal [41, 42].

Pradhan Mantri Surakshit Matritva Abhiyan (PMSMA)

Pradhan Mantri Surakshit Matritva Abhiyan (PMSMA) was launched in 2016 to ensure quality antenatal care and high-risk pregnancy detection among pregnant women. Pregnant women can visit designated healthcare centres for checkups, tests, and doctor consultations on the 9th of every month. The programme ensures that pregnant women get proper care, helping to detect, and treat any health problems early. It is particularly useful for women in rural and low-income areas. ANC services are provided by OBGY specialists/radiologists/physicians with support from private sector doctors to supplement the efforts of the government sector. One of the critical components of the Abhiyan is the identification and follow-up of high-risk pregnancies [43].

The scheme targets to ensure that all pregnant women receive at least one complete ANC checkup done by a specialist in second or third trimester of pregnancy. The comprehensive checkup includes physical examination, laboratory investigations, TT immunization, IFA supplementation, and nutrition counselling. High-risk women are identified by a sticker system and linked to intensive follow-up and referral services [43].

Monthly PMSMA clinics are held at over 16,000 government health services where both public and private sector providers offer ANC services. Early ANC registrations and regular checkups are facilitated by community outreach and IEC/BCC campaigns. A strong monitoring and reporting framework support provides insights into the programme and guidance [43].

Since the inception of the programme, PMSMA has reached over 4.7 crore pregnant women, ensuring that majority of them get at least one ANC checkup done by a skilled provider. This has helped in improving the ANC coverage and identifying high-risk pregnancy at an early stage contributing to better maternal and neonatal health outcomes [43, 44].

Implementation Gaps

Some of the challenges identified in implementation of the programme include delayed disclosure of pregnancy, low availability of medical personnel, logistic issues and lack of infrastructure in remote or rural areas, and occasional shortages of medical supplies. Monitoring and evaluation of the programme needs to be strengthened along with spreading awareness about the programme among pregnant women.

Many women still face barriers and have limited access to PMSMA services due to geographical disparities, lack of awareness, or poor connectivity to health facilities. Some areas report low participation rates on designated PMSMA days. The quality of care provided can vary significantly between different facilities. Issues such as overcrowding, insufficiently trained staff, and inadequate laboratory infrastructure impact service delivery. Data show that only about one-third of pregnant women receive all recommended ANC components under PMSMA. Postnatal follow-up care remains inadequate in many regions. Data collection and management systems need to be improved to monitor service utilization effectively and assess the programme's overall impact on maternal health outcomes [44, 45].

LaQshya

MoHFW has launched LaQshya—Labour room quality improvement initiative in 2017, a focused and targeted approach to strengthen key processes related to labour rooms. Its main aim is to reduce preventable maternal and newborn deaths, morbidity and still births by improving the quality of care around child birth in labour rooms and maternity operation theatres. This programme is suitable for high delivery load facilities like medical colleges, district hospitals, etc. [46].

LaQshya's strategy includes infrastructure upgradation, ensuring essential equipment, adequate and skilled human resources, capacity building through regular training and simulations, and strict adherence to clinical protocols like essential newborn care, infection prevention, and maternity care. All these facilities are assessed using National Quality Assurance Standards (NQAS) and depending on the score, the facilities are awarded badges [46].

LaQshya's delivery model is phased and systematic: it starts with facility assessment and gap analysis, implements targeted interventions and rapid improvement cycles, builds capacity through training and simulations, and mandates continuous monitoring and audits through web-based dashboard and real-time reporting. Dedicated high-dependency units have been operationalized in higher-level facilities. A total of 283 obstetric high-dependency unit (HDU) /Intensive care unit (ICU) have been approved in high caseload tertiary care facilities including Government Medical College hospitals and district hospitals, across the country. This scheme has contributed to tangible improvements in quality of care and health outcomes. Facilities with certifications have shown reduced stillbirth rates and improved management of complications [47, 48].

Implementation Gaps

LaQshya fails to measure all issues of harmful practices and evidence-based care during labour, mistreatment of mothers or newborns during childbirth and support for women during childbirth. Lack of all measures to assess management of high-risk cases and birth complications in mothers and newborns is a concern. It also does not include performance-based measures to assess leadership, governance, and staff motivation [48].

Insufficient training and support for healthcare providers, lack of infrastructure to support comprehensive care, variability in the quality of implementation, and resistance to change among some healthcare providers have been some challenging issues in the implementation. Field assessments highlight gaps in infrastructure maintenance, periodic shortages of drugs and consumables, and inconsistent availability of trained staff, especially in remote and high-burden districts. Staff rotation and turnover disrupt continuity and team cohesion in labour rooms. Some facilities struggle to sustain improvements post-certification due to limited follow-up and refresher training. Beneficiary feedback reveals that communication and privacy standards are not uniformly met [47, 48].

Surveillance Systems for MCH

Information System for Maternal Health: For any programme to be successful, monitoring is instrumental not only in formulating programmes and policies but also in evaluating compliance and assessing their effectiveness. The Government of India has initiated various such surveillance systems related to monitoring maternal and child health.

Maternal Death Surveillance and Response (MDSR) has been implemented and institutionalized since 2017. All states have been provided with guidelines and tools for conducting community-and-facility-based MDSR and reporting deaths along with causes of death.

Name-based tracking of pregnant women has been initiated on the RCH portal/ MCTS Portal as a policy decision by the Government of India. This is to ensure appropriate MNCH services such as timely ANC, institutional delivery, and PNC along with immunization and other related services.

Maternal and child protection card (MCP Card)*:* An MCP card has been launched for documenting and monitoring services for antenatal, intranatal, and postnatal care of pregnant women, immunization, and growth monitoring of infants. This card helps empower women with knowledge about MCH services, recognizing danger signs, and ensuring access to essential healthcare resources to promote the health and well-being of both mother and child.

Apart from MoHFW, the Ministry of Woman and Child Development (MoWCD) is also working towards holistic development of the mother–child dyad, especially those belonging to the lower socio-economic strata. Many programmes, plans, guides, etc., have been formulated by the MoWCD. Some of their programmes for maternal well-being are discussed here.

Pradhan Mantri Matru Vandana Yojana (PMMVY)

Pradhan Mantri Matru Vandana Yojana (PMMVY), launched in 2017, aims to provide financial support to socially and economically disadvantaged pregnant women and lactating mothers to improve their health and nutrition. The primary objectives of PMMVY include financial assistance to compensate for wage loss, to enable women to rest adequately before and after childbirth, promoting better health outcomes for both the mother and the child, encourage institutional deliveries and post-delivery vaccination of the infant [49].

The scheme encourages families to prioritize the health of the girl child by offering additional incentives for families with female children. Eligible women receive cash benefit of Rs 5000/- for the first live birth and again for the second child in case of a girl child. The benefit is transferred to the woman in 3 instalments and is linked to achieving health milestones—pregnancy registration and first ANC, child birth registration and completion of first cycle of immunization [49].

The scheme is implemented through a digital platform (PMMVY-CAS), where the frontline workers (Anganwadi Workers, ASHAs, ANMs) help in beneficiary identification, registration, and documentation. Payments are processed via Direct Benefit Transfer (DBT) into Aadhaar-linked bank or post office accounts, ensuring transparency and reducing leakages. The implementation guidelines emphasize timely processing and verification at each administrative level, with monitoring through a web-based Management Information System (MIS) [49].

Studies indicate that this scheme has helped in increasing the utilization of services like antenatal care, institutional deliveries, and childhood immunization. This has improved the health of both the mother and child, reduced their financial burden and is helping in their behaviour change towards using free medical facilities [50, 51].

Implementation of this scheme has raised many challenges such as delays in cash transfer, issues with the DBT system, reaching remote or isolated areas as well as lack of awareness among beneficiaries. Many women in, especially in rural areas, are still unaware of the scheme or face difficulty in arranging the documents as they are illiterate. Studies show that both monitoring system and grievance redressal mechanisms are weak and inadequate which leads to dissatisfaction among beneficiaries [50, 51].

POSHAN Abhiyan

POSHAN stands for Prime Minister's Overarching Scheme for Holistic Nutrition. Launched on March 8, 2018, POSHAN Abhiyan (National Nutrition Mission) aims to reduce malnutrition, i.e. stunting, wasting, underweight and anaemia prevalence in India, especially among children under six years, pregnant women, and lactating mothers. POSHAN Abhiyan uses a multi-ministerial approach and focuses on eliminating malnutrition, using technology for robust monitoring and improve service delivery. The programme encourages community participation through events and awareness campaigns to educate people about nutrition and healthy eating habits. The POSHAN tracker app allows monitoring, verification of the beneficiary and helps in transparent distribution of take-home rations [52, 53].

The scheme aligns with Mission Saksham Anganwadi and POSHAN 2.0 integrating health and nutrition along with community efforts in the form of Jan Andolan, POSHAN Maah/Pakhwada, and behavioural change at the grassroots. A helpline number has also been created along with SMS alerts for ration delivery accountability and beneficiary feedback [53].

The scheme now covers almost all states and UTs. The Jan Andolan activities have catalysed nutrition-related behaviour change thus promoting good healthcare services. The NFHS 5 data show that there is decline in stunting, wasting, and underweight prevalence among children under 5 years in some states. However, populous states have shown rise in stunting and underweight prevalence. All beneficiaries may not be covered due to lack of staff or proper training. Deep rooted cultural practices affect the interventions adversely [53, 54].

POSHAN Abhiyan 2.0

POSHAN Abhiyan 2.0 also known as Mission Saksham Anganwadi was launched in 2021. It builds on the original programme by integrating various nutrition-related schemes—Anganwadi services, POSHAN Abhiyan, Scheme for Adolescent Girls—under one umbrella for better coordination. This phase emphasizes maternal nutrition, infant feeding practices, and treatment for malnutrition, creating a more comprehensive approach to tackling nutritional issues [53, 55].

The main aim of POSHAN 2.0 is to enhance the nutritional status of vulnerable groups namely—Children (0–6 years), pregnant women, lactating mothers, and adolescent girls (14–18 years) while ensuring better delivery of services through improved governance and capacity-building efforts in aspirational districts and all districts of north east region. POSHAN 2.0 includes strategies such as improving maternal nutrition, infant and young child feeding practices, food diversity, promoting traditional food practices, and using digital tools for tracking nutritional outcomes. It emphasizes on Early Childhood Care and Education (3–6 years); and Anganwadi infrastructure including modern and upgraded Saksham Anganwadi. Similar to the first phase, this programme encourages community involvement through awareness campaigns and events that promote good nutrition practices [53, 55].

Some Key Features for Maternal Well-Being Under Poshan 2.0 Include

- *Focus on Maternal Nutrition:* POSHAN 2.0 emphasizes maternal nutrition as a critical factor in reducing anaemia and improving health outcomes. It includes interventions like Iron Folic Acid (IFA) supplementation to combat deficiencies, supplementary nutrition to pregnant women and lactating mothers, ensuring they receive essential nutrients.
- *Community Engagement:* The programme promotes community involvement through awareness campaigns and events like Poshan Maah, fostering a supportive environment for maternal health.
- *Integrated Services:* By combining Anganwadi Services and the Scheme for Adolescent Girls, POSHAN 2.0 ensures that mothers receive comprehensive care, including health education, and access to healthcare services.
- *Monitoring and Evaluation:* The use of digital tools like the Poshan Tracker allows for real-time monitoring of beneficiaries, ensuring effective delivery of services and timely interventions [53, 55].

The facilities provided under POSHAN 2.0 include supplementary nutrition for the beneficiaries which includes provision of hot-cooked meals, take-home rations and quality-tested food. Programmes like Jan Andolan, Poshan Maah, and Poshan Pakhwada are organized with specific themes for mass mobilization and behaviour change. The CAS tracker helps in real-time beneficiary tracking and addressing their problems. Functionaries at block, district, and state levels monitor and discuss progress and issues across various departments [53].

The NFHS 5 data show that stunting, wasting, and underweight among children under five has reduced significantly. There is transparency in beneficiary verification and transparent ration distribution through POSHAN tracker. By March 2025, the scheme covered the entire country. Renovation and modernization of Anganwadi centres is going on with focus on infrastructure, digital tools, and quality assurance.

Implementation Challenges

ICDS being universalized all over India has a huge coverage which also brings about several implementational challenges. Inadequate infrastructure, staff, and insufficient training are serious concerns. The availability of suitable infrastructure in all the implementation areas is a big challenge. Since the programme is holistic, it involves coordination between different service providers, which sometimes becomes difficult, leading to problems like inconsistent supply of nutrition, uneven access to health care, etc. [53, 54].

Conclusion and Way Forward

The strategies which may work to improve maternal health during pregnancy have to be multi-faceted in the Indian context, where complications including anaemia, morbidity, and mortality in the mother–child dyad are quite high. Some key interventions which may contribute to improving maternal health during pregnancy include the following:

- *Iron and Folic Acid (IFA) Supplementation to Begin in Adolescence:* Apart from giving IFA supplementation to pregnant women, there is a need to focus on women before they conceive. Thus, we need to have a preconception programme targeting women of reproductive age, including adolescent girls for either continuous or intermittent IFA supplementation.
- *Dietary Diversification:* Enhancing diet diversity by promoting the consumption of a variety of food groups will ensure the intake of all nutrients in appropriate amounts throughout the year and will also help to overcome micronutrient deficiencies among pregnant women and their offspring.
- *Behavioural Change Communication (BCC) Campaigns*: Such campaigns at PHCs, Anganwadis, and community centres will help to generate awareness of healthy eating practices among pregnant women and adolescent girls. These campaigns should focus on dietary improvement and early detection of anaemia or any other pregnancy-related complications as well as planning and managing a healthy pregnancy.
- *Food Fortification: Double-fortified salt (DFS),* which is fortified with both iron and iodine, should be made easily accessible so as to improve the iron intake of women. The fortification of staple foods like wheat flour and rice with iron and other micronutrients can easily integrate into the daily diets of women during pregnancy or even before conception without requiring significant dietary changes. Including DFS or iron fortified rice through government programmes like the Public Distribution System (PDS), or in ICDS should be encouraged.

- *Screening and Early Detection:* Routine screening for malnutrition including underweight, anaemia, and obesity in adolescent girls and women of reproductive age should be done. This will help detect and treat any complications before conception and reduce those during pregnancy.
- *Access to Health Services*: Improving access to healthcare for women through PHCs especially in rural areas will ensure early detection and management of risk factors during pregnancy as well as institutional deliveries. Mechanisms should be put in place to discourage caesarean deliveries unless warranted by medical reasons.
- *Subsidized Seasonal Foods:* The high cost of nutritious foods, especially vegetables, prevents their adequate intake. Subsidizing seasonal perishable food items and fortified non-perishable ones can help improve the nutritional status of pregnant women.
- *Support for Women in Rural Areas:* Initiatives like facilitating health workers' home visits and mobile health units can help in improving the health of pregnant women in difficult-to-access areas.
- *Addressing Mental Health:* Stress, anxiety, and depression can affect both the mother and the baby. Addressing mental health is another aspect which should be mandatory for all pregnant women as a part of an antenatal checkup.

These strategies must be integrated into broader public health frameworks and supported by government programmes, making it easier for women to access the necessary resources for combating any complications during pregnancy or before conception. Further, increasing focus on nutrition of adolescent girls, improving access to nutrient rich foods, biofortification, and a better public distribution system can help improve maternal nutrition outcomes, including positive intergenerational effects.

References

1. International Institute for Population Sciences (IIPS) & ICF. (2021). *National Family Health Survey (NFHS-5), 2019–21*, India.
2. Bhaskar, S. (2022). *First 1000 Days of Life: Importance of Maternal and Child Nutrition During Pregnancy and up to Two Years of Age.* https://swachhindia.ndtv.com/first-1000-days-of-life-importance-of-maternal-and-child-nutrition-during-pregnancy-and-up-to-two-years-of-age-50895/
3. Likhar, A., & Patil, M. S. (2022). Importance of Maternal Nutrition in the First 1000 Days of Life and Its Effects on Child Development: A Narrative Review. *Cureus, 14*(10), Article e30083. https://doi.org/10.7759/cureus.30083
4. Khekade, H., et al. (2023). Preconception Care: A Strategic Intervention for the Prevention of Neonatal and Birth Disorders. *Cureus, 15*(6), Article e41141. https://doi.org/10.7759/cureus.41141
5. Singh, T. (2023). *The State of Maternal Health in India. Economic and Political Weekly.* https://www.epw.in
6. UNICEF. (2024). *India: Maternal Mortality and Health Disparities.* UNICEF India. https://www.unicef.org/india

7. Nguyen, P. H., et al. (2021). Maternal Diets in India: Gaps, Barriers, and Opportunities. *Nutrients, 13*(10), 3528. https://doi.org/10.3390/nu13103528
8. Hamal, M., et al. (2020). Social Determinants of Maternal Health: A Scoping Review of Factors Influencing Maternal Mortality and Maternal Health Service Use in India. *Public Health Reviews, 41*(1), 13. https://doi.org/10.1186/s40985-020-00125-6
9. https://nhm.gov.in/index1.php?lang=1&level=3&sublinkid=1024&lid=388
10. Khapre, M., Shewade, H. D., Kishore, S., Ramaswamy, G., & Dongre, A. R. (2020). Understanding Barriers in Implementation and Scaling up of Weekly Iron and Folic Acid Supplementation (WIFS) Programme Among Adolescent Girls in a City of North India: A Mixed-Method Study. *Journal of Family Medicine and Primary Care., 9*(3), 1497–1509.
11. Sudfeld, C. R., et al. (2020). Population-Level Effective Coverage of Adolescent Weekly Iron and Folic Acid Supplementation is Low in Rural West Bengal, India. *Journal of Family Medicine and Primary Care, 9*(3), 1497–1509. https://doi.org/10.4103/jfmpc.jfmpc_1144_19
12. Shah, T., Prajapati, B., & Shah, V. (2022). Situational Analysis of Rashtriya Kishor Swasthya Karyakram at One of the Districts of Gujarat. *Indian Journal of Community Medicine, 47*(4), 543–548. https://doi.org/10.4103/ijcm.ijcm_18_22
13. Khapre, M., et al. (2022). Understanding Barriers in Implementation and Scaling Up WIFS from Providers' Perspective: A Mixed-Method Study, Rishikesh, India. *Indian Journal of Community Medicine, 47*(4), 543–548. https://doi.org/10.4103/ijcm.ijcm_370_22
14. National Health Mission. (n.d.). *Operational Framework for Weekly Iron and Folic Acid Supplementation (WIFS).* https://nhm.gov.in/images/pdf/programmes/wifs/operational-framework-wifs/operational_framework_wifs.pdf
15. https://nhm.gov.in/images/pdf/programmes/RKSK/RKSK_Operational_Framework.pdf
16. National Health Mission, Assam. (n.d.). *Rashtriya Kishor Swasthya Karyakram (RKSK).* https://nhm.assam.gov.in/schemes/detail/rashtriya-kishore-swasthya-karyakram-rksk
17. Barua, A., Watson, K., Plesons, M., et al. (2020). Adolescent Health Programming in India: A Rapid Review. *Reproductive Health, 17*(1), 87.
18. National Health Mission, Ministry of Health and Family Welfare, Government of India. (2020). *School Health & Wellness Programme.* https://nhm.gov.in/index1.php?lang=1&level=3&sublinkid=1384&lid=746
19. UNESCO. (2025). *15 million Learners, One Mission: School Health and Wellness Programme.* UNESCO. https://www.unesco.org/en/articles/15-million-learners-one-mission-school-health-and-wellness-programme
20. Ministry of Health and Family Welfare & Ministry of Human Resource Development. (2018). *Operational Guidelines on School Health Programme under Ayushman Bharat Health and Wellness Ambassadors Partnering to Build a Stronger Future.* In Operational Guidelines [Report]. https://nhm.gov.in/New_Updates_2018/NHM_Components/RMNCHA/AH/guidelines/Operational_guidelines_on_School_Health_Programme_under_Ayushman_Bharat.pdf
21. National Health Mission. (n.d.). https://nhm.hp.gov.in/rksk/school-health-wellness-ambassador-shwa
22. Jain, N., Bahl, D., & Mehta, R., et al. (2022). Progress and Challenges In Implementing Adolescent and School Health Programmes in India: A Rapid Review. *BMJ Open, 12*, e047435. https://doi.org/10.1136/bmjopen-2020-047435
23. Anemia Mukt Bharat. (n.d.). https://anemiamuktbharat.info/
24. International Institute for Population Sciences (IIPS) and ICF. (2017). *National Family Health Survey (NFHS-4), 2015–16: India.* IIPS.
25. Joe, W., Rinju, N. P., Alambusha, R., Kulkarni, B., Yadav, K., & Sethi, V. (2022). Coverage of Iron and Folic Acid Supplementation in India: Progress Under the Anemia Mukt Bharat strategy 2017–20. *Health Policy and Planning, 37*(5), 597–606. https://doi.org/10.1093/heapol/czac015
26. Neogi, S. B., Babre, A., Varghese, M., et al. (2022). Improving the Approach to Assess Impact of Anaemia Control Programs During Pregnancy in India: A Critical Analysis. *BMC Pregnancy and Childbirth, 22*, 966. https://doi.org/10.1186/s12884-022-05248-z
27. Mission Indradhanush. https://missionindradhanush.in/

28. Intensified Mission Indradhanush-Operational Guidelines. https://nhm.gov.in/New_Updates_2018/NHM_Components/Immunization/Guildelines_for_immunization/Mission_Indradhanush_Guidelines.pdf
29. Ministry of Health & Family Welfare, Update on Mission Indradhanush. https://mohfw.gov.in/?q=en/pressrelease-168
30. Gurnani, V., Haldar, P., Aggarwal, M. K., Das, M. K., Chauhan, A., Murray, J., Arora, N. K., Jhalani, M., & Sudan, P. (2018). Improving Vaccination Coverage in India: Lessons from Intensified Mission Indradhanush, a Cross-Sectoral Systems Strengthening Strategy. *BMJ*, k4782. https://doi.org/10.1136/bmj.k4782
31. National Health Mission. (2020). Surakshit Matritva Aashwasan (SUMAN) standard operating guidelines. Ministry of Health and Family Welfare, Government of India. https://nhm.gov.in/New_Updates_2018/NHM_Components/RMNCHA/MH/Guidelines/SUMAN%20Guideline%202020%20Web%20Version.pdf
32. Ministry of health and Family Welfare. Surakshit Matritva Aashwasan (SUMAN) https://suman.mohfw.gov.in/
33. Verma, R., & Singh, S. (2024). Barriers to Utilization of the SUMAN Scheme Among Pregnant Women in Rural India: A Cross-Sectional Study. *Indian Journal of Public Health, 68*(1), 45–51.
34. National Health Mission (Ministry of Health & Family Welfare, Government of India. (n.d.). *Janani Suraksha Yojana*. https://www.nhm.gov.in/index1.php?lang=1&level=3&lid=309&sublinkid=841
35. Dangi, M. K., Keerti, Upadhyay, M., Prajapati, J., Choudhary, S., & Nagal, R. (2024). A study to assess the awareness and uptake of Janani Suraksha Yojana among the women attending a tertiary care hospital. *International Journal of Community Medicine and Public Health, 11*(12), 4869–4874. https://doi.org/10.18203/2394-6040.ijcmph20243657
36. Mishra, P. S., Kumar, P., & Srivastava, S. (2021). Regional Inequality in the Janani Suraksha Yojana Coverage in India: A Geo-Spatial Analysis. *International Journal for Equity in Health, 20*, 24. https://doi.org/10.1186/s12939-020-01366-2
37. National Health Systems Resource Centre. (2021). *Evaluation of the Janani Suraksha Yojana (JSY) Program: A Report on the Findings*. https://nhsrcindia.org/sites/default/files/2021-03/JSY%20Programme%20Evaluation.pdf
38. National Health Mission. (2021). *Guidelines for Implementation of the Janani Suraksha Yojana (JSY) Program*. https://nhm.gov.in/WriteReadData/l892s/7861979062147487 2646.pdf
39. National Health Mission (MoHFW). (2025). *Janani Shishu Suraksha Karyakaram (JSSK)*. New Delhi. https://nhm.gov.in/index1.php?lang=1&level=3&sublinkid=842&lid=308#:~:text=Janani%20Shishu%20Suraksha%20Karyakaram%20(JSSK)%20launched%20on%201st%20June%2C,expense%20delivery%2C%20including%20caesarean%20section
40. Press Information Bureau. (2020). *Janani Shishu Suraksha Karyakaram*. Ministry of Health and Family Welfare, Government of India. https://www.pib.gov.in/PressReleasePage.aspx?PRID=1606211#:~:text=Janani%20Shishu%20Suraksha%20Karyakaram%20(JSSK,all%20kinds%20of%20User%20Charges
41. Chaudhary, S., et al. (2017). Evaluation of Janani Shishu Suraksha Karyakram Scheme and Out-of-pocket Expenditure in a Rural Area of Northern India. *Journal of Family Medicine and Primary Care, 6*(3), 477–481. https://doi.org/10.4103/2249-4863.222010
42. Joshi, U., Shah, T., Gohil, V., Sharma, R. Y., & Shah, V. R. (2025Apr 23). Strengths, Weaknesses, Opportunities, and Challenges of Conditional Cash Transfers Under the Janani Shishu Suraksha Karyakram in India: A Narrative Review. *Cureus, 17*(4), Article e82874. https://doi.org/10.7759/cureus.82874
43. Ministry of Health & Family Welfare, Government of India. (2016). *Pradhan Mantri Surakshit Matritva Abhiyan (PMSMA) Operational Guidelines*. MoHFW, Maternal Health Division. https://pmsma.mohfw.gov.in/about-scheme/
44. Press Information Bureau (2024). *Update on Pradhan Mantri Surakshit Matritva Abhiyan (PMSMA)*. Government of India, Ministry of Health and Family Welfare. https://pib.gov.in/Pressreleaseshare.aspx?PRID=2040949

45. Dandona, R., Majumder, M., Akbar, M., Bhattacharya, D., Nanda, P., Kumar, G. A., & Dandona, L. (2022). Assessment of Quality of Antenatal Care Services in Public Sector Facilities in India. *British Medical Journal Open, 12*(12), Article e065200. https://doi.org/10.1136/bmjopen-2022-065200
46. Ministry of Health & Family Welfare, Government of India. (2017). *LaQshya—Labour Room Quality Improvement Initiative: Guidelines.* National Health Mission, MoHFW. https://www.nhm.gov.in/index1.php?lang=1&level=3&sublinkid=1307&lid=690
47. Press Information Bureau (PIB), Government of India. (2018). *Press Release: LaQshya Initiative Showing Tangible Impact on Maternal and Newborn Outcomes.* PIB.
48. Singh, S., Hasan, Z., Sharma, D., et al. (2024). Appraising LaQshya's Potential in Measuring Quality of Care for Mothers and Newborns: A Comprehensive Review of India's Labor Room Quality Improvement Initiative. *BMC Pregnancy and Childbirth, 24*, 239. https://doi.org/10.1186/s12884-024-06450-x
49. National Institute of Rural Development & Panchayati Raj (NIRDPR). (2021). *PMMVY-CAS: Implementation Guidelines for Pradhan Mantri Matru Vandana Yojana.* NIRDPR. https://nirdpr.org.in/crru/docs/health/PMMVY%20Scheme%20Implemetation%20Guidelines.pdf
50. Jagannath, R., & Chakravarthy, V. (2025). The Impact of Pradhan Mantri Matru Vandana Yojna Scheme on Access to Services Among Mothers and Children and Their Improved Health and Nutritional Outcomes. *Frontiers in Nutrition, 11*, 1513815. https://doi.org/10.3389/fnut.2024.1513815
51. Shruthi, M. V., Dakshayini, S., & Dharmoji, T. Y. (2024). *Performance of Pradhan Mantri Matru Vandana Yojana: An Empirical Evaluation in Karnataka. The Economics Journal*, 7(1), 126–131. https://doi.org/10.33545/26179210.2024.v7.i1.273
52. Ministry of Women and Child Development, Government of India. (n.d.). *POSHAN Abhiyaan.* https://poshanabhiyaan.gov.in/
53. Ministry of Women and Child Development, Government of India. (n.d.). https://wcd.gov.in/offerings/nutrition-mission-saksham-anganwadi-and-poshan-2-0-mission-saksham-anganwadi-poshan-2-0
54. Dhingra, S., & Chandna, H. (2021, February 24). Modi govt's POSHAN scheme needs attention, states used only 40 % funds, NITI Aayog says. *ThePrint.* https://theprint.in/india/governance/modi-govts-poshan-scheme-needs-attention-states-used-only-40-funds-niti-aayog-says/610521
55. Ministry of Women and Child Development, Government of India. *Mission Saksham Anganwadi and Poshan 2.0.* Scheme guidelines https://cdnbbsr.s3waas.gov.in/s34c144c47ecba6f8318128703ca9e2601/uploads/2024/12/202412111663461918.pdf

Chapter 9
Child Nutrition in India: Understanding the Policy Ecosystem

Ananya Awasthi and Shoba Suri

Introduction

A discussion on India's nutrition policy should rightly begin with the constitutional mandate of the country. While the Indian constitution contains legal provisions that directly address health and nutrition, the "Directive Principles of State Policy" stands out in this regard. Article 47 states: "The State shall regard the raising of the level of nutrition and the standard of living of its people and the improvement of public health as among its primary duties …". Thereafter, successive "Five Year Plans" by the Planning Commission, which is India's nodal authority for policy planning, did acknowledge the need for addressing wide-spread undernutrition among pregnant women and young children. The stated objective of the seventh Five Year plan was to enhance the labor force's productivity and reduce infant and maternal mortality. Historically, from a policy perspective, nutrition has been perceived and understood more for its "instrumental" role rather than its "intrinsic" value [28].

Moreover, for many decades in post-independent India, nutrition was predominantly viewed through the lens of food security. Food policy, especially with the advent of the "Green Revolution" and "Public Distribution Systems (PDS)", prioritized self-sufficiency of staple grains like rice and wheat, rather than adopting a more holistic approach to nutrition. Consequently, food policy historically emphasized calorie sufficiency, leaving much to be desired in promoting balanced diets, micronutrient sufficiency, and nutrition security [29].

A. Awasthi (✉)
Anuvaad Solutions, New Delhi, India
e-mail: awasthi@anuvaad.org.in

S. Suri
Observer Research Foundation, New Delhi, India
e-mail: shoba.suri@orfonline.org

S. Suri (ed.), *Child Health and Nutrition from Conception to Age Two*,
https://doi.org/10.1007/978-981-95-7868-9_9

Evolution of Nutrition Policy in India

Establishment of the Integrated Child Development Services (ICDS) in 1975 marked a significant milestone in early childcare. Initially launched in select blocks, it was later expanded nationwide, becoming a leading government program in delivering comprehensive services for childcare, health and nutrition, and early education. The program primarily targets women and children, with services delivered through dedicated Anganwadi Centers [23].

A notable milestone in the evolution of the policy landscape in India is the launch of National Nutrition Policy in 1993. The policy document highlights that a very progressive approach was taken back then to demonstrate multi-factorial causality of malnutrition and highlight its inter-linkages with the agricultural and food systems. Moreover, this policy document also emphasized addressing the socio-economic determinants of malnutrition [18].

From a policy perspective, the next major milestone was launch of the "National Nutrition Strategy" by NITI Aayog in 2017, which highlighted a "target-driven approach" for improving nutritional outcomes. Some of the key monitorable targets included reduction in child undernutrition and prevalence of anemia, both in young children and adolescents and in women of reproductive age [31]. In 2018, this evolved into the launch of GOI's flagship program called the Poshan Abhiyaan or POSHAN (Prime Minister's Overarching Scheme for Holistic Nutrition) which aimed at improving the nutritional outcomes of children, adolescents, and pregnant and lactating women. Major highlights of Poshan Abhiyan included a focus on mapping high impact nutrition interventions targeting the first thousand days, leveraging technology for delivery of these interventions, investing in capacity building of front-line workers, promoting multi-sectoral convergence, and driving behavior change communication [1].

A key aspect of the nutrition landscape in India is the placement of the nutrition mission and programs within the Ministry of Women and Child Development (MoWCD). This dedicated ministry is responsible for formulating and implementing policies and programs that promote the welfare and development of women and children. In addition to the nutrition program, the MoWCD also oversees programs such as the Beti Bachao Beti Padhao for promoting the welfare of the girl child, the Pradhan Mantri Matru Vandana Yojana (PMMVY) that provides maternity benefit transfers, and various other programs focused on child protection, women's safety, and women's empowerment [19].

Mission Saksham Anganwadi and Poshan 2.0

After the launch of Poshan Abhiyaan, MoWCD in 2022 merged the erstwhile Poshan Abhiyaan with the ICDS program into an integrated nutrition support program (INSP) called Mission Saksham Anganwadi and Poshan 2.0.

Elaborating on the rationale behind the new guidelines, Poshan 2.0 highlights that nutrition policies have remained unchanged over the years, showing limited progress toward adopting a more integrated approach to nutritional security. The guidelines state that past interventions have not been sufficient in delivering quality services, focusing primarily on ensuring calorie sufficiency while often neglecting dietary diversity and the promotion of large-scale behavioral changes to improve nutritional outcomes. Consequently, the current calorie-driven approach has resulted in a noticeable absence of micronutrients in both Take-Home Rations (THR) and Hot Cooked Meals (HCM). Furthermore, the guidelines highlight that traditional knowledge related to nutrition remains underutilized, and the scheme's implementation has been hindered by limited involvement of beneficiaries and local stakeholders, reflecting inadequate community ownership of Anganwadi activities. A critical challenge flagged by Poshan 2.0 is the poor implementation of the nutrition program, marked by the absence of last-mile tracking.

The stated vision of the Mission Poshan 2.0 guidelines is to align India's development trajectory with the UN Sustainable Development Goals (SDGs). Poshan 2.0 guidelines particularly highlighted the need for contributing toward the achievement of SDG 2 on zero hunger and SDG 4 on quality education. The major stated objectives of the Poshan 2.0 guidelines are:

- Contribute to human capital development.
- Address the challenges of malnutrition.
- Promote nutrition awareness and good eating habits.
- Address nutrition-related deficiencies.

Poshan 2.0 consolidates existing schemes into four primary verticals: (1) Nutrition support for POSHAN through the Supplementary Nutrition Programme (SNP), (2) Early childhood care and education, (3) Anganwadi Infrastructure with upgraded Saksham Anganwadis, and (4) Poshan Abhiyaan. These verticals aim to streamline efforts and enhance the effectiveness of the integrated nutrition support initiatives. The target beneficiaries of Poshan 2.0 continue to be children in the age group of 0–6 years, pregnant women (PW) and lactating mothers (LM). In addition, adolescent girls (14–18 years) residing in high burden "aspirational districts" and Northeastern states have now been included as a target beneficiary.

Additionally, Poshan 2.0 identifies several focus areas—maternal nutrition, Infant and Young Child Feeding (IYCF) norms, treatment of moderate acute malnutrition (MAM) and severe acute malnutrition (SAM), and wellness through Ayurveda, Yoga, Naturopathy, Unani, Siddha, and Homeopathy (AYUSH). Additionally, the guidelines outline several core strategies to combat malnutrition, including interventions to correct "nutrition related deficiencies", initiatives to raise awareness and encourage healthy dietary habits for "sustainable health and well-being", communication strategies and building "green eco-systems" and "Poshan Vatikas" [12].

Anganwadi Services

The Anganwadi Services, formerly known as ICDS, have long been a cornerstone in provision of early childcare in India. The key services covered under the Anganwadi services include, supplementary nutrition, health and nutrition education, immunization and supplementation, health check-ups, and referral services and preschool education [23].

Supplementary Nutrition Program

The Supplementary Nutrition Program (SNP) represents the most critical component of Anganwadi Services. With the goal of meeting the Recommended Dietary Allowance (RDA) as against the Average Daily Intake (ADI), SNP is delivered in three major formats: Take-home Rations (THR), Hot Cooked Meals (HCM), and Morning Snacks. According to Poshan 2.0 guidelines, beneficiaries who are entitled to receive the supplementary nutrition include, pregnant women, lactating mothers, children between the ages of 6 months to 3 years, children with acute malnutrition (SAM category) and adolescent girls aged 14–18 years (where applicable). Whereas older children between the ages of 3–6 years are mandated to receive HCM and morning snacks in their local AWC. Moreover, supplementary nutrition must be provided for at least 300 days a year, averaging 25 days per month. Eligibility to receive SNP is restricted to beneficiaries registered at the AWC.

Most importantly, Poshan 2.0 guidelines mandate that THR must be distinguished from raw rations like provision of rice or wheat. To achieve this distinction, Poshan 2.0 provides several recommendations for diversifying the THR and HCM preparations by encouraging the inclusion of green vegetables, fruits, cereals, pulses, millets, nuts, fats, medicinal plants and herbs. It mandates that millets may be included in the SNP preparations, at least once a week. The guidelines also advocate for replacing the white sugar with other alternatives like jaggery for sweetening and promoting the consumption of healthy nuts and oilseeds [12].

Nutrient Norms for SNP

SNP is provided to beneficiaries in accordance with the nutritional norms outlined in Schedule II of the National Food Security Act, 2013. These norms were updated on 25 January 2023. A detailed description of nutrition norms for SNP is provided in Tables 9.1 A and 1 B [17].

Table 9.1 SNP norms for macronutrients

Category	Type of SNP	Calories (Kcal)	Protein (g)	Fat (g)	Carbohydrate (g)
Children (6–12 months)	THR	200	8–10	10–12	20
Children (1–3 years)	THR	400	15–20	15–20	40
Children (3–6 years)	Morning snack and HCM	400	15–20	15–20	55
Undernourished children (6–12 months)	THR	400	15–20	15–18	35
Undernourished children (1–3 years)	THR	700	25–30	25–30	70
Undernourished children (3–6 years)	Morning snack, HCM and THR	800	25–30	25–30	70
Adolescent girls (14–18 years)	THR	600	18–20	–	-
Pregnant women and lactating mothers	HCM and THR	600	22–25	22–25	80

Source National Food Security Act (2023)

Cost Norms for SNP

Cost norms for the Supplementary Nutrition Programme continue to follow the rates approved in 2017, with unit costs ranging from ₹8 per day for children, ₹9.5 per day for pregnant and lactating women, and up to ₹12 per day for children in the acutely malnourished category [12]. Recent economic analyses suggest that while diversification of food baskets is mandated by the new policy guidelines, the *economic feasibility* of achieving dietary diversity through social safety programs like ICDS remains low, given the current budgetary allocations [26].

Health and Nutrition Education

It is a key activity which focuses on empowering new mothers with essential knowledge, health-seeking behaviors and practices that promote the well-being of mother and child. Anganwadi Workers (AWWs), through interpersonal counseling, group sessions, and home visits, educate mothers about exclusive breastfeeding and complementary feeding, which are crucial for the proper development of their newborns. Counseling also aids in the management of children with SAM; ensuring mothers are well equipped to address these critical health concerns. Home visits facilitate interpersonal communication and nutrition promotion, reinforcing adherence to evidence-based practices for maternal and child nutrition.

Three other Anganwadi Services are provided in convergence with the Ministry of Health and Family Welfare (MoHFW) through a concerted effort by community

Table 9.2 SNP norms for micronutrients

Category	Type of Meal	Calcium (mg)	Zinc (mg)	Iron (mg)	Dietary Folate (µg)	Vitamin A (µg)	Vitamin B6 (mg)	Vitamin B12 (µg)
Children (6–12 months)	THR	100	0.7	0.7	24	57	0.17	0.33
Children (1–3 years)	THR	135	1.0	2.0	35	60	0.27	0.33
Children (3–6 years)	Morning snack and HCM	150	1.5	3.0	40	80	0.33	0.67
Undernourished children (6–12 months)	THR	200	1.5	1.5	50	115	0.35	0.66
Undernourished children (1–3 years)	THR	270	2.0	4.0	70	120	0.55	0.66
Undernourished children (3–6 years)	Morning snack, HCM and THR	300	3.0	6	80	160	0.66	1.24
Pregnant women and lactating mothers	HCM and THR	335	4.0	7	160	240	0.63	0.73

Source National Food Security Act (2023)

health workers—AWWs, ASHAs (Accredited Social Health Activists), and ANMs (Auxiliary Nurse Midwives).

Immunization and Supplementation

Safeguarding the health of children by preventing serious and potentially life-threatening diseases relies heavily on immunization and supplementation. Primary immunization for children, bi-annual Vitamin A supplementation for those aged 9 months to 5 years, and the provision of IFA (Iron Folic Acid) syrup twice a week for children aged 6 months to 5 years are part of the standard protocol for services available at the AWCs. Additionally, bi-annual deworming tablets are given to children between the ages of 1 and 5 years. For pregnant women, IFA supplements are administered from the fourth month of pregnancy until six months postpartum, along with two tetanus toxoid shots to ensure both maternal and neonatal health. In addition, monthly Village Health Sanitation and Nutrition Days (VHSND) are organized to provide comprehensive health services.

Health Check Ups

Another key service provided at the AWCs is the health check-up of children. This includes identification and special management of acutely malnourished children, antenatal care for expectant mothers, postnatal care of nursing mothers, and diarrhea management by providing ORS and Zinc supplementation.

Health Services and Referral

For providing comprehensive care to mothers and children, health services and referrals play a crucial role. This includes antenatal and postnatal care, counseling for pregnancy, lactation, and infant feeding, managing SAM and MAM children, providing access to medicines for common ailments such as fever, cold, and worm infestations, as well as first aid. For severely malnourished or sick children, newborns, and pregnancy complications, referrals are made to appropriate health facilities to ensure they receive the necessary medical attention.

Anganwadi Centers

Delivery of the Anganwadi services is facilitated through a network of over 13,96,000 Anganwadi Centers (AWCs) spread across the country [32]. AWCs are government-owned or rented buildings in local areas where nutrition, health, and early childhood education services are provided to intended beneficiaries. According to Mission Poshan 2.0 any beneficiary registered at their nearest Anganwadi Center can avail these services free of cost. Each AWC is managed by an Anganwadi Worker (AWW) with assistance from an Anganwadi Helper (AWH).

A key goal of the Poshan 2.0 guidelines is to improve the infrastructure and quality of Anganwadi Centers (AWCs) by transforming them into Saksham Anganwadi. As per the guidelines, approximately 50,000 AWCs shall be constructed from 2021–22 to 2025–26, at a rate of 10,000 per year. The provision of internet/Wi-Fi connectivity, LED screens, rainwater-harvesting systems, water purifiers/RO machines, and advanced learning aids for early childhood development are covered in the scope of refurbishment requirements. It is important that AWCs should provide onsite drinking water and toilet facilities. The guidelines also recommend that AWCs operating in rented spaces with inadequate infrastructure be relocated to nearby government primary schools. In urban slums where permanent buildings are unavailable, mobile AWCs are expected to be established [12].

Implementation Framework for Poshan 2.0

Policy guidelines for Poshan 2.0 provide a detailed implementation framework for the nutrition program at the center, state, district, block, and community level. At the central level, the guidelines suggest the establishment of a Central Empowered Programme Committee (CEPC) anchored by the Ministry of Women and Child Development. CEPC is suggested to be a technical body with participation from different convergent ministries and technical institutions.

Similarly, at the state level, the Chief Secretary of the States/UTs are made responsible for leading inter-departmental convergence, through the State Steering Committee (SEC). Additionally, secretaries of various departments are expected to use this platform to promote convergence between various schemes and to raise large-scale awareness about addressing malnutrition [12].

A crucial element of the guideline is the designation of the **District Magistrate** (DM)/Collector as the nodal authority to oversee district's nutritional status and monitor the quality of service delivery. Moreover, MoWCD recently issued new national guidelines for **District Nutrition Committees (DNCs)** to all states and UTs. According to the new guidelines, districts are now mandated to organize DNCs under the chairpersonship of the DMs with the support of District Program Officers (DPOs). The terms of reference for DNCs include periodic review of nutrition indicators, monitoring the delivery of Supplementary Nutrition Program, development of a District Nutrition Plan, reviewing the performance using data from Poshan Tracker, promoting inter-departmental convergence, and providing a platform for overall administration and governance of the nutrition program. Also, the guidelines have defined the District Programme Officers as the process owners of DNC meetings and the custodians of district level nutrition data. Their role includes, reviewing progress based on the Block Convergence Action Plan and Monthly Progress Reports (MPR), ensuring the uninterrupted supply of ICDS services, and regularly monitoring the data from Poshan Tracker Dashboard to take corrective actions as needed [22].

Effective implementation of nutrition and childcare programs relies heavily on the coordinated efforts of various functionaries in the field. Therefore, Poshan 2.0 also provides detailed roles and responsibilities of different ICDS functionaries that implement the program at the block and community level.

The **Child Development Project Officer (CDPO)** serves as the primary official responsible for overseeing and executing the ICDS program at the block level. The key responsibilities of CDPO include coordinating and evaluating the delivery of nutrition services, within the project jurisdiction, especially for children with SAM or MAM. The CDPO conducts periodic monitoring, including surprise checks and quality testing of supplementary nutrition, while ensuring food safety and hygiene, and monitoring stock distribution. CDPOs also lead the preparation and implementation of the Block Convergence Action Plan. In addition, the CDPO also conducts joint field visits and monthly reviews with medical officers, compiles and shares monthly progress reports with the state, and is expected to participate in VHSND meetings and community events to motivate beneficiaries.

The **Lady Supervisor (LS)** oversees the work of about 15–25 AWCs and monitors the work of AWWs, thus ensuring project implementation at the cluster level. The lady supervisor reports to the Child Development Project Officer (CDPO) of the respective block. The duties of a Lady Supervisor include supervising the work at AWCs and reporting any shortages and requirements at AWCs to CDPO. They support AWWs in conducting home visits for pregnant women and severely malnourished children and supporting community mobilization. They also compile reports of AWWs, reviewing child health outcomes and recommend interventions.

The role of an **Anganwadi Worker (AWW)** is multifaceted, focusing on the well-being of children and mothers within the community. An AWW is responsible for organizing supplementary nutrition feeding programs for mothers and children. They offer health and nutrition education, counsel mothers on breastfeeding, complimentary feeding, and other infant and young child feeding (IYCF) practices. Regular monitoring of children's growth is a critical task, with AWWs routinely weighing children aged 0 to 6 years and maintaining their growth charts. Additionally, AWWs input relevant beneficiary data into the Poshan Tracker app to ensure accurate monitoring and reporting. They also conduct home visits to pregnant women and new mothers, providing guidance on nutrition, immunization, regular health check-ups, IYCF practices, and distributing nutritional supplements. AWWs coordinate with ASHAs (Accredited Social Health Activists) and ANMs (Auxiliary Nurse Midwives) for health check-ups and referral services, identifying children with special needs and referring them to appropriate health centers. AWWs also organize Poshan Panchayats, Village Health, Sanitation and Nutrition Days (VHSND), and other community-based events to promote health and nutrition. Their efforts are vital in generating ground level awareness about nutrition and facilitating access to the Anganwadi services [12].

Poshan Tracker

Poshan Tracker, launched by the MoWCD through the technical support of the National e-Governance Division, is an ICT platform that monitors comprehensive delivery of Anganwadi services to the beneficiaries and enables real-time analytics for the implementation of the Poshan program [24]. As one of the largest government-led nutrition surveillance systems, Poshan Tracker monitors the nutritional status of over 80 million children on a monthly basis [16]. In addition to entering monthly growth status data of children, AWWs are also mandated to input regular data on the last-mile delivery of services such as THR or HCM and even tracking home visits. Additionally, the Poshan Tracker also monitors the status of Anganwadi Centers and the availability of infrastructure such as access to toilets and clean drinking water.

Furthermore, monthly data on numerous services tracked by the Poshan Tracker can be accessed through open-access Poshan Tracker dashboard, providing comprehensive insights into the program's reach and impact. The dashboard is available in public domain and can be accessed at https://www.poshantracker.in/statistics.

Jan Andolan *and Community Mobilization*

A big focus of the nutrition program is the promotion of social and behavioral change to enlist wider public participation and transform the demand for improved nutrition services into a mass movement known as *"Jan Andolan"*. This initiative includes a range of activities designed to foster community engagement and awareness about nutrition and health. Community-based Events (CBEs) are organized twice a month at AWCs, where important public health nutrition messages are communicated. These messages emphasize the importance of handwashing and sanitation, anemia prevention, nutritious food, and dietary diversity. Cultural platforms like *"Annaprashan Diwas"*, which marks the initiation of complementary feeding, and *"Suposhan Diwas"*, which targets husbands or fathers to take greater ownership of the family's nutritional well-being, are utilized to convey these messages effectively. Additionally, nationwide campaigns like the *"Rashtriya Poshan Maah"* in September, and *"Poshan Pakhwada"*, in March, are observed annually.

Mission Poshan 2.0 guidelines also introduce the concept of **"Poshan Panchayats"**—a platform led by women beneficiaries of Anganwadi services, promoting community-driven accountability.These Panchayats are expected to act as local change-makers, raising awareness and monitoring nutrition services through participatory methods.With mandated inclusion of vulnerable groups, Poshan Panchayats are suggested to conduct social audit of Anganwadi services to improve transparency and grassroots oversight at Anganwadi Centers.

Additionally, the "Streamlining Guidelines" issued by the MoWCD in 2021 mandate for the establishment of **"Poshan Vatikas"**, or nutri-gardens to cultivate fresh food products for local consumption [20]. The Poshan 2.0 guidelines reaffirm this commitment, proposing the creation of Poshan Vatikas at AWCs, government schools, gram panchayat lands, or any other available village land. Poshan Vatika aims to provide locally grown fruits, vegetables, and medicinal plants, fostering dietary diversity for pregnant women, lactating mothers, and the wider community. They may also incorporate poultry and fishing units where culturally appropriate. Oversight for these gardens is entrusted to the DMs and the DNCs. in collaboration with departments such as Forest, Agriculture, Horticulture, Panchayati Raj Institutions (PRIs), Rural Development, and AYUSH [12].

The **Pradhan Mantri Matru Vandana Yojana (PMMVY)** is another key program implemented under the supervision of MoWCD. PMMVY is a maternity benefit program that offers direct benefit transfer (DBT) to women for supporting childbirth and childcare of the first born. The programme also promotes positive behavioral change toward the girl child, by providing extra incentives if the second born is a girl [19].

Interministerial Convergence for Nutrition

Malnutrition is a result of the interplay between multiple socio-economic, cultural, and environmental factors that can directly or indirectly influence the health and nutrition outcomes of vulnerable population, especially women and children. Review of evidence demonstrates the multi-sectoral nature of nutrition and how key determinants such as care and feeding practices, dietary intake, sanitation, food environment, resources mobilization, governance, and cultural norms can influence the nutritional outcomes of the population [39].

Since multiple determinants of nutrition are often interconnected, it is important to understand how multi-sectoral convergence in policy and program action can effectively address the problem of malnutrition in India. From a policy perspective, MoWCD's Poshan 2.0 identifies "convergence" as a key strategy for adopting an integrated approach to improve population-level nutritional outcomes. The guidelines also provide a "convergence matrix" to promote intervention-driven convergence across 18 ministries and departments. This coordinated approach aims to address undernutrition at the household level effectively [12]. *Relevant cross-sectoral programs that promote convergent action to address malnutrition have been briefly described below.*

Ministry of Health and Family Welfare (MoHFW), through the **National Health Mission** is the nodal Ministry responsible for providing "equitable", "affordable", "accountable", and "quality" healthcare to all. NHM covers the entire spectrum of public health services, including maternal and child health, vaccination, communicable and non-communicable disease prevention and control, sanitation, hygiene, and nutrition. NHM integrates reproductive, maternal, newborn, child, and adolescent health services to deliver comprehensive care throughout the life course [9]. Anaemia Mukt Bharat (AMB) is a key initiative under NHM program that directly aims to addresses malnutrition by providing a comprehensive policy strategy for anemia management. AMB focuses on anemia prevention through iron and folic acid (IFA) supplementation, testing, screening, treatment, and awareness generation [27].

Recently, MoHFW and MoWCD released a protocol for Community-based Management of Malnutrition (CMAM). CMAM protocol lists 10 detailed steps for the management of children with acute wasting (low weight for height), particularly those falling in the category of SAM and MAM. Additionally, the CMAM protocol provides details on screening children requiring medical attention and referral to nutrition rehabilitation centers [21].

The **Swachh Bharat Mission (SBM)**, also known as the Clean India Mission is the world's largest sanitation drive, aimed at achieving an Open Defecation Free India [10]. Research has shown a clear link between poor sanitation and diarrhea leading to malnutrition. Diarrheal diseases, intestinal worms, and repeated exposure to such diseases reduces body's ability to absorb nutrients from the food ingested. Thus, improvements in hygiene components including promotion of handwashing with soap, use of safe water, and proper sanitation are important along with nutritional interventions to improve malnutrition [2, 35]. The SBA is a vital public health program that promotes access to toilets and encourages behavior change for improved hygiene, thereby potentially enhancing the nutritional outcomes of the population.

According to the principle of "right to food", the **National Food Security Act (NFSA),** enacted in July 2013, aims to ensure that eligible beneficiaries receive a specified quantity of food grains at affordable prices, thus ensuring food security for all in India. NFSA identifies two types of beneficiaries—priority households where every person is entitled to receive 5 kgs of food grains each month at subsidized costs, and Antyodaya Anna Yojana (AAY) households who represent the poorest families and are eligible for 35 kgs of food grains every month at highly subsidized prices [6]. In response to the COVID-19 pandemic, the government also launched the **Pradhan Mantri Garib Kalyan Anna Yojana (PMGKAY)** which provided an additional 5 kg of free food grains to approximately 800 million beneficiaries across the country. Some of these additional entitlements have continued well beyond the pandemic [7].

Building on the food security net**,** the Mid-Day Meal Scheme is an important central scheme led by the Ministry of Human Resource Development. Recently renamed as **Pradhan Mantri Poshan Shakti Nirman (PM POSHAN)**, the scheme provides free cooked meals to children in government schools. By providing school meals aimed at addressing hunger and nutrition, the scheme encourages regular school attendance among disadvantaged sections and enhances their ability to concentrate on classroom activities [8].

The affordability of healthy diets and food insecurity are other key determinants that have long been associated with malnutrition. Global evidence shows that addressing poverty and structural inequalities through financial support to vulnerable households can be a pivotal strategy for combating malnutrition [4]. In this regard, India's **MGNREGA** (Mahatma Gandhi National Rural Employment Guarantee Act) program stands out as an important social safety net program that provides right to work for a minimum of 100 days per year to every adult in a rural household who wants to undertake unskilled manual work [11].

Global Nutrition Agenda and Commitments over the Decades

The global nutrition agenda has evolved significantly over the past few decades. In the mid-twentieth century, the focus was primarily on combating hunger and severe forms of undernutrition, particularly in developing countries. Efforts were driven by international organizations like the United Nations (UN), which established programs to address food security and provide emergency food aid [41]. The establishment of the United Nations World Food Programme (WFP) in 1961 marked a significant step toward addressing global hunger through food aid [47]. The Green Revolution, which started in the 1960s, introduced high-yield crop varieties and modern farming techniques, aimed to increase food production, and reduce hunger, particularly in Asia and Latin America [37].

The 1990s marked a turning point with broader understanding about the nutrition burden, recognizing the hidden hunger caused by micronutrient deficiencies. The World Health Organization (WHO) and the Food and Agriculture Organization (FAO) began to emphasize the importance of micronutrients, leading to global initiatives like the International Conference on Nutrition in 1992, which set the stage for a more holistic approach to addressing malnutrition [3]. The turn of the century brought increased global attention to nutrition through the Millennium Development Goals (MDGs), which aimed to eradicate "extreme poverty" and "hunger" by 2015 and reduce undernutrition as a key development priority [40]. During this period, the global nutrition agenda began to address the double burden of malnutrition, including both undernutrition and NCDs like obesity emerging from poor diets. This recognition led to more integrated strategies that addressed both ends of the malnutrition spectrum. The Global Strategy on Diet, Physical Activity and Health launched in 2004 aimed to reduce the global burden of NCDs by promoting healthy diets and physical activity [48]. It was followed by the Lancet Series on Maternal and Child Undernutrition in 2008, which underscored the critical importance of nutrition in the first 1000 days of life and advocated for targeted interventions to reduce stunting and wasting [38].

The Scaling Up Nutrition in 2010 was launched to accelerate global and national efforts for combating undernutrition [34]. It encouraged a collaborative, multisectoral strategy by engaging governments, civil society, the private sector, and international agencies to expand efforts for both nutrition-specific and nutrition-sensitive interventions. In 2015, the Sustainable Development Goals were announced marking a significant milestone in the global nutrition agenda [42]. Goal 2, "Zero Hunger", specifically aims to "end hunger" by 2030. The SDGs represent a comprehensive commitment to addressing nutrition as part of broader efforts to achieve sustainable development. The UN Decade of Action on Nutrition (2016–25) was declared to prevent all forms of malnutrition in the world [45]. This decade-long initiative aims to accelerate the implementation of nutrition policies and programs across all sectors, including agriculture, health, education, and social protection.

The outbreak of the COVID-19 pandemic marked a major setback for global nutrition efforts, as it intensified food insecurity across many parts of the world [13]. It has highlighted the vulnerability of global food systems and the need for resilience in nutrition programs. Thereafter, global conflicts like the war in Ukraine too have exposed the vulnerability of global food supply chains, exacerbating challenges in regions already struggling with malnutrition [46]. The recent reductions in international aid by the United States government pose a growing challenge to the long-term sustainability of global nutrition assistance programs [14]. It will be important to closely assess the impact of these funding cuts.

Despite various challenges, the current global nutrition agenda emphasizes the importance of equity, ensuring that vulnerable and marginalized populations have access to the nutrition they need [5]. This includes a focus on gender equality, social protection, and inclusive policies to address malnutrition. Advances in technology, including digital health tools, biofortification, and data-driven decision-making, are increasingly being integrated into nutrition programs [44]. These innovations have the potential to scale up the impact of global nutrition efforts. There is growing recognition of the intersection between climate change and nutrition. The global nutrition agenda now includes strategies to promote climate-resilient food systems and sustainable diets that can withstand environmental challenges while improving nutritional outcomes [43].

Thus, the global nutrition agenda has significantly evolved over the decades, reflecting a deeper understanding of the multiple complexities of malnutrition with a stronger commitment to addressing malnutrition. As a country with one of the highest burden, India has aligned its national policies with global commitments. Over time, India has transitioned from focusing solely on food security to adopting a more integrated and comprehensive approach that addresses the multiple determinants of malnutrition.

India's Response: Progress, Challenges, and Opportunities

India, home to one of the world's largest populations affected by malnutrition, has aligned its national policies with global nutrition goals. The country has shifted from a food security-centric approach to a more comprehensive framework that addresses multiple determinants of malnutrition.

India's journey in formulating and implementing nutrition policies has been marked by significant milestones, from the establishment of ICDS in 1975 to the recent launch of Mission Poshan 2.0 by the MoWCD. These initiatives underscore the government's commitment to addressing malnutrition and improving the health outcomes of its population, particularly women and children. Poshan 2.0 represents a comprehensive attempt to address these challenges by integrating various programs and emphasizing intersectoral convergence. The focus on leveraging cultural practices, promoting dietary diversity, monitoring the quality of THR, using technology for tracking service delivery, and improving the infrastructure of Anganwadi Centers are commendable steps toward achieving better nutrition outcomes India's nutrition policies have made substantial progress over the years; however, critical challenges remain that must be systematically addressed to ensure the effective implementation and impact of the national nutrition policies and programs.

Progress and Impact on Nutrition Outcomes

Comparing the two most recent rounds of the National Family Health Survey indicates a notable improvement in the utilization of ICDS services for child beneficiaries, rising from 58% in 2015 to nearly 71% in 2019–21. Over the same period, the prevalence of underweight children—an important indicator of undernutrition—declined by 5%. Analysis of national level data suggests that increased utilization of ICDS services has contributed to approximately 9–12% of this reduction. Nevertheless, nearly one-third of children in India continue to experience undernutrition [36].

Budgetary Allocation for Poshan

Although MoWCD's share in the central government's overall expenditure has steadily declined—from 0.96% in 2015–16 to 0.5% in 2025–26—the nutrition program still dominates the MoWCD's budget, with Mission Poshan 2.0 accounting for nearly 82% of its central allocation in the 2025–26 budget [33]. Despite the policy prioritization of nutrition through the merger of ICDS and Poshan Abhiyaan under the integrated Mission Poshan 2.0, allocations for the nutrition program remain nearly equivalent to the combined allocations of the earlier sub-schemes. For example, in the Revised Estimates (RE) for FY 2019–20, the total allocation for the sub-schemes stood at ₹21,255 crore—₹701 crore more than the allocation for Poshan 2.0 in FY 2023–24 [15]. The allocations in 2025 are also not significantly different, though slightly higher at ₹21,960 crore. It is worth noting that in the latest budget, the government announced its intention to increase financial allocations to revise the cost norms under the Supplementary Nutrition Programme [30].

Use of Data for Decision Making

One of the critical challenges highlighted by Poshan 2.0 is the poor implementation of nutrition programs in the past, particularly the absence of effective tools to monitor last-mile delivery. While Poshan Tracker has been introduced to improve data collection and monitoring at the grassroots level, ensuring that the data collected is used effectively for programmatic adjustments and decision-making is essential. This can include scaling up governance mechanisms like the District Nutrition Committees or state and central level convergence committees, which can utilize data from Poshan Tracker for monitoring the implementation of the Poshan program. Alternatively, actionable nudges, prompts, or decision alerts can be integrated into the Poshan Tracker App, thus enabling supervisory staff such as LSs, CDPOs, and DPOs to use real-time data to identify implementation bottlenecks and take timely action.

Convergence with Health Systems

Given the placement of the Poshan policy mandate within the MoWCD, effective integration between nutrition and health programs remains limited. Improved coordination between the MoWCD and MoHFW and their field counterparts is essential, particularly in areas such as growth monitoring of the newborns, management of SAM/MAM children, prevention of anemia, and promotion of IYCF practices. A key strategy could be integrating health data with the nutrition data in Poshan Tracker using a common unique ID, enabling data sharing, and fostering service convergence.

Human Resource and Infrastructure

Another long-standing issue plaguing the Anganwadi services has been underinvestment in HR leading to high vacancies of officers and field functionaries. As on 30 September 2022, there were 30% vacancies for the CDPO positions at the national level and 36% vacancies for the position of Anganwadi supervisor [15]. Moreover, training and capacity building of Anganwadi workforce continues to be a challenge. Even though the Poshan 2.0 guidelines prioritize the development of Saksham Anganwadis with state-of-the-art infrastructure, government data from the Poshan Tracker reveals that as of June 2025, only 48% Anganwadi Centers have their own buildings, 25% lack functional toilets, and around 9% do not have a drinking water source [25].

People's Participation

Most importantly, while Poshan 2.0 emphasizes behavior change communication, greater efforts are required to engage communities and promote ownership of nutrition interventions. Strengthening platforms like VHSNDs and Poshan Panchayats can boost local accountability and support for nutrition initiatives. Demand generated by panchayats, self-help groups, field functionaries, and especially the direct beneficiaries of Anganwadi services indeed has the potential to drive change at the grassroots. It can ensure transparent delivery of services like THR and HCM, while empowering communities to actively engage in decision-making processes.

Conclusion

India stands at a crucial juncture in its nutrition journey. While the global nutrition agenda has evolved to embrace equity, resilience, and innovation, India has made significant strides in aligning its policies with these priorities—reflected in the launch of Mission Poshan 2.0 and the renewed emphasis on convergence, data, and community engagement. Yet, the persistent burden of undernutrition, coupled with systemic challenges such as inadequate financing, fragmented implementation, and gaps in infrastructure and human resources, underscores that progress has been uneven. As India continues to refine its nutrition ecosystem, the path forward must be rooted in three principles: **adequate investment**, **institutional accountability**, and **people-centric delivery**. Bridging the divide between intention and implementation will require sustained political will, coordinated inter-ministerial action, and genuine participation from the communities most affected.

References

1. NITI Aayog. (2020). Abhiyaan monitoring report. https://www.niti.gov.in/sites/default/files/2020-10/AbhiyaanMonitoringReport.pdf.
2. Black, R. E., Morris, S. S., & Bryce, J. (2003). Where and why are 10 million children dying every year? *The Lancet, 361*(9376), 2226–2234.
3. FAO. (n.d.). The international conference on Nutrition. https://www.fao.org/4/v7700t/v7700t02.htm
4. FAO, IFAD, UNICEF, WFP, & WHO. (2021). The state of food security and nutrition in the world 2021: Transforming food systems for food security, improved nutrition, and affordable healthy diets for all. *FAO*. https://doi.org/10.4060/cb4474en
5. Global Nutrition Report. (n.d.). *Introduction: Towards global nutrition equity*. https://globalnutritionreport.org/reports/2020-global-nutrition-report/introduction-towards-global-nutrition-equity/
6. Government of India, Ministry of Consumer Affairs, Food and Public Distribution. (2013). *National Food Security Act (NFSA)*. https://nfsa.gov.in/
7. Government of India, Ministry of Consumer Affairs, Food and Public Distribution. (n.d.). *Pradhan Mantri Garib Kalyan Anna Yojana (PMGKAY)*. https://dfpd.gov.in/Home/ContentManagement?Url=pmgka.html&ManuId=3&language=2
8. Government of India, Ministry of Education, Department of School Education & Literacy. (2022). *Pradhan Mantri Poshan Shakti Nirman (PM POSHAN) guidelines*. https://pmposhan.education.gov.in/Files/Guidelines/2023/Guidelines%20on%20PM%20POSHAN%20SCHEME.pdf
9. Government of India, Ministry of Health and Family Welfare, National Health Mission. (n.d.). *NHM Components: RMNCAH+N: Nutrition*. https://nhm.gov.in/index1.php?lang=1&level=2&sublinkid=1446&lid=796
10. Government of India, Ministry of Rural Development. (2005). *Mahatma Gandhi National Rural Employment Guarantee Act (MGNREGA)*. https://nrega.nic.in/MGNREGA_new/Nrega_home.aspx
11. Government of India, Ministry of Rural Development. (2005). *Mahatma Gandhi National Rural Employment Guarantee Act (MGNREGA)*. https://nrega.nic.in/MGNREGA_new/Nrega_home.aspx

12. Government of India, Ministry of Women and Child Development. (2022). *Mission Saksham Anganwadi and Poshan 2.0 scheme guideline.* https://wcd.gov.in/pregnant-lactating-women-children/nutrition-mission-saksham-anganwadi-and-poshan-2-0
13. HLPE Joint Steering Committee. (2021). Impacts of COVID-19 on food security and nutrition: Developing effective policy responses to address the hunger and malnutrition pandemic. https://openknowledge.fao.org/server/api/core/bitstreams/5d230f39-ad95-47c4-a23e-471c07953223/content.
14. Hussein, S., & Samet, J. M. (2025). Measuring population health impact of the trump administration's withdrawal from WHO and cuts to USAID: Time to start counting. *Population Health Metrics, 23*(13). https://doi.org/10.1186/s12963-025-00376-y
15. Accountability Initiative. (2023). Mission Saksham Anganwadi and Poshan 2.0: Budget *briefs 2023.* https://accountabilityindia.in/wp-content/uploads/2023/02/Mission-Saksham-Anganwadi-and-Poshan-2.0-Budget-Briefs-2023.pdf
16. Jaacks, L. M., Awasthi, A., & Kalra, A. (2024). India's Poshan tracker: Data-driven tool for maternal and child nutrition. *The Lancet Regional Health–Southeast Asia, 25*, 100381.
17. Ministry of Consumer Affairs, Food, and Public Distribution. (2023). *Amendment in Schedule II of the National Food Security Act.* https://dfpd.gov.in/notifications/en
18. Ministry of Human Resource Development, Government of India. (1993). *National Nutrition Policy.* https://wcd.nic.in/sites/default/files/nnp_0.pdf
19. Ministry of Women and Child Development, Government of India. (2017). *Pradhan Mantri Matru Vandana Yojna.* https://wcd.gov.in/women/pradhan-mantri-matru-vandana-yojna
20. Ministry of Women and Child Development, Government of India. (2021). *Streamlining guidelines on quality assurance, roles and responsibilities of duty holders, procedure for procurement, integrating AYUSH concepts.* https://wcd.gov.in/images/uploaded/1706599962_xAnW5QNvwB.pdf
21. Ministry of Women and Child Development, Government of India. (2023). Protocol for management of malnutrition in children under Mission Poshan 2.0. https://wcd.gov.in/offerings/schemes-services-mission-poshan-2-0-portals-protocol-for-management-of-malnutrition-in-children
22. Ministry of Women and Child Development, Government of India. (2024). *National guidelines for district nutrition committees.* https://drive.google.com/file/d/1f2D0JOqCviLBSJ6yXs1DYORcsDb4QFa9/view
23. Ministry of Women and Child Development, Government of India. (n.d.). *Integrated Child Development Services: Broad framework.* https://wcd.php-staging.com/documents/uploaded/ICDS%20Mission%20Broad%20Framework.pdf
24. Ministry of Women and Child Development, Government of India. (n.d.). *About us: Poshan Tracker.* https://www.poshantracker.in/aboutus
25. Ministry of Women and Child Development, Government of India. (n.d.). *Statistics–Poshan Tracker.* https://www.poshantracker.in/statistics
26. Mittal, S., Sharma, M., Walters, D., & Varghese, M. (2023). *Advances in Agri-food systems* (Vol. II, Ch. 12).
27. National Health Mission. (2018). Anemia Mukt Bharat operational guidelines. https://www.nhm.gov.in/images/pdf/Nutrition/AMB-guidelines/Anemia-Mukt-Bharat-Operational-Guidelines-FINAL.pdf.
28. Panda, M. (2024). Evolution of India's policy response to hunger, nutrition, and food security since independence. In S. M. Dev, A. Ganesh-Kumar, & V. L. Pandey (Eds.), *Achieving zero hunger in India (India studies in business and economics).* Springer. https://doi.org/10.1007/978-981-99-4413-2_2
29. Pingali, P., Mittra, B., & Rahman, A. (2017). The bumpy road from food to nutrition security: Slow evolution of India's food policy. *Global Food Security, 15*, 77–84. https://doi.org/10.1016/j.gfs.2017.05.002
30. Press Information Bureau. (2025). Highlights of union budget 2025–26. https://www.pib.gov.in/PressReleaseIframePage.aspx?PRID=2098353.

31. Press Information Bureau, Government of India. (2017). *NITI Aayog calls renewed focus on nutrition, launches the National Nutrition Strategy*. https://pib.gov.in/PressReleaseIframePage.aspx?PRID=1508602
32. Press Information Bureau, Government of India. (2023). *Total 13.96 lakh Anganwadis registered under the Poshan Tracker application*. https://pib.gov.in/PressReleasePage.aspx?PRID=1943759
33. PRS Legislative Research. (2025). *Demand for grants 2025–26: Analysis–Ministry of Women and Child Development*. https://prsindia.org/files/budget/budget_parliament/2025/DFG_Analysis_2025-26-WCD.pdf.
34. Scaling Up Nutrition (n.d.). *History*. https://scalingupnutrition.org/about/what-we-do/history
35. Shrestha, A., Six, J., Dahal, D., Marks, S., & Meierhofer, R. (2020). Association of nutrition, water, sanitation, and hygiene practices with children's nutritional status, intestinal parasitic infections and diarrhea in rural Nepal: A cross-sectional study. *BMC Public Health, 20*, 1–21.
36. Singh, S. K., Chauhan, A., Alderman, H., Avula, R., Dwivedi, L. K., Kapoor, R., et al. (2024). Utilization of integrated child development services (ICDS) and its linkages with undernutrition in India. *Maternal & Child Nutrition, 20*(3), e13644. https://doi.org/10.1111/mcn.13644
37. Social Science Research Council. (n.d.). *The 1960s: The Green Revolution*. https://100.ssrc.org/1960s-the-green-revolution/
38. The Lancet. (2008). The Lancet series on maternal and child Undernutrition. https://www.thelancet.com/series/maternal-and-child-undernutrition.
39. UNICEF. (2020). *UNICEF conceptual framework: Maternal and child nutrition*. https://knowledge.unicef.org/resource/unicef-conceptual-framework-maternal-and-child-nutrition
40. United Nations. (2015). Millennium Development Goals report: 2015.
41. United Nations. (n.d.). *Research guides: Food security and nutrition—A global issue: UN milestones*. https://research.un.org/en/foodsecurity/un-milestones
42. United Nations. (n.d.). *The 17 goals|Sustainable Development*. https://sdgs.un.org/goals
43. United Nations. (n.d.). *Mid-term review foresight paper*. https://www.who.int/docs/default-source/nutritionlibrary/departmental-news/mid-term-review---un-decade-of-action-on-nutrition/nutrition-decade-mtr-foresight-paper-en.pdf
44. United Nations System Standing Committee on Nutrition, Costa Coitinho Delmuè, D., Granheim, I. D. O., & Oenema, S. (2020). UNSCN Nutrition 45: Nutrition in a digital world. UNSCN.. https://www.unscn.org/uploads/web/news/UNSCN-Nutrition-45-WEB.pdf
45. UNSCN. (n.d.). *The Decade of Action on Nutrition 2016–2025*. https://www.unscn.org/en/topics/un-decade-of-action-on-nutrition
46. Vos, R. (2024). The war in Ukraine continues to undermine the food security of millions. *IFPRI Blog.*. https://www.ifpri.org/blog/war-ukraine-continues-undermine-food-security-millions/
47. World Food Programme. (n.d.). *History*. https://www.wfp.org/history
48. World Health Organization. (2004). Global strategy on diet, physical activity and health. https://apps.who.int/gb/ebwha/pdf_files/WHA57/A57_R17-en.pdf.

Part IV
Intervention and Support

Chapter 10
Role of Government Programs and Recommendations for Policy Improvement

Priya Rampal

Introduction

Undernutrition remains a critical global challenge, contributing to nearly 45% of all deaths among children under five [1, 2]. It weakens immunity, making children more susceptible to diseases such as acute respiratory infections, diarrhea, and malaria [3, 4]. Beyond immediate health concerns, undernutrition hinders both physical and cognitive development, contributing significantly toward the global burden of disease and restricting children from reaching their full potential [5, 6].

Research consistently highlights that the first 1,000 days from conception are pivotal for a child's growth and future health outcomes [7]. Most growth retardation originates within the first thousand days from conception [8–11]. During this period, maternal malnutrition can lead to intrauterine growth retardation (IUGR), increasing the likelihood of stunting, wasting, and underweight conditions [12–14]. Without adequate nutrition, children face lifelong impairments, perpetuating cycles of malnutrition across generations [15]. This phase—often termed the 'window of opportunity'—plays a vital role in ensuring proper nutrition and fostering healthy early interactions [16–20]. Conversely, repeated shocks—such as disease, poor nutrition, or lack of emotional support—can hinder development [21, 22]. The first 1,000 days are a period of both great opportunity and vulnerability for growth and development.

Efforts to combat undernutrition in early-childhood yield substantial long-term benefits, not only in health but also in education and economic productivity [23, 24]. The interplay between 'nature' and 'nurture' shapes a child's nutritional outcomes: while genetic predisposition influences baseline health, environmental interventions—including access to food, healthcare, and education—determine overall well-being [25]. Supportive investments in child health and nutrition right from birth might help prevent undernutrition.

P. Rampal (✉)
Oxford Policy Management India Pvt Ltd, Delhi, India
e-mail: priya.rampal@opml.co.uk

S. Suri (ed.), *Child Health and Nutrition from Conception to Age Two*,
https://doi.org/10.1007/978-981-95-7868-9_10

India has implemented key supportive investments to improve child nutrition, including:

- **Integrated Child Development Services (ICDS)**), which provides food, preschool education, and healthcare. These services are provided from Anganwadi centers established mainly in rural areas and staffed with frontline workers at the correct time for the infants.[1]
- **Universal Immunization Programme (UIP)**), offering vaccines against critical childhood diseases.[2] The national immunization policy includes vaccines for diseases such as tuberculosis, diphtheria, pertussis, tetanus, polio, measles, hepatitis B, and more recently, rotavirus, pneumococcal conjugate vaccine (PCV), and human papillomavirus (HPV) vaccine.
- **Public Distribution System (PDS)**), ensuring food security through subsidized staples like wheat and rice. The Food Corporation of India manages the PDS, which focuses on ensuring food security.
- State-driven programs, such as **Indira Kranti Patham (IKP)**), also known as Velugu, which is a significant rural poverty reduction initiative implemented in Andhra Pradesh, India. The program aims to empower the rural communities, particularly the poorest households, by improving their livelihoods and quality of life through self-sustainable institutions.[3]
- Infrastructure improvements, including sanitation and healthcare facilities, alongside income-support programs like **MGNREGA**).[4]

Figure 10.1 gives the challenges and recommendations of major government programs in the states of Andhra Pradesh and Telangana.

Despite these efforts, data gaps persist in monitoring long-term nutritional trends and socioeconomic characteristics of individuals over a span of time. The Young Lives project provides valuable longitudinal insights, following children in Andhra Pradesh and Telangana to assess the impact of early-life nutrition on future health outcomes [26]. Owing to the timing of the first two rounds, it is possible to examine the nutritional status of a child inside the WoO (in the year 2002) and outside it (in the year 2006). The data is purposefully analyzed for the cohort born in 2000–2001 to determine whether the cohort can catch up in nutritional status outside the WoO. The

---

[1] The young lives do not specifically mention or collect information on the Integrated Child Development Services (ICDS) in its data collection. However, it does ask whether children receive food at preschool or crèche. Information on mid-day meals has been collected formally and has been used to draw conclusions for the younger cohort in 2006.

[2] For more information on the immunization programme, refer to: https://www.nhm.gov.in/index1.php?lang=1&level=3&sublinkid=944&lid=378.

[3] For more information on IKP, refer to https://documents.worldbank.org/curated/en/948991468258858710/pdf/WPS6841.pdf; https://www.icrw.org/wp-content/uploads/2018/11/Velugu-SERP-Model-Documentation.pdf.

[4] MGNREGA's primary aim is to enhance the livelihood security of rural households by providing at least 100 days of guaranteed wage employment in a financial year to every household whose adult members volunteer to do unskilled manual work. For more information refer to https://nrega.nic.in/MGNREGA_new/Nrega_home.aspx.

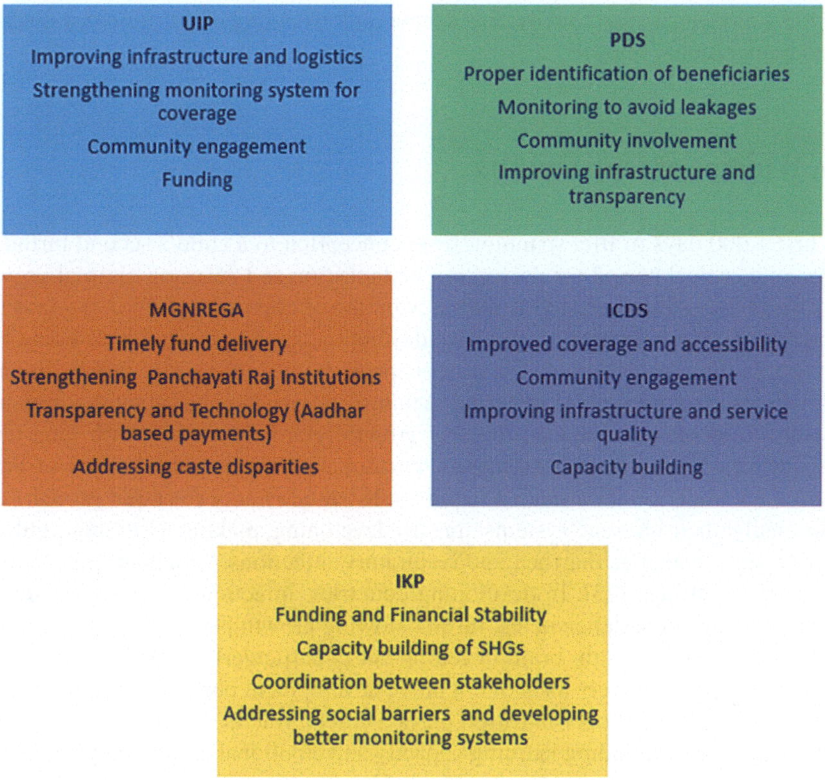

Fig. 10.1 Challenges and recommendations for government programs

nutritional indices or anthropometric measures used to conduct the analysis over the two years are stunting (low height-for-age), wasting (low weight-for-height), and underweight (low weight-for-age). This chapter addresses two main questions: whether early-life nutritional status affects future nutritional status relative to the other factors, and whether it depends on neonatal status and prenatal care. Using the UNICEF framework, the study employs linear and logit regressions to assess the WoO's impact on later nutritional status. Previous studies using Young Lives data [27, 28] have explored this relationship, but this study extends the analysis with Shapley value decomposition to evaluate the contribution of explanatory variables, including government programs. Findings indicate that 70% of nutritional variation beyond the 'window of opportunity' is shaped by early-life nutrition by weight-for-age and 64% by height-for-age, reinforcing the importance of prenatal care and maternal health. Prenatal care and maternal health significantly influence a child's nutritional status at birth, with smaller birth size correlating with lower infancy nutritional indicators. This chapter explores the lasting effects of early nutrition and how government programs contribute to child health improvements. By leveraging updated data and analytical models, it aims to provide a deeper understanding of nutritional status and its intergenerational impact.

The Window of Opportunity

The first 1,000 days of life, spanning from conception to a child's second birthday, represent a critical period for preventing malnutrition and ensuring optimal growth [2]. This phase—often referred to as the 'window of opportunity' (WoO)—lays the foundation for lifelong health, cognitive development, and physical well-being [7]. During this time, growth rates are at their peak, both in utero and during infancy [16]. Adverse factors such as maternal malnutrition, inadequate infant feeding, and exposure to infections can lead to early growth retardation, often with long-term consequences [15]. Infants have higher nutritional demands per kilogram of body weight than adults, as their bodies require substantial energy for rapid growth [24] Additionally, their immune systems are still developing, making them more vulnerable to diseases such as diarrhea and respiratory infections, which are prevalent in low-resource settings [23]. In developing countries, infectious diseases frequently exacerbate nutritional deficiencies, further slowing growth [11].

Beyond physical health, brain development is particularly sensitive during this period, with approximately 85% of cognitive development occurring within the first 1,000 days [22, 29].[5] Proper nutrition plays a crucial role in determining long-term cognitive abilities, including learning capacity and emotional regulation [20]. Childhood growth and development are crucial indicators of nutritional status, influenced by genetic and environmental factors [30]. Preschool children worldwide exhibit similar growth patterns under optimal nutrition and socioeconomic conditions [31].

However, not all children experience optimal growth trajectories. In developing countries, growth rates often falter before one year of age in poor and vulnerable children leading to malnutrition due to inadequate dietary intake and poor health, which reinforce each other. These children often come from households with food insecurity, inadequate maternal and childcare, and poor access to health services [30–32]. Studies indicate that weight faltering begins around three months of age, continues through the first year, and gradually slows around 18–19 months [28]. Meanwhile, height-for-age deficits emerge immediately after birth and persist through the first two to three years, while weight-for-height declines during the first 15 months before stabilizing [19].

When faced with nutritional stress, the body prioritizes weight maintenance over height, leading to stunting—a condition with long-term implications for health and development [17, 33, 34]. Acute illnesses or dietary deficiencies can halt linear

[5] From conception to adulthood, growth can be divided into various phases: intrauterine, infancy, childhood and adolescence. Prenatal growth and infancy are the most rapid growth periods. These are also the years when the child is most vulnerable to malnutrition (Goulet, 2010). However, the first 24 months are referred to as the window of opportunity for prevention of malnutrition.

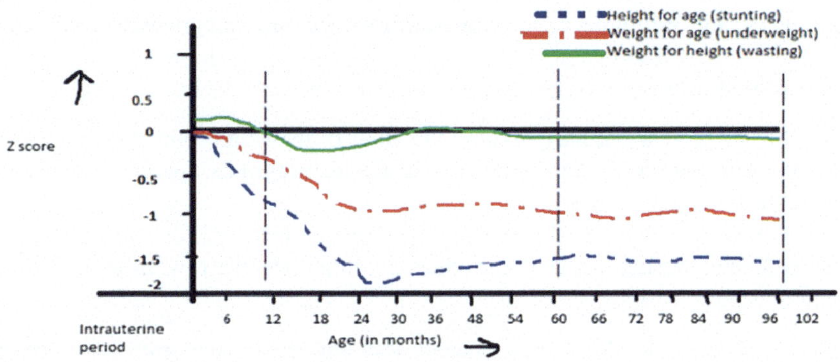

Fig. 10.2 The window of opportunity. *Source* Stylized figure based on Shrimpton et al. (2001) and Victora et al. (2010)

growth, forcing children into a vulnerable cycle of malnutrition and delayed recovery [36, 37]. Persistent inadequate nutrition and recurrent infections prevent catch-up growth, resulting in lasting height deficits that extend into adulthood. Recognizing the importance of early intervention, policies and programs must focus on maternal nutrition, infant feeding practices, and healthcare accessibility to ensure that children receive the nutritional support necessary to thrive during this crucial window [12, 25]. Figure 10.2 gives a stylized diagram of the WoO.

Methods

In a rapidly changing world, nutrition remains one of the most defining factors of a child's growth, development, and future potential. For children born between 2000 and 2001, this study examines how the Window of Opportunity (WoO)—the first 1,000 days from conception to two years—compares to later compensatory and supportive factors in shaping nutritional outcomes.

Rather than viewing childhood nutrition in isolation, this analysis embraces a holistic perspective, acknowledging that environmental investments, government programs, and economic shifts all play a role. The central question is: Can interventions after infancy compensate for early-life disadvantages, or does the WoO hold a unique influence that cannot be undone?

Framing the Study

Across multiple districts in India, thousands of children grow up facing varying levels of food security, maternal care, and access to healthcare. While some benefit from government safety nets and improved infrastructure, others endure economic constraints and environmental shocks that threaten their development.

To explore these patterns, two pivotal moments in a child's life are analyzed:

1. Infancy (1–2 years, 2002): Examining how birth weight and prenatal factors compare to supportive mechanisms like health programs, income growth, and sanitation improvements.
2. Toddlerhood (4–5 years, 2006): Investigating whether a child's nutritional status at birth and during infancy continues to influence their well-being, despite external interventions.

By tracing these trajectories, this chapter seeks to go beyond statistics, offering insights into how social structures shape nutritional outcomes.

Understanding the Interplay of Nature and Nurture

Every child's growth is determined by a balance between genetics (nature) and environmental influences (nurture). To disentangle these relationships, the study adopts the UNICEF framework [20, 36] reinforced further by Black et al. [35], a model that identifies:

- Basic causes of undernutrition, including economic hardship, political conditions, and household dynamics.
- Immediate contributors, such as dietary intake, recurrent illnesses, and healthcare access.
- Supportive and Compensatory factors, including nutrition programs, infrastructure improvements, and food distribution systems.

The UNICEF framework is adapted for the analysis in three ways in this work. First, prenatal factors are included. Second, since the framework is established for a point in time, health or nutritional investments made in the past are considered. For instance, better health and sanitation facilities need to be considered while analyzing the nutritional status of a child, both within and outside the WoO. Third, various compensatory or supportive investments such as government programs are included in the analysis.

A Story Told Through Data

Consider two children, born in the same year in rural Andhra Pradesh. One is raised in a household with stable food access and government-supported nutrition programs. The other, despite a similar start, lives in an area affected by climatic shocks and limited healthcare accessibility.

While both children begin their lives shaped by prenatal conditions, their trajectories diverge based on external interventions, economic shifts, and environmental stressors. The question is: Which factor holds the greatest influence—early nutrition or later investments?

Modeling Nutritional Impact

To quantify these effects, a **nutrition production function** is developed[6]: Like the health production function, the nutrition production function can also potentially be endogenous [36, 37]. There is a measurement error associated with measuring the height and weight of the child which is used to calculate the *z*-scores for height-for-age and weight-for-age. The nutritional status of the child in the current period is assumed to be a function of the child's nutritional status in the past period [38]. This chapter works with the caveat that the nutritional status might be biased.

$$\mathrm{HAZ_{WoO}} = \beta_o + \beta_1 \mathrm{HAZ_{neo}} + \Sigma\beta_c X_c + \Sigma\beta_h X_h + \Sigma\beta_g X_g + \xi_i \tag{10.1}$$

$$\mathrm{HAZ_{neo}} = \alpha_o + \alpha_1 \mathrm{HAZ_{pre}} + \Sigma\alpha_c X_c + \Sigma\alpha_h X_h + \Sigma\alpha_g X_g + \xi_i \tag{10.2}$$

where:

- $\mathrm{HAZ_{WoO}}$ represents **height-for-age in toddlerhood** (2006).
- $\mathrm{HAZ_{neo}}$ refers to height-for-age during infancy (2002).
- $\mathrm{HAZ_{pre}}$ accounts for prenatal conditions, including birth weight and maternal nutrition.
- X_c covers child variables such as age and gender and child health variables like recent illness and immunization history.
- X_h captures household characteristics, including parental education, maternal weight, household size, social group, fuel type, and sanitation type as well as a proxy for household X_h also accounts for location-specific factors like whether the child resides in rural or urban area and the district of residence (Srikakulum, West Godavari, Anantpur, Cuddapah, Mahaboobnagar, Karimnagar, Hyderabad).
- X_g represents compensatory and supportive mechanisms, such as government food programs, employment schemes, and early-childhood feeding initiatives. These include access to government programs such as MGNREGA (whether the household participates in National Rural Employment Guarantee Act which guarantees 100 days of work in a year at minimum wages), Public Distribution

[6] This is a linear specification of the model. Regressions of quadratic, cubic, log-linear and linear-log specifications and the findings remain consistent across all specifications. The linear specification in the main text offers the advantage of exploring results using the Shapley value decomposition [39].

Equations for height-for-age are written with the same explanatory variables, they are modified for weight-for-age (underweight) and weight-for-height (wasting).

System (for rice, dal, kerosene, and sugar), Indira Kranti Patham (IKP)[7] and whether a child receives food at preschool, crèche, or mid-day meals.[8]

Environmental Disruptions

Beyond nutrition-specific factors, environmental events like climatic shocks can permanently alter a child's developmental path [40–42]. To account for these, three variables capture rainfall fluctuations:

1. Total deficit rainfall—tracking years with below-average precipitation (2002–2005 for infancy, 2006–2009 for toddlerhood).
2. Total excess rainfall—summing above-average precipitation for the same periods.
3. Average rainfall over a decade—offering insights into long-term weather patterns affecting food security.

Additionally, weight-for-age is adjusted for seasonal variations, recognizing that short-term nutritional fluctuations often correlate with food availability.

Predicting Undernutrition

Since the WHO defines undernourished children as those with *z*-scores below −2 SD, logistic regression models estimate the likelihood of a child falling into this category:

In 2006, probability of a child being undernourished is represented as $P(\mathrm{HAZ}_{\mathrm{WoO}} < -2)$

$$P(\mathrm{HAZ}_{\mathrm{WoO}} < -2) = F(\beta_o + \beta_1 \mathrm{HAZ}_{\mathrm{neo}} + \Sigma\beta_c X_{ct} + \Sigma\beta_h X_{ht} + \Sigma\beta_g X_{gt} + \xi_i) \tag{10.3}$$

In 2002, probability of a child being undernourished is represented as $P(\mathrm{HAZ}_{\mathrm{neo}} < -2)$

$$P(\mathrm{HAZ}_{\mathrm{neo}} < -2) = F(\alpha_o + \alpha_1 \mathrm{HAZ}_{\mathrm{pre}} + \Sigma\alpha_c X_{ct} + \Sigma\alpha_h X_{ht} + \Sigma\alpha_g X_{gt} + \xi_i). \tag{10.4}$$

where F(.) is a standard normal distribution function.

---

[7] IKP is a state-wide poverty reduction project to enable the rural poor to improve their livelihoods and quality of life through their own organizations.

[8] The young lives do not specifically mention or collect information on the Integrated Child Development Services (ICDS) in its data collection. However, it does ask whether children receive food at preschool or crèche. Information on mid-day meals has been collected formally and has been used to draw conclusions for the younger cohort in 2006.

A Comprehensive Examination

To ensure a balanced analysis, Shapley value decomposition is used to break down the R-squared (model goodness-of-fit measure) [39, 43]. Starting with the full model, the method successively removes regressor variables, one by one according to a particular ordering of the variables. The difference in R-squared associated with the elimination of a variable can be regarded as the variable's marginal contribution within this specific ordering of the regressors. Treating all orderings equally probable, the Shapley value of a variable equals the variable's average marginal contribution across all possible orderings. This technique distributes predictor significance across multiple regressors, identifying which factor—birth conditions, household investments, or government programs—exerts the strongest influence.

Beyond Numbers: The Human Perspective

Ultimately, this study aims to go beyond statistical modeling. It seeks to answer an essential question: Can later interventions truly compensate for early nutritional deficits, or does the Window of Opportunity lock in developmental advantages and disadvantages?

By weaving data, policy insights, and real-world experiences, this chapter offers a contextualized, narrative-driven analysis, providing a compelling case study on the interplay between early nutrition and later interventions.

Data and Variables

The erstwhile Andhra Pradesh comprised three distinct agro-climatic zones—Coastal Andhra, Rayalaseema, and Telangana—each shaped by unique natural resources, historical legacies, and institutional structures. The state is home to diverse social and religious groups, with communities categorized into Scheduled Castes (SC), Scheduled Tribes (ST), Backward Classes (BCs), and Other Castes (OC). SC and ST are constitutionally recognized as historically disadvantaged groups, while BCs include aboriginal tribes, Vimukhti Jatis, and vocational communities.

The Younger Cohort, born in 2001–2002, was surveyed over three waves—2002, 2006, and 2009—to track demographic variables. The initial sample included 2,011 children (1,081 boys and 930 girls), with minor attrition reducing the cohort to 1,950 in 2006 and 1,936 in 2009. Gender representation remained slightly skewed toward males, while regional distribution stayed stable across the three zones, with Coastal Andhra consistently having the highest female representation and Telangana maintaining the highest male ratio. The caste breakdown mirrored broader social hierarchies, where Backward Classes formed the largest group, followed by

Scheduled Castes, Scheduled Tribes, and Other Castes. A rural bias was evident, with three-fourths of the cohort residing in rural areas throughout all three waves, reflecting Andhra Pradesh's broader demographic composition in the early 2000s. The cohort's age progression aligned with expectations, averaging 12 months in 2002, 64 months in 2006, and 96 months in 2009, ensuring a consistent longitudinal dataset for developmental analysis.

Nutritional trends in the cohort, drawn from Young Lives data, reveal a worsening trajectory over time. In 2002, 25.68% of children were stunted, 29.03% were underweight, and 21.07% were wasted, with urban children experiencing lower undernutrition rates compared to their rural counterparts. The contrast was particularly stark in stunting—16.27% in urban areas compared to 29.03% in rural regions. Gender disparities persisted, as boys showed higher rates across all indicators, most notably underweight (31.78% vs. 25.87%). The largest social group represented was Backward Classes (48%), followed by Other Castes (21%), Scheduled Castes (18%), and Scheduled Tribes (13%), mirroring the caste-based disparities in nutritional outcomes. These are in line with NFHS data [44, 45].

By 2006, these indicators deteriorated, with stunting rising to 33.08% and underweight to 41.44%. Undernutrition was significantly worse in rural areas, where 37.62% of children were stunted and 45.60% underweight, compared to urban levels of 19.72 and 29.48% respectively. The state-level NFHS-3 data further underscores these disparities, reporting 41% of rural children underweight versus 29% in urban areas, with corresponding stunting rates of 42 and 30%, respectively. While gender gaps narrowed slightly since 2002, boys continued to exhibit higher stunting and underweight rates, reinforcing persistent vulnerabilities.

Economic inequalities played a decisive role in nutritional disparities, with children from the lowest wealth quartile facing the highest levels of stunting (34.89%) and underweight (38.13%) in the year 2002, whereas those in the highest quartile experienced significantly lower rates of undernutrition. This gap widened by 2006, when the poorest quartile saw stunting rise to 43.58% and underweight to 52.45%, reflecting deepening socioeconomic inequities. Social group disparities remained pronounced, as Scheduled Tribes (ST) and Scheduled Castes (SC) recorded the highest rates of undernutrition, with nearly 49% of ST children underweight and over 39% stunted, whereas Other Castes (OC) consistently showed the lowest prevalence across all indicators.

A comparative analysis of 2002 and 2006 reveals a steady deterioration in child nutrition, particularly for rural, economically disadvantaged, and socially marginalized groups. Stunting rose from 25.68% in 2002 to 33.08% in 2006, while underweight prevalence increased from 29.03 to 41.44%, underscoring worsening child nutritional status. Rural children remained the most vulnerable, with stunting escalating from 29.03 to 37.62% and underweight from 28.48% to 45.60%. Although gender gaps narrowed slightly, both boys and girls faced rising malnutrition rates. The interwoven influences of caste, wealth, and location demonstrate the structural inequities shaping child health outcomes, reaffirming the critical need for equity-driven interventions to mitigate long-term consequences of nutritional deficits.

The average household size was 5.52 members, suggesting that many children were growing up in larger families, which may stretch household resources. Parental education levels were low, particularly for mothers (mean of 4.48 years), and maternal anthropometric indicators—average weight of 44 kg and height of 147 cm—further point to intergenerational malnutrition risks. Access to government programs varied: while 81% had access to PDS rice, access to other key nutritional supplements like dal (2%) was extremely limited. Participation in flagship social protection schemes like NREGA and IKP was moderate (34% each), and only 8% had access to crèches, despite 87% attending preschool. Encouragingly, immunization coverage was very high, with over 95% of children receiving BCG, measles, DPT, and OPV, though uptake of HiB vaccine was lower (41%). Sanitation (33%) and clean cooking fuel (27%) access remained poor, potentially exacerbating health risks. Lastly, subjective health perceptions showed that while 37% of caregivers felt their child's health had improved, 12% reported worsening, and 29% expressed fear of child mortality, highlighting persistent concerns despite programmatic coverage. These multidimensional patterns underscore the importance of addressing both structural determinants and service delivery gaps to reverse worsening nutritional outcomes.

Measuring Early-Life Conditions and Household Wealth

Assessing the nutritional status of a child requires an understanding of both biological and socioeconomic factors. Since direct birth weight data is unavailable, perceived birth size serves as a proxy measure, capturing maternal insights into early-life health. Additionally, antenatal care—whether the mother attended prenatal visits, took iron supplements during pregnancy, or her recorded weight in 2006—acts as an indirect indicator of maternal health during gestation.

One of the most influential determinants of childhood nutrition is household income, shaping access to adequate food, healthcare, and living conditions. However, income information was not collected in the survey, necessitating an alternative approach, and therefore we used the wealth index. A wealth index was created separately for rural and urban households, incorporating regional variations in asset ownership.

The Young Lives dataset provides a detailed breakdown of economic indicators, highlighting differences between urban and rural wealth accumulation. In urban areas, household wealth is typically associated with housing stability and consumer goods, including ownership of a home, radio, refrigerator, bicycle, TV, motorbike, car, mobile phone, landline, sewing machine, almirah, clock, table-chair, bed, and fan. In contrast, rural households often derive economic stability from agricultural assets and farming equipment. Therefore, the rural wealth index also incorporates tractors, pumps, livestock, bullock carts, threshers, and land ownership—elements that are vital for economic sustainability in agricultural settings.

To ensure accuracy, Principal Component Analysis (PCA) was used to construct separate wealth indices for round one and round two, adjusting for regional disparities across Andhra Pradesh and Telangana. This methodology helps capture the economic landscape, offering a contextualized understanding of how wealth influences early-life nutrition and developmental outcomes.

Results and Discussion

The analysis, using both linear and logit regressions, highlights the extent and probability of a child being undernourished. Given that both methods yield similar conclusions, the discussion primarily focuses on the linear regression findings, while logit regressions are used to reinforce key arguments.

The Window of Opportunity: Discussion

Regression results underscore the crucial role of the WoO in shaping later nutritional outcomes (Table 10.1). Since the first 1,000 days begin at conception, the initial 270 days in utero set the foundation for infant health and growth trajectories. To assess this impact, the study first examines infant and neonatal nutrition in 2002.

Table 10.1 Linear regressions for HAZ and logit regressions for whether stunted in 2006

	HAZ in 2006	HAZ in 2006	Whether stunted in 2006	Whether stunted in 2006
Past Nutritional Status				
HAZ in 2002	0.324***	0.321***	0.803***	0.789***
	(0.016)	(0.016)	(0.061)	(0.059)
	WAZ in 2006	WAZ in 2006	Whether underweight in 2006	Whether underweight in 2006
Past Nutritional Status				
WAZ in 2002	0.461***	0.463***	1.168***	1.165***
	(0.018)	(0.018)	(0.077)	(0.077)
Other controls				
Child characteristics	Yes	Yes	Yes	Yes
Household characteristics	Yes	Yes	Yes	Yes
District	Yes	No	Yes	No
Shocks	No	Yes	No	Yes

Children born smaller than their peers show significantly lower nutritional indicators in infancy.[9] Alongside breastfeeding practices, birth size accounts for 20% of the variation in weight-for-age, 11% for height-for-age, and 17% for weight-for-height (Table 10.2). This demonstrates the enduring influence of early-life conditions on physical development. Additionally, maternal prenatal care—including antenatal visits, iron intake during pregnancy, place of birth, and mode of delivery—contributes between 2.5 and 5% to the variation across nutritional indicators.

By toddlerhood (2006), the nutritional status outside the WoO remains strongly linked to the child's early-life nutritional condition (2002). These findings align with existing literature highlighting the long-term implications of early nutrition on later health [38, 46, 47]. Leveraging Shapley decomposition, the study quantifies the persistence of early-life nutritional effects, revealing that nutritional status in infancy (2002) explains 70% of weight-for-age variation and 64% of height-for- age variation in 2006 (Table 10.2). This reaffirms the idea that nutritional disadvantages in early life are difficult to reverse, emphasizing the importance of the first 1,000 days as the most critical period for growth and development [8, 34].

Case Study Connection: The Role of Early Nutrition in Shaping Futures

Consider the case of two children born in Andhra Pradesh in 2000–2001—one with access to maternal health services, early nutrition interventions, and household stability, while the other faces poor prenatal care, low birth weight, and food insecurity.

By infancy (2002), the first child benefits from antenatal care, reflecting in adequate weight and height measures, while the second struggles with lower birth size and delayed growth markers.

Fast forward to toddlerhood (2006)—the first child maintains a steady growth trajectory, bolstered by early breastfeeding, adequate maternal nutrition, and stable food access. Meanwhile, the second child exhibits persistent undernutrition, a consequence of early-life deficits that were not fully mitigated by later interventions.

This case reflects the study's findings—nutritional status during the WoO overwhelmingly dictates growth potential, reaffirming the need for targeted interventions within infancy rather than relying solely on later compensatory mechanisms.

---

[9] This variable is collected by asking the caregiver about the perception of a child's birth size in comparison to other children in the community. Since 80% of the sample does not have the actual birth weight of the child, we use this variable to gauge a child's nutritional status at birth.

Table 10.2 Shapley–Owen values for infancy and toddlerhood (percentage of R^2)

		Infancy (1–1.5 years)			Toddlerhood (4.5–5.5 years)	
Group	Regressor	Weight-for-age	Height-for-age	Weight-for-height	Weight-for-age	Height-for-age
1a	**Indicators of In utero Health (WoO in the first 270 days)**					
	Prenatal care	3.79	2.39	5.06		
	Perception of birth size and breastfeeding	18.92	10.14	16.54		
1b	**WoO at 365–547 days (infancy)**					
	Past nutritional status				70.99	62.48
2	**Indicators of prenatal and postnatal care**					
	Health better	27.22	11.37	24.94	2.39	1.63
	Vaccination	0.96	1.22	2.85	2.00	2.93
3	**Compensatory and supportive investments**					
	Government programs PDS, IKP, DWRCA				3.76	5.86
	Sanitation, fuel, and drinking water	4.72	4.53	2.43	2.57	4.90
	Wealth index	8.63	6.55	3.19	3.73	6.37
4	**Child characteristics**					
	Child age, social group, gender	21.80	33.59	11.54	9.46	8.24
5	**Community level characteristics**					
	Location (type of site and district)	11.87	29.19	29.53	5.10	7.60
6	**Bad event**			2.09	0.11	4.33

The Intergenerational Link: How Maternal Health Shapes Child Growth

The study also finds maternal health—especially maternal weight—significantly influences child nutrition, reinforcing the importance of maternal well-being from conception onwards. These findings are in line with past research linking maternal malnutrition to low birth weight [46, 48, 49].

A growing body of evidence suggests that a mother's nutritional deprivation as a child can be passed down to her newborn, affecting the child's growth potential in non-genetic ways [50]. For instance, studies on California birth records show that low birth-weight mothers are more likely to give birth to low birth-weight infants, with intergenerational transmission particularly strong in high-poverty zones [51]. Similarly, children born in adverse socioeconomic conditions face heightened risk from poor maternal health, deepening existing inequalities [52].

Data from rural Vietnam further suggests that both maternal and paternal height significantly correlate with child height-for-age, reflecting the cumulative impact of parental health on child development [53]. This highlights why investing in maternal nutrition, particularly in resource-poor settings, can break the cycle of intergenerational malnutrition.

Compensatory or Supportive Investments: Discussion

While the first 1,000 days lay the foundation for a child's nutritional trajectory, compensatory investments—such as government programs, improved health services, sanitation, and household wealth—have the potential to mitigate nutritional deficiencies. However, their effectiveness depends on when and how interventions are implemented.

One study highlights that environmental factors vary across individuals, and the combined effect of genetic predispositions and external conditions—referred to as 'etiologic heterogeneity'—can influence whether malnutrition manifests in a child [50]. This raises a fundamental question: Can interventions introduced beyond infancy compensate for nutritional disadvantages experienced in early life?

Case Study Connection: The Role of Compensatory Investments in Mitigating Early Deficits

Returning to the case of the two children born in Andhra Pradesh, their nutritional trajectories diverged significantly in the first 1,000 days.

- The first child, raised in a household with better access to early nutrition and healthcare, entered toddlerhood with adequate height and weight-for-age measures.
- The second child, whose mother had poor prenatal care and limited postnatal support, exhibited stunted growth by infancy, raising concerns about long-term nutritional impacts.

However, by 2006, the second child benefited from targeted interventions—including mid-day meals at school, improved sanitation, and government safety-net programs like PDS and IKP. While these interventions provided some relief, they did not fully compensate for the early-life deficits, aligning with the study's findings that nutritional status in infancy explains 70% of weight-for-age variation in toddlerhood (Table 10.2).

The Role of Sanitation and Environmental Factors

Research consistently links poor sanitation, open defecation, and high population density to persistent child malnutrition [54, 55]. In countries with high rates of open defecation, stunting prevalence often exceeds 35%, highlighting the critical need for sanitation reforms. In India, where population density is high, the negative health effects of poor sanitation are amplified [56].

Despite this well-established link, sanitation variables appear insignificant in this analysis. However, other household infrastructure investments, including drinking water improvements and access to cleaner cooking fuel, show positive associations with nutritional status. Sanitation and fuel quality account for approximately 5% of the variation in stunting and underweight in 2002 and explain 3–5% of the variation in 2006 (Table 10.2).

The Impact of Mid-Day Meals and Social Safety Nets

By toddlerhood, government-supported programs—especially mid-day meals in schools—begin to positively influence nutritional status. Since infants are too young to benefit from these interventions, their effect is measurable only after early childhood. Studies confirm that mid-day meal programs act as safety nets, significantly improving child health and nutritional indicators [57].

Similarly, social security initiatives like PDS and IKP help stabilize household food access and economic conditions, indirectly supporting child nutrition [58]. These compensatory programs collectively account for around 5% of the R-squared for weight-for-age and height-for-age during toddlerhood.

Wealth and Nutrition: A Persistent Relationship

Household wealth continues to be a major determinant of child nutrition, reinforcing existing research linking income and per capita consumption expenditure to nutritional status [36, 37, 59]. The analysis finds a strong positive effect of wealth index on z-scores across all indicators for both rounds of data collection.

- In infancy (2002), wealth index explains 9% of the variation in weight-for-age, 6.5% for height-for-age, and 3.1% for weight-for-height.
- In toddlerhood (2006), it contributes 4 and 6.3% of the R-squared for weight-for-age and height-for-age, respectively (Table 10.2).

These findings reinforce that while wealth can enhance nutritional opportunities, early-life deficits are difficult to reverse solely through later economic improvements.

Other Controls: Household and Environmental Influences

Beyond nutrition-specific interventions, a range of household and environmental factors shape a child's nutritional trajectory. The analysis confirms that parental education, household size, socioeconomic background, and environmental shocks play crucial roles in determining growth outcomes.

Parental Education and Household Size

Among household-level influences, father's education is found to be a key determinant of child nutrition. When the father is the primary earner and decision-maker, higher educational attainment often translates into greater awareness of health and dietary needs, leading to improved nutritional status for children [60].

Conversely, larger households exhibit poorer nutritional outcomes, likely due to resource constraints. Families with limited financial means may struggle to adequately distribute food and healthcare among multiple members, contributing to growth deficits.

Case Study Connection: How Household Factors Shape Outcomes

In the case study of the two children born in Andhra Pradesh, household dynamics further influenced their nutritional trajectories.

- The first child, raised in a smaller household with an educated father, benefited from greater food security and parental awareness, supporting healthy growth patterns.
- The second child, born into a larger family with fewer educational and economic resources, faced nutritional deficits, reinforcing findings that household size and parental education directly impact child development.

Caste and Social Disparities in Nutrition

The study finds significant variations in nutritional outcomes across caste groups. In infancy (2002), children from Scheduled Castes (SCs), Scheduled Tribes (STs), and Backward Classes (BCs) displayed poorer nutritional indicators than those from Other Castes (OCs). By toddlerhood (2006), BC children showed particularly high rates of stunting, consistent with broader research highlighting unequal health and nutrition access across caste groups [61].

Environmental Shocks and Seasonal Nutritional Variability

Extreme weather conditions—particularly excess rainfall—negatively impact weight-for-age and height-for-age z-scores. Seasonal analysis further reveals that children interviewed during summer months tend to exhibit lower weight-for-age indicators compared to those measured in winter [62, 63].

This aligns with agricultural cycles, where summer represents a low point in food availability and household income, potentially leading to reduced dietary intake for children. Rural communities are especially vulnerable, with rural children consistently exhibiting poorer nutritional indicators compared to their urban counterparts.

Urban Versus Rural Nutritional Disparities

The study reinforces regional disparities in child nutrition, with rural areas experiencing higher rates of undernutrition. At an aggregate level, 50% of rural children were classified as underweight, compared to 38% in urban locations [44, 45].

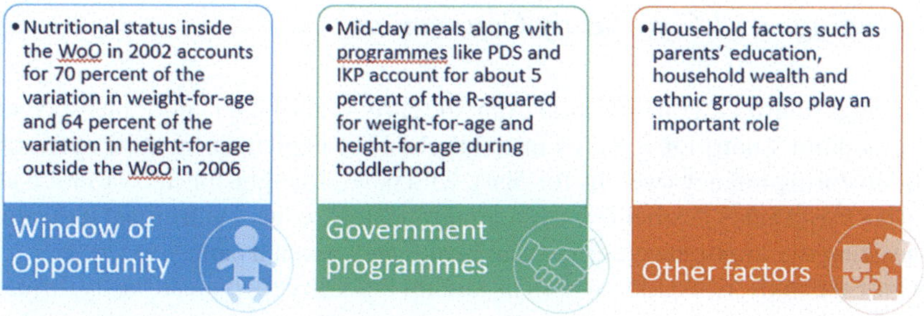

Fig. 10.3 Snapshot of important findings

Bringing It Together: Case Study Implications

The findings illustrate that nutrition is shaped by a complex interplay of household education, socioeconomic conditions, and environmental shocks. In the case study:

- The first child, growing up in an urban setting with stable food access, was less affected by seasonal and environmental disruptions.
- The second child, born in a rural location with exposure to excess rainfall and financial instability, experienced prolonged undernutrition, reflecting the real-life impact of rural disadvantage.

These disparities reaffirm the need for targeted interventions, ensuring children in low-resource households and rural areas receive support beyond infancy, mitigating long-term nutritional deficits. Figure 10.3 gives a snapshot of important findings.

Conclusion

Strengthening Early Nutrition for Long-Term Impact

This chapter set out to determine the extent to which early-life nutrition influences long-term nutritional status, relative to other environmental factors. By analyzing data at two key points—infancy (2002) and toddlerhood (2006)—it examined the impact of prenatal conditions, birth size, and maternal health, alongside compensatory mechanisms such as improved sanitation, government programs, and infrastructure investments. Using a cohort of approximately 2,000 children, the study adapted the UNICEF framework to identify critical drivers of nutritional status both inside and outside the Window of Opportunity (WoO).

Key Findings and Case Study Connection

The findings reinforce a fundamental truth: the early years matter enormously. Nearly 70% of a child's nutritional status in toddlerhood is explained by their nutritional condition during infancy (weight-for-age), with 64% of height-for-age variation also traced back to infancy. A smaller birth size significantly reduces nutritional indicators, emphasizing the importance of maternal health and prenatal care.

In the case study, two children born in Andhra Pradesh experienced vastly different trajectories:

- The first child, born with adequate birth weight, received prenatal care and consistent breastfeeding, supporting healthy development.
- The second child, born with lower birth weight and inadequate maternal nutrition, faced early-life growth deficits—which persisted despite later interventions.

This reflects the study's core finding—that compensatory and supportive investments such as mid-day meals, PDS, and improved sanitation, while helpful, only account for 5–6.5% of variation in nutritional status. These measures cannot fully counteract deficits experienced within the first 1,000 days.

Policy Implications: Prioritizing Early Interventions

From a policy perspective, the findings make a compelling case for early nutritional interventions—particularly within the first 270 days in utero. Since maternal nutrition directly influences birth weight, prenatal care must be strengthened, with targeted policies ensuring expectant mothers receive adequate nourishment. Addressing maternal health in pregnancy is critical to disrupting intergenerational cycles of malnutrition.

Additionally, while compensatory programs offer valuable nutritional support, they must be enhanced to increase their impact. There is potential to shift from nutrition-sensitive to nutrition-specific interventions, ensuring programs explicitly focus on early nutrition rather than broader socioeconomic factors.

Challenges and the Path Forward

Despite existing government initiatives, gaps remain in identifying beneficiaries, funding allocations, administrative efficiency, and infrastructure development. Strengthening monitoring systems, improving community engagement, and expanding program coverage would significantly enhance effectiveness.

Greater collaboration between stakeholders—including the private sector, civil society, and policymakers—will be essential in crafting holistic solutions. Long-term success lies in not just treating malnutrition but preventing it, ensuring every child receives the nutritional foundation needed for a healthy future.

References

1. WHO. (2024). *Factsheets.* Accessed at Fact sheets—Malnutrition (who.int).
2. UNICEF. (2023). *Malnutrition in Children—Global Data.* Retrieved from https://data.unicef.org/topic/nutrition/malnutrition/
3. WHO. (2025). *Malnutrition in Children.* Retrieved from https://www.who.int/data/nutrition/nlis/info/malnutrition-in-children
4. USAID. (2020). *Multi-Sectoral Nutrition Strategy Technical Brief: Implementation Guidance for Preventing Child & Maternal Death.* Accessed at Role of Nutrition in Preventing Child and Maternal Deaths (usaid.gov) in August 2024.
5. Fishman, S. M., et al. (2004). *Childhood and Maternal Underweight.* Accessed at http://www.who.int/publications/cra/chapters/volume1/0039-0162.pdf in The Comparative Quantification of Health Risks.
6. Vats, H., et al. (2025). *Determinants of Malnutrition Among Children Under Five Years of Age in India: A Review.* Retrieved from https://www.researchgate.net/publication/371291310_DETERMINANTS_OF_MALNUTRITION_AMONG_CHILDREN_UNDER_FIVE_YEAR_OF_AGE_GROUP_IN_INDIA_A_REVIEW
7. NITI Aayog. (2023). *Transforming Child Nutrition: State-Level Approaches and Practices for Community-Based Comprehensive Care and Management of Acute Malnutrition.* Retrieved from https://www.niti.gov.in/sites/default/files/2023-12/CMAM-report-NITI-Aayog.pdf
8. Martorell, R. (1985). Child Growth Retardation: A Discussion of Its Causes and Its Relationship to Health in Nutritional Adaptation in Man. In K. Blaxter & J. C Waterlow (Eds.). (pp. 13–29). John Libbey.
9. Martorell, R., Rivera, J., & Kaplowitz, H. (1990). Consequences of Stunting in Early Childhood for Adult Body Size in Rural Guatemala. *Annales Nestle, 48*, 85–92.
10. Dornan, P., & Georgiadis, A. (2015). *Nutrition, Stunting and Catch-Up Growth* (Young Lives Policy Brief No. 27). Retrieved from https://www.younglives.org.uk/sites/www.younglives.org.uk/files/YL-PolicyBrief-27_Nutrition%20Stunting%20and%20Catch-up%20Growth.pdf
11. Scott, J. A. (2020). The First 1,000 Days: A Critical Period of Nutritional Opportunity and Vulnerability. *Nutrition & Dietetics, 77*, 295–297. Retrieved from https://doi.org/10.1111/1747-0080.12617SCOTT.
12. UNICEF. (2024). *Improving Maternal Nutrition: An Acceleration Plan to Prevent Malnutrition and Anaemia During Pregnancy.* Retrieved from https://www.unicef.org/media/153581/file/Maternal%20nutrition%20acceleration%20plan.pdf
13. Xu, T., et al. (2024). Global Burden of Maternal Disorders Attributable to Malnutrition from 1990 to 2019 and Predictions to 2035: Worsening or Improving? *Frontiers in Nutrition, 11*, Article 1343772. https://doi.org/10.3389/fnut.2024.1343772
14. Flores, R. & Frongillo, E. A. (2001). Levels and Trends in Growth Failure in Developing Countries in Nutrition and Growth. In R. Martorell & F. Haschke (Eds.), *Nestle Nutrition Workshop Series, Pediatric Program*, 47.
15. Pandit, P., Galande, S., & Iris, F. (2021). Maternal malnutrition and Anaemia in India: Dysregulations Leading to the 'Thin-Fat' Phenotype in Newborns. *Journal of Nutritional Science, 10*, e91. https://doi.org/10.1017/jns.2021.83
16. Shrimpton, S., Victora, C. G., de Onis, M., Lima, R. C., Blossner, M., & Clugston, G. (2001). Worldwide Timing of Growth Faltering: Implications Nutritional Interventions. *Pediatrics, 107*(5), 1–7.

17. Victora, C. G., et al. & the Maternal and Child Undernutrition Study Group. (2008). Maternal and Child Undernutrition: Consequences for Adult Health and Human Capital. *Lancet, 371*(9609), 340–357.
18. Suryawan, A., et al. (2022). Malnutrition in Early Life and Its Neurodevelopmental and Cognitive Consequences: A Scoping Review. *Nutrition Research Reviews, 35*(1), 136–149. Retrieved from https://doi.org/10.1017/S0954422421000159.
19. Martorell, R. (1999). The Nature of Child Malnutrition and Its Long-Term Implications. *Food and Nutrition Bulletin, 20*, 288–292.
20. UNICEF. (2024). *Early Childhood Nutrition*. Retrieved from https://www.unicef.org/nutrition/early-childhood-nutrition
21. UNICEF. (2024). *Nutrition for Every Child—Global Annual Results Report*. Retrieved from https://clearinghouse.unicef.org/sites/ch/files/ch/sites-PD-Nutrition-Child%20Nutrition%20and%20Development%20KU-UNICEF_2023_GARR_Nutrition-for-every-chil-8.0.pdf
22. National Scientific Council on the Developing Child (CDC). (2007). *The Timing and Quality of Early Experiences Combine to Shape Brain Architecture* (Working Paper #5). Retrieved from http://developingchild.harvard.edu/resources/reports_and_working_papers/working_papers/wp5/.
23. National Health Mission, NHM. (2025). *Child Health in India—National Health Mission*. Retrieved from https://www.nhm.gov.in/index1.php?lang=1&level=2&sublinkid=819&lid=219
24. Vir, S. C., & Suri, S. (2023). Young Child Undernutrition: Crucial to Prioritize Nutrition Interventions in the First 1,000 Days of Life. *Indian Journal of Pediatrics, 90*(1), 85–94. Retrieved from https://doi.org/10.1007/s12098-023-04732-4.
25. Jain, A., Kim, R., Swaminathan, S., & Subramanian, S. V. (2024). Socioeconomic Inequality in Child Health Outcomes in India: Analyzing Trends Between 1993 and 2021. *International Journal for Equity in Health, 23*, Article 149 Retrieved from https://doi.org/10.1186/s12939-024-02218-z
26. Sehgal, M., Jatrana, S., Johnson, L., et al. (2024). Assessing Child Health in India: Development and Validation of a Comprehensive Child Health Index. *Child Ind Res, 17*, 657–682. https://doi.org/10.1007/s12187-024-10112-x
27. Schott, W. B., Crookston, B. T., Lundeen, E. A., Stein, A. D., & Behrman, J. R., and the Young Lives Determinants and Consequences of Child Growth Project Team. (2013). Periods of Child Growth up to Age 8 Years in Ethiopia, India, Peru and Vietnam: Key Distal Household and Community Factors. *Social Science & Medicine, 97*, 278–287.
28. Lundeen, E. A., et al. (2014). Growth Faltering and Recovery in Children Aged 1–8 Years in Four Low and Middle Income Countries: Young Lives. *Public Health Nutrition, 17*(9), 2131–2137.
29. Best Start Resource Centre (BSRC). (2011). *Early Brain Development: Parent Knowledge in Ontario*. Retrieved from http://www.beststart.org/resources/hlthy_chld_dev/pdf/Early_brain_development_fnl.pdf
30. Goulet, O. (2010). Growth Faltering: Setting the Scene. *European Journal of Clinical Nutrition, 64*, S2–S4.
31. UNICEF. (2012). Programming Guide: Infant and Young Child Feeding.
32. UNICEF. (United Nations Children's Fund). (1990). *Strategy for Improved Nutrition of Children and Women in Developing Countries*. New York: A Policy Review.
33. Richard, S. A., Black, R. E., & Checkley, W. (2012). Revisiting the Relationship of Weight and Height in Early Childhood. *American Society for Nutrition and Advances in Nutrition, 3*, 250–254.
34. Victora, C. G., de Onis, M., Hallal, P. C., Blössner, M., & Shrimpton, R. (2010). Worldwide Timing of Growth Faltering: Revisiting Implications for Interventions. *Pediatrics, 125*(3), e473–e480.
35. Black, R. E., et al. (2008). Maternal and Child Undernutrition Group. Maternal and Child Undernutrition: Global and Regional Exposures and Health Consequences. *Lancet, 371*, 243–260.

36. Strauss, J., & Thomas, D. (1998). Health, Nutrition and Economic Development. *Journal of Economic Literature, 36*(2), 766–817.
37. Glewwe, P., & Miguel, E. A. (2008). The Impact of Child Health and Nutrition on Education in Less Developed Countries. In T. P. Schultz & J. Strauss (Eds.), *Handbook of Development Economics* (Vol. 4, pp. 3561–606). Elsevier Publisher.
38. Strauss, J. & Thomas, D. (1995). Human Resources: Empirical Modeling of Household and Family Decisions. In J. R. Behrman & T. N. Srinivasan (Eds.), *Handbook of Development Economics* (Vol. 3). North Holland Press.
39. Shorrocks, S. A. (2013). Decomposition Procedures for Distributional Analysis: A Unified Framework Based on the Shapley Value. *Journal of Economic Inequality, 11*, 99–126.
40. Hoddinott, J., & Kinsey, B. (2001). Child Growth in the Time of Drought. *Oxford Bulletin of Economics and Statistics, 63*(4), 409–436.
41. Alderman, H., Hoddinott, J., & Kinsey, B. H. (2006). Long Term Consequences of Early Childhood Malnutrition. *Oxford Economic Papers, 58*(3), 450–474.
42. Mendiratta, V. (2015). *Impact of Rainfall Shocks on Child Health: Evidence from India.* (PSE Working Papers 33). Accessed at https://hal.archives-ouvertes.fr/halshs-01211575/document in November 2015.
43. Huettner, F., & Sunder, M. (2012). Rego: Stata Module for Decomposing Goodness of Fit According to Owen and Shapley values. United Kingdom Stata Users' Group Meetings 2012, Stata Users Group 17, Stata Users Group.
44. IIPS and Ministry of Health and Family Welfare. (2000). National Family Health Survey-2, Andhra Pradesh, 1998–99, International Institute for Population Sciences, Mumbai.
45. IIPS and Macro International. (2007). National Family Health Survey-3 (NFHS-3), 2005–2006, International Institute for Population Sciences, Mumbai.
46. Fedorov, L., & Sahn, D. (2005). Socioeconomic Determinants of Children's Health in Russia: A Longitudinal Survey. *Economic Development and Cultural Change, 53*(2), 479–500.
47. Cebu Study Team. (1992). A Child Health Production Function Estimated from Longitudinal Data. *Journal of Development Economics, 38*, 323–351.
48. Alderman, H. (2005). Linkages Between Poverty Reduction Strategies and Child Nutrition: An Asian Perspective. *Economic and Political Weekly, 40*, 4837–4842.
49. FOCUS. (2006). Focus on Children Under Six, Citizen's Initiative for the Rights of Children Under Six (CIRCUS).
50. Hernandez, L. M., & Blazer D. G. (2006). *Genetics and Health Chapter in Genes, Behaviour and the Social Environment.* Accessed at http://www.ncbi.nlm.nih.gov/books/NBK19932/#_ncbi_dlg_citbx_NBK19932 in November 2015.
51. Currie, J., & Moretti, E. (2007). Biology as Destiny? Short- and Long-Run Determinants of Intergenerational Transmission of Birth Weight. *Journal of Labor Economics, 25*(2), 231–263. Retrieved from https://doi.org/10.1086/511377.
52. Bhalotra, S., & Rawlings, S. (2013). Gradients of Intergenerational Transmission of Health in Developing Countries. *Review of Economics and Statistics, 95*(2), 660–672.
53. Venkataramani, A. S. (2011). The Intergenerational Transmission of Height: Evidence from Rural Vietnam. *Health Economics, 20*(12), 1448–1467.
54. S pears, D. (2011). *How Much International Variation in Child Height Can Sanitation Explain?* [Working paper]. Retrieved from http://www.princeton.edu/rpds/papers/Spears_Height_and_Sanitation.pdf.
55. Chambers, R., & Madeazza, G. V. (2013). Sanitation and Stunting in India: Undernutrition's Blind Spot. *Economic & Political Weekly, 48*(25), 15–19.
56. Spears, D. (2012). Height and Cognitive Achievement Among Indian Children. *Economics & Human Biology, 10*(2), 210–219.
57. Singh, A., Park, A., & Dercon, S. (2012). School Meals as a Safety Net: An Evaluation of the Midday Meal Scheme in India. *Economic Development and Cultural Change, 62*(2), 275–306.
58. Narayanan, S., & Gerber, N. (2015). *Social Safety Nets for Food and Nutritional Security in India* (Working paper IGIDR). Retrieved from http://www.igidr.ac.in/pdf/publication/WP-2015-031.pdf.

59. Glick, P., & Sahn, D. (2000). Schooling of Girls and Boys in a West African Country: The Effects of Parental Education, Income, and Household Structure. *Economics of Education Review, 19*(1), 63–87.
60. Ali, S. S., Karim N., & Haider S. S. (2005). Association of Literacy of Fathers with Malnutrition Among Children Under Three Years of Age in Rural Area of District Malir, Karachi. *Medical Channel, 11*(1), 26–29.
61. Babar, N. F., Muzaffar, R., Khan, M. A., & Imdad, S. (2010). Impact of Socioeconomic Factors on Nutritional Status in Primary School Children. *Journal of Ayub Medical College, Abbottabad, 22*(4), 15–18.
62. Rao, S., Kanade, A. N., Yajnik, C. S., & Fall, C. H. D. (2009). Seasonality in Maternal Intake and Activity Influence Offspring's Birth Size Among Rural Indian Mothers—Pune Maternal Nutrition Study. *International Journal of Epidemiology, 38*(4), 1094–1103.
63. Hillbruner, C., & Egan, R. (2008). Seasonality, Household Food Security, and Nutritional Status in Dinajpur, Bangladesh. *Food and Nutrition Bulletin, 29*(3), 221–231.

Chapter 11
Role of Health Professionals and Community Workers in Monitoring Child Development

Sebanti Ghosh

Introduction

Enabling young children to reach their full developmental potential is both a child rights issue and a crucial requirement for achieving sustainable development goals. Global Strategy for Women's, Children's and Adolescents' Health 2016–30, provide the overarching framework for children to survive and thrive to achieve their full potential. Optimal health and development from preconception to adulthood are crucial for future human capital formation. The Convention on the Rights of the Child, highlights the importance of early child development, stating that a child has the right to develop to "the maximum extent possible" (Article 6), and that "States Parties recognize the right of every child to a standard of living adequate for the child's physical, mental, spiritual, moral and social development" (Article 27).The immense benefits of investing in early childhood development (ECD) and nurturing caring practices by parents and caregivers for improved learning, productivity, long-term health, and social well-being along the life course is well emphasized by The Lancet series 2017 on Advancing Early Childhood Development: From Science to Scale.

ECD is defined in a standard manner as the process of cognitive, physical, language, temperament, socio-emotional, and motor development of children that starts at the time of conception until 8 years of age. The earliest years as well as pregnancy period are particularly important, for being the time of rapid brain development, and enhanced sensitivity and impact of nurturing care interventions related to health, nutrition, development support, safety, and early learning opportunities as was elaborated in The Lancet Series in 2017.

S. Ghosh (✉)
Public Health (MNCAH) and Nutrition Expert, Delhi, India
e-mail: sebantisonu@gmail.com

S. Suri (ed.), *Child Health and Nutrition from Conception to Age Two*,
https://doi.org/10.1007/978-981-95-7868-9_11

This chapter focuses on the importance of providing nurturing support through healthcare professionals for child development from preconception till two years of age.

The importance of ECD as a central component of global and national development has been recognized through the inclusion of a dedicated target 4.2 (all girls and boys have access to quality early childhood development, care and pre-primary education so that they are ready for primary education) and indicator 4.2.1 (Proportion of children aged 24–59 months who are developmentally on track in health, learning and psychosocial well-being, by sex) within the Sustainable Development Goals (SDGs), demonstrating a high level global commitment toward equitable access to quality early childhood development for all children. A single dollar investment in early childhood development has the potential to give a return as high as three dollars [1].

Yet an estimated 250 million i.e., 43% children under five years are at risk of not achieving their developmental potential in the first five years of life in low- and middle-income countries (LMICs).

Policy Landscape

Global Policy In 2018, WHO, UNICEF and the World Bank Group, in collaboration with the Partnership for Maternal, Newborn and Child Health (PMNCH) and the Early Childhood Development Action Network, launched the Nurturing Care Framework for ECD to support health and relevant sectors and stakeholders in aligning their commitments and develop a coordinated roadmap for action to provide good health, adequate nutrition, safety and security, responsive caregiving, and opportunities for early learning to ensure full development potential of every child [1].

Over the next five years, this has resulted in improved understanding and recognition of the importance of early childhood development among multiple sectors including health and stakeholders together, with a forty eight percent increase in the number of low- and middle-income countries implementing policies and services early childhood development to ensure a greater number of children are on track for optimal development [2]. WHO and UNICEF, in the 2021 document Investing in Our Future: A Comprehensive Agenda for the Health and Well-being of Children and Adolescents reiterates the importance of healthy development as a cumulative continuous process, broadening the focus from survival to thriving and well-being of children. Improving Early Childhood Development: WHO Guidelines 2020 emphasized on provision of responsive care and early learning activities during the first three years of life through parents and caregivers along with the need for empowering parents in responsive care giving and integrating psychosocial interventions to support maternal mental health.

India Policy Landscape Nearly half, i.e., 45% of India's young children are at risk of poor development [3]. Despite the remarkable progress in child survival, India still faces a very high burden of chronic child malnutrition and anemia which adversely affects optimal child development in the country. Currently 35% of children below five years are stunted, 19% wasted, 32% underweight and 67% of 6–59 months old children anemic in India according to National Family Health Survey (NFHS) 5 2019–21. Moreover, inter-generational transmission of poor development is marked with 19% women in the reproductive age group being underweight, 12% having short stature and 57% anemic and a high burden of 18% low birth weight babies.

India has made significant progress in policy and programming pertaining to optimal child development. Multiple policies across Ministry of Health and Family Welfare (MoHFW) and Ministry of Women and Child Development (MWCD) have integrated and prioritized Care Beyond Survival: Thriving and Development agenda for infants and young children as reflected in the India Newborn Action Plan (INAP) 2014, National Early Childhood Care and Education (ECCE) Policy, 2013, Rashtriya Bal Swasthya Karyakram (RBSK) 2014, Home-based care for young child (HBYC) 2018, PAALAN 1000 Campaign 2022, and Family Participatory Care Guidelines [4]. The above mentioned policies and guidelines promote multi-sectoral actions focusing on delivering integrated health, nutrition, age-appropriate play and communication, development milestone tracking, screening of development delays/disabilities and appropriate referral for management, growth monitoring & promotion services and counselling as well as early learning activities by frontline health and nutrition workers and generating awareness and improving knowledge and skills of mothers & family members including fathers, grandparents to provide responsive and nurturing care along with family participatory developmentally supportive care for small and sick newborn in health facilities [4]. In addition the Integrated Child Development Scheme (ICDS) under MWCD is one of the largest community-based programs in the world aimed at improving health, nutrition, optimal child development, and early childhood care and education to children below six years [5]. Moreover to enable socioeconomically vulnerable families to access and provide quality, nurturing child-care key complementary actions in sectors like social protection include the Maternity Benefits (Amendment) Act 2017 with provision of paid maternity and childcare leave and workplace creches for children, Pradhan Mantri Matru Vandana Yojana offering conditional cash support for maternal nutrition and well-being, and National Creches Scheme to provide high-quality childcare services for children 6 months to 6 years, of working mothers [5–8].

Understanding Child Development and the Risks

Early childhood development (ECD) is a maturational and iterative process involving an ordered progression of motor, cognitive, language, socio-emotional and self-regulatory skills, and capacities across the first few years of life. While early childhood development covers children aged 0–8 years, the Nurturing Care Framework focuses on the period from pregnancy till three years since the first 1,000 days of life is a very sensitive period for brain development [1].

The major threats to optimal child development include extreme poverty, violence and conflict, gender inequities, environmental hazards, poor mental health and undernutrition [9]. The five key nutrition risk factors which have been identified for poor ECD are: poor maternal nutrition, iodine deficiency during pregnancy, iron deficiency, poor linear growth, and severe acute malnutrition [10]. Despite progress made toward reduction in risks to optimal child development according to the 2023 estimates by World Bank, almost 700 million people or 8.5% are living in extreme poverty with one out of six children living in extreme poverty. The multiple conflict, climate crises, and COVID pandemic had triggered reversal of the gains in child survival, development, and well-being. Globally, while under five year mortality rate and the neonatal mortality rate have declined to 37 and 17 respectively in 2022 [11], at the same time, 148 million children under five across the globe are stunted, and 45 million suffered from wasting [12]. The Lancet Maternal and Child Undernutrition Series, 2021 shows that the incidences of stunting and wasting which are well identified risk factors for poor child development, remain highest during first six months of life in low- and middle-income countries, reinforcing the importance of focusing on first 1,000 days. Poor maternal nutrition leads to low birth weight (LBW), which is associated with poor developmental outcomes. LBW infants are at significant developmental risk—including lower cognitive scores, poorer problem-solving skills, and behavioral issues.

The quality of a child's early experiences makes a critical difference as their brains develop, providing either strong or weak foundations for learning, earnings health and behavior, earnings health and behavior adult social relationships, well-being and throughout life. It has been noted that even babies born in underprivileged families who receive all the components of nurturing care—good health, adequate nutrition, safety and security, responsive parenting, and opportunities for early learning show an increase in their developmental potential. National investment in ECD is a cost-effective measure to promote inclusive economic growth, eradicate extreme poverty, and break inter-generational cycles of inequity [13] (Table 11.1).

Child Developmental Monitoring and Counselling

Wide variations in children's development have been observed. There are multiple socio-economic, cultural, gender, environment, and other factors which influence developmental trajectories at the individual, family, and community levels. In this context, focusing solely on tracking milestones without taking into account the socio-economic-cultural-gender and environmental determinants of child development is insufficient to identify children at risk of suboptimal development.

Child development monitoring should be multi-dimensional to include various components such as (i) milestone-based development tracking, identification of any developmental delay & individualized counselling, (ii) growth monitoring, & contextualized counselling using WHO Growth Charts to assess age-appropriate growth and detection of early growth faltering, (iii) assessment of child diets and

Table 11.1 Factors influencing child development in first 1,000 days

Influencing factors	Pathways of influence
Preconception health and nutrition care for parents	Preconception care is important for reducing the risks of premature births, low birthweight, birth defects, or other birth-related conditions that could hinder optimal development Studies have identified the mechanisms through which poor metabolic and mental health in parents before pregnancy can impact their children's development, both during infancy and beyond [14–17]
Adolescent health & well-being Support	Interventions like helping girls complete schooling, promoting healthy diets, delaying pregnancy, and supporting healthy timing and planning for it contribute to minimizing the probability of low birthweight or stunting [18]
Exposure to tobacco smoke	Parental tobacco use including maternal smoking during pregnancy and passive smoke exposure during pregnancy are linked to adverse fetal development and perinatal outcomes including a 23% increased risk of stillbirth and 13% increased risk of congenital malformation severely compromising the development potential of the unborn child [19, 20]. Parental smoking and exposure of infants/young children to tobacco smoke in their immediate environment pose a higher risk of asthma, respiratory infections, and meningococcal disease, leading to increased mortality [20]
Exposure to environmental toxins	An infant or young child who is exposed to environmental pollutants from sources like unsafe drinking water, air pollution, or chemicals, and also the child who lacks access to spaces for outdoor physical activity and exploration is at higher risk of both non-communicable diseases (NCDs), infectious diseases (such as pneumonia and diarrhea) and developmental delays that can reduce their lifelong cognitive, socio-emotional, and physical potential [21]
Positive parenting	Scientific findings from neuroscience and developmental psychology highlight the benefit of caregiver and child interactions for early childhood development, including formation of neural connections in the child's brain. A lack of positive relationships and inadequate supervision and engagement with children are strongly associated with a child's increased risk for behavioral and emotional problems [22]
Role of fathers	Interventions that engage fathers to improve their knowledge, related maternal and infant nutrition and encourage their active support and participation can contribute to improved exclusive breastfeeding rates and better nutrition for both infants and their mothers. Men's care and direct interaction with their young children improve infants and toddlers' cognitive, social, and emotional development, and enhance their mental health and well-being, school readiness and subsequent educational achievements. It can also help to develop children's empathy for others [23]

feeding practices, (iv) health check-ups for review of immunization status (v) assessments for detection and identification of any congenital anomalies and birth defects, diseases/infection, deficiencies, and disabilities, and appropriate referral (vi) review of the socio-economic-cultural conditions of the family/community (vii) assessment of exposure to environmental toxins including smoking/tobacco use in parents & second hand smoke and (viii) review of psychosocial health of mothers & care givers including risks for poor mental health [24]. Assessment of these socio-economic-cultural-gender factors should become an integral part of developmental and growth monitoring and providing counselling services in community-based and primary health care services. Currently such review of the socio-economic-cultural-gender factors is a weak or missing link in the current child development monitoring processes. Current development monitoring is mostly focused on tracking developmental milestones and growth monitoring using the WHO growth charts. Developmental milestones indicate the developmental abilities in various domains of physical, motor, cognitive, language, social, and emotional development that children are expected to acquire on average at a certain age, sometimes within a range. In addition, a more in-depth individual assessment is needed for children with signs of developmental delay or regression, congenital defects and disability and appropriate referral needs to be ensured for adequate management of such infants to maintain a safe continuum of care. Family participation is crucial in the holistic child development monitoring process so that the family—parents and other care givers are counselled, supported and enabled to provide age appropriate, stimulating, and nurturing care in the child's daily life [24].

The multi-component comprehensive development monitoring and active engagement of parents and family remains fragmented and suboptimal in the current scenario of child development monitoring along with gaps in quality, capacities of health and child development service providers both at community and at facility level and in monitoring of the services provided. There are inter country and intra country inequities in coverage and quality of holistic multi-dimensional child development monitoring.

Services to track and support early childhood development must be organized across the continuum-of-care. Firstly universal support for delivering nurturing care focused optimal health, nutrition, development & growth monitoring and early learning interventions should reach every child, through health promotion and prevention services at home/community and primary health acre level. Secondly, specialized support is required for families with infants and children with additional needs for specialized services. These include families with small and sick newborn, infants with birth defects or congenital anomalies, infants/children with developmental delays and developmental difficulties, disabilities undernourished children (underweight, stunted, and moderately/severely acute malnourished, HIV infected or exposed children, children of mothers suffering from depression, children in domestic violence, and young children without caregivers. There is also an emerging need for developmentally supportive nurturing in inpatient care for the survival and optimal thriving of small and sick newborns.

Role of HealthCare Professionals

The health sector has an important leading role and responsibility to provide nurturing childhood development related care interventions in close coordination with relevant sectors of nutrition, social protection, education, etc. Many interventions starting from preconception care, maternal, newborn, and child health and nutrition, mental health promotion, and HIV prevention and care have a direct impact on child development.

Firstly, the healthcare professionals both facility and community-based providers are expected to reach the newborn, infant and young children and their mothers/caregivers and families in the first three years of life through multiple home/community and facility-based to provide evidence-based maternal health and nutrition interventions during the antenatal period, childbirth, & postnatal period, essential newborn care at birth, infant/child immunization,, growth monitoring and developmental milestone tracking, and nutrition and health counselling. In addition, the facility-based healthcare providers undertake care of small and sick newborn, child immunization, screening for birth defects/congenital anomalies, developmental delays & difficulties, disabilities and diseases, growth monitoring, and prevention & management of childhood illnesses like diarrhea and pneumonia during this important and sensitive period of child development. Thus it is obvious health services are uniquely positioned to implement components of various nurturing care, for example, facilitating immediate skin to skin contact, early and exclusive breastfeeding promotion, responsive age-appropriate feeding, milestones and growth monitoring, health and nutrition counselling, early detection and management of birth defects, developmental delays, disabilities, growth faltering, management of severe acute malnutrition and integrated management of childhood illness. These nurturing care practices reduce risks of childhood mortality morbidity and poor development outcomes. However, while nurturing care approaches are gradually getting integrated in health care with updating of policy and program guidelines regarding the same, these services can be further strengthened by prioritizing nurturing care elements through enhancing the knowledge and skills of both frontline community-based and facility-based providers [25, 26]. In addition, the health sector can play a strong role in leveraging partnerships across sectors within government and also with private sector to support families and young children including those most vulnerable through provision of comprehensive, interdisciplinary and nurturing care to support optimal development and well-being of each child [27] (Table 11.2).

Table 11.2 Role community & facility-based health workers

Role of community-based health workers	Role of facility-based health workers
• Improve outreach and accessibility to early childhood development and care by mobilization of communities and linking to timely health, nutrition, early learning and social protection services and counselling • Identify vulnerable families and communities including the socio-economic condition, household environment, incidence of violence where children are at increased risk of suboptimal development or maltreatment and prioritize them for support • Provide home or community-based services as follows: tracking and counselling on developmental milestone related progress using checklist including identifying early warning signals; growth monitoring and promotion using growth charts to identify early growth faltering, provide immunization, assessment of feeding practices and diets undertake individualized health & nutrition counselling and facilitate timely referral for infants/children identified with any risk • Provide contextualized counselling to empower parents and family members with knowledge and skills on child development milestones and identification of delays, importance of growth monitoring, age-appropriate play & stimulation, responsive parenting, and optimal health and nutrition practices at each contact. Engage actively with both parents, grandparents, other family members and caregivers during counselling Engage actively with both parents, grandparents, other family members and caregivers during counselling • Identification and referral of high risk newborn children for adequate management and follow-ups services. High risk newborns include infants with low birth weight, preterm born, sick newborn, infants with birth defects, infants/young children with developmental delays and difficulties, children with disability and moderate and severe acutely malnourished (MAM/SAM) children • Assess mother/parent child interactions and bonding, in every health service contact and provide necessary guidance and counselling including age appropriate, play, stimulation & communication and responsive parent giving • Assess mother's and caregiver's mental health using appropriate screening checklist and facilitate support/referral as needed • Undertake social mobilization and actively engage with community leaders, panchayat members, school teachers, self- help group members to promote nurturing care and optimal child development	– Adopt evidence-based approaches to monitor children's growth and development comprehensively during every child consultation, including immunization contacts, well-child and sick child visits – Provide evidence-based developmentally supportive nurturing inpatient care for small and sick neonates using a family centered-approach – Identify and provide evidence-based management of high risk newborn—low birth weight/preterm/ sick newborn, birth defects, developmental delays & difficulties, disabilities, moderate and severe acutely malnourished (MAM/SAM) children with or without medical complications – Provide counselling to empower mothers and caregivers with knowledge and skills on child development, responsive parenting and nurturing care and optimal health and nutrition practices at each contact – Observe and assess parent child interaction and provide necessary guidance and counselling including age appropriate, play, stimulation & communication and responsive parent giving – Assess mother's and caregiver's mental health using appropriate screening checklist and provide appropriate services & support/and facilitate referral as needed – Collaborate with community-based workers across all levels of healthcare as well as other sectors to ensure a continuum of nurturing care-based child health and development care

Challenges and Gaps in Monitoring Child Development

Policy Related

Suboptimal prioritization in integrating early child development and nurturing care interventions including screening and early identification of birth defects, developmental delays and/or difficulties, disabilities, deficiencies, along with appropriate referral and management within ongoing maternal, newborn, child health, and nutrition program plans and implementation.

Program and Systems Related

1. There is no standardized guidance on evidence-based approaches for comprehensive multi-dimensional assessment and monitoring of early childhood development and growth in primary care services, apart from the use of developmental milestone tracking, and growth monitoring using anthropometric assessments in child health & nutrition services [24].
2. In many situations, parents and caregivers are not able to provide strong nurturing environments without help from local, regional, national, and international agencies owing to socio-economic and cultural constraints including poverty, migration, conflict, disasters, low social status, lack of education, minimal access to health, and nutrition services, gender-based violence. The impact of social-cultural, gender, and economic barriers impacting child development is often missed out in child development planning, implementation, and monitoring. The health care professionals are inadequately equipped to address socio-economic-cultural-gender determinants of child development.
3. Insufficient and limited capacity of community and facility-based healthcare providers to engage with and enable parents to understand developmental milestones and markers of progress, early signs of poor development and/or difficulties, provide responsive caregiving, and age-appropriate communication and stimulation to support optimal child development.
4. Community-based health workers are often poorly oriented and trained to identify signs of developmental delays and birth defects, provide individualized counselling and referral for needed services. They do not often have optimal capacity to undertake early identification, provide referral and follow-up support services and guidance to the parents counsel and support parents with at-risk babies.
5. Nurturing care is crucial for optimizing health, nutrition and development of premature, low birthweight babies and babies with congenital conditions who are often deprived of the same due to limited skills of facility-based healthcare providers to provide developmentally supportive nurturing care, and actively engage parents in inpatient caregiving processes.

6. Child development and humanitarian context: Adversities faced by children in conflict, disaster and displacement conditions result in a greater risk of impaired development, with minimal access to quality health, nutrition, and development monitoring services for parents and families. Around 250 million children are living in countries affected by armed conflict, while 160 million are very likely to suffer from famine and crises of food security [28]. Around 2% of global humanitarian funding is spent on education, however, early childhood development accounts for only a tiny fraction of that [28].
7. Measurement of early childhood development is complex and difficult. Approaches to measuring ECD at scale, have traditionally been based on screening and diagnostic tests where highly trained professionals are required. Standardized frameworks and institutional mechanisms to holistically track child development and nurturing care-related indicators remain suboptimal. The lack of standardized indicators and institutional mechanisms adversely affects regular monitoring and progress of ECD interventions.
8. Currently a multi-faceted early child development index (ECDI) has been designed by UNICEF to assess whether children (36–59 months of age) are "on track" in domains of literacy-numeracy, motor skills, approaches to learning, and social-emotional development [29].

Community Related

Limited awareness, understanding, and skills among parents, caregivers, and family members regarding child development—particularly early childhood developmental milestones—along with recognizing early warning signs of risk conditions or poor development, and practicing responsive caregiving, including age-appropriate play, communication, and stimulation.

Successful Community-Based Programs in India, South Asia, and Globally

1. Integrated nutrition and ECD program: Integrated nutrition and ECD interventions have greater potential for impact on nutrition and ECD outcomes in comparison to a single intervention [3]. Scientific evidence indicates that provisioning responsive care and early stimulation to stunted children helps them achieve better catch up growth similar to the level of their non-stunted peers [30, 31].

Some key examples of integrated ECD and nutrition programs:

- **Intensified ECD and Nutrition services through Integrated Child Development service (ICDS) Andhra Pradesh, India** piloted intensifying counselling on responsive IYCF practices and developmental stimulation (responsive feeding

and stimulating toys) within the routine ICDS services for children aged 3–15 months which improved the cognitive development scores, increased diversity in the children's diet, and increased their intake of key nutrients [32].
- **Bangladesh Responsive IYCF programming**: An intensive, large-scale intervention package aimed at improving IYCF in Bangladesh resulted in improvements in development achievements among children aged 6–23.9 and 24–47.9 months for language development and among children aged 6–23.9 month for gross motor development in addition to the large, significant impact on IYCF practices [33].
- **Chile Bundling of ECD and anemia prevention interventions**: The home-based ECD interventions and iron supplementation in Chile improved mental and socio-emotional development in anemic children [34].

2. Combined intervention programming including community mobilization, home visits, and creche facilities

Community-based interventions comprising of participatory learning and action with women's groups, counselling through home visits and setting up of crèche facilities for child care for working mothers in selected rural areas of Jharkhand and Odisha in India positively impacted child development by reducing undernutrition among children under three years [35].

3. Comprehensive Intersectoral Early Childhood Development and Care Programs

- **Meghalaya State Early Childhood Development Mission**: The state government of Meghalaya has launched Early Childhood Development Mission as integrated inter sectoral mission with Health, Education, Social Welfare, Community and Rural Development Departments with the aim to ensure that children aged 0–6 years receive nurturing care for their growth and early childhood development (ECD) in the state. Strategic actions include capacity building of frontline health and nutrition workers, strengthening SHGs and other community institutions, setting up helplines to support and guide frontline workers and parents. engaging & empowering parents through mobilization of parent groups and organization of community-based events to generate awareness on the importance of ECD [36]
- **Integration of nurturing care and child development in HIV care and prevention programs in Africa:** Several initiatives in African countries have shown encouraging results in integrating child development and nurturing care within maternal and child health and HIV care and prevention programs. The initiatives like Botswana's Early Moments Matter, South Africa's Side-by-Side campaigns, Rwanda's Community Insurance for Child Care focused on enhancing health-care worker capacity, intensifying social and behavior change communication campaigns, adopt child-friendly social protection policies, and promote strategic use of high-quality data including HIV disaggregated data in program decision making [37].

4. Empowering parents through engagement of local frontline health workers to promote early childhood development

Box 1: Results of Aarambh Project

Aarambh Project in Maharashtra. The third-party evaluation findings indicate the relevance of the project in successfully capacitating frontline health workers on responsive parenting and nurturing care for early childhood development. Improvements in nutrition status of children was noted with the decline in underweight, stunting and wasting from 39.1%, 42.8% and 17.4%, respectively in Nov–Dec 2018, to 32.5%, 41.0% and 12.4%, respectively in 2019) It is now being scaled up in a phased manner by the state government. During the same period, there was a significant improvement in the mean development quotient measured by Development Screening test and mean social quotient using the Vineland Social Maturity [38]

– **Aarambh Project, Maharashtra India** is a successful community-based model for delivering nurturing care interventions through individual, group and community-based engagement of parents and family members, creation of parent gatherings and enablement of parents and family members through frontline health and nutrition workers for promoting optimal health, nutrition and development stimulation play and communication. The project was implemented by Mahatma Gandhi Institute of Medical Sciences (MGIMS), Sewagram in collaboration with Department of Health and Family Welfare (DoHFW), Integrated Child Development Scheme (ICDS) of Department of Women and Child Development (DWCD) with the support of UNICEF in selected districts of Maharashtra. The Aarambh model leveraged the routine contact points with parents and other caregivers to build their capacities and support them to adopt nurturing care practices.

– **Kenya Group-Based Parenting Interventions to Promote Child Development**

A multi-arm, cluster-randomized community effectiveness trial in rural Kenya demonstrated that large group-based parenting interventions, including responsive stimulation and play for development and nutrition education involving Kenya's network of community health volunteers, successfully promoted child development which included improved child cognitive & receptive language, and socio-emotional development outcomes. These interventions showed no reduction in effectiveness compared to an intervention model using more personalized counselling of parents during home visits. The latter model was more expensive, human intensive and time-consuming. Thus the model of community-based parenting interventions offers greater potential for scalability in low resource settings [39].

Successful Facility-Based Interventions for Monitoring Child Development

1. Developmentally supportive family centered intensive inpatient care for small and sick newborn

– **Mother-neonatal intensive care unit (M-NICU) in India**: In 2017, Safdarjung Hospital, a premier government tertiary care facility in New Delhi demonstrated the feasibility of keeping the mother with their sick and newborn 24 × 7 by establishing a mother-neonatal intensive care unit (M-NICU) and providing developmentally supportive inpatient critical care. This resulted in better response and survival outcomes, improved breastfeeding rates, no increase in any adverse event like nosocomial infection and ensured quality continuum of care at home and regular follow-up as mothers were actively engaged in the care giving process. The Government of India has endorsed this initiative guidance has been disseminated [40].

– **Family Participatory Care in Neonatal Intensive Care Units in Tertiary and Secondary Care Hospitals**

A randomized controlled trial at the intensive neonatal care unit of a tertiary care Ram Manohar Lohia Hospital in New Delhi, involving mothers & caregivers demonstrated the benefits of Family Participatory Care (FPC) approach which empowers parents in responsive caregiving of their sick newborn during the hospital stay. This resulted in generated positive response from parents who got the opportunity to bond with their sick newborn and learn the skills to provide supportive nurturing care, and reduced their anxiety and stress, FPC also helped at-risk neonates to have a smooth transition from hospital to home, ensuring a safe continuum-of-care as parents had acquired necessary knowledge and skills for continuing and adhering to the responsive care protocols that increases their chance of surviving and thriving after discharge [41].

The Norway–India Partnership Initiative scaled this approach across 85 neonatal care units in three states with funding from the state governments. The results were promising with 75% mother and family members receiving capacity building FPC sessions; 86% newborns below 2 kg provided with kangaroo mother care until disch/arge; exclusive breastfeeding rate at 86%, and continuation of kangaroo mother care at home at 75%. The results also showed decline in mortality rate post-discharge from 7% to 2.7% in the implementing districts [42].

Bundling of Community and Facility-Based Interventions

Delivering integrated early childhood development interventions at community level and in primary health care facilities: Aga Khan Development Network (AKDN), implemented Early Childhood Development (ECD) programs in several states of India to ensure children get a smart start in life. In Uttar Pradesh, AKDN works closely with the government and local partners to promote the health, nutrition, and cognitive and social-emotional development of young children through capacity building of parents, teachers, and frontline health workers, enhancing their abilities to provide nurturing and responsive care at home and during outreach/community-based service deliver. At the same time the initiative promoted and worked closely with primary health care facilities to create developmentally supportive child-friendly environment in government health facilities for example in the OPDs for children and Nutrition Rehabilitation Centres for treatment of severely acute malnourished children (SAM) while orienting and training the facility-based providers (Table 11.3).

Emerging Recommendations

This is the time for consolidating and building on the learnings from the policy and programmatic achievements till date, address the current gaps based on evidence and expand & accelerate ongoing efforts to ensure sustained progress at scale.

The following issues merit attention and strengthening in policy and program implementation:

Robust national and sub-national multi-sectoral coordination mechanism is essential to ensure coordinated and coherent policy and program actions to strengthen the survive and thrive agenda for each child. It is important to consolidate existing experiences, identify what is working well and the constraints/challenge to improve strategy using evidence, update the roles and responsibilities of each sector and strengthen the convergent delivery of the interventions for child development in a comprehensive manner at the individual child and family level.

The need of the hour is to prioritize and embed child development interventions in existing reproductive, maternal newborn and child health and nutrition programs and budgets to facilitate improved coverage with quality and equity.

It is essential to shift from a narrow focus on developmental milestone monitoring to a broader inclusive approach to understanding multifactorial socio-economic, cultural and environmental risks. Concerted efforts are required to be made for addressing the additional or specialized requirement for children with clear signs of developmental delays and/or difficulties including multi-domain assessment, assure referral services for appropriate management, often requiring interdisciplinary care and follow-up support services.

The shift toward an interdisciplinary inclusive care also entails that child development and care services address the mental and psychosocial health of mothers/parents and address the social determinants of early childhood development.

It is vital to strengthen the capacity of systems to deliver quality care and support to children, including those requiring additional support.

(i) This requires policy and program for prioritized investment in training programs along with post training mentoring and supportive supervision to equip both health facility-based and community workers with the necessary

Table 11.3 Box summarizing learnings from key successful interventions [30–42]

Type of Successful Interventions	Key Strategic Approaches which worked well	Key outcomes
Community-based interventions		
1. Integrated nutrition & ECD services in Andhra Pradesh, India, Bangladesh Chile 2. Inter sectoral State ECD Mission, Meghalya India, 3. Integrated ECD in crèche services Odisha, Jharkhand 4. Integration of ECD in HIV& AIDS prevention & management program 5. ECD friendly primary health care facilities 6. Parenting interventions – Aarambh Project Maharashtra, India – Group parenting interventions Kenya	Multi-sectoral whole-of-government led whole-of-society approach Integrating ECD in nutrition interventions child care services, & HIV prevention & care, through both existing government program and non-government organizations Empowering parents and family members including grandparents in responsive nurturing care giving through engagement of frontline health & nutrition workers Parent to parent support network	Increased capacities of frontline health workers on responsive nurturing care focused ECD interventions Increased knowledge & skills of parents in responsive and nurturing parenting and caregiving Improved nurturing care practices—responsive feeding and health care at home Improvements in nutrition status of children—decline in underweight, stunting and wasting Improvements in cognitive development scores Improvements in development—language skills, & gross motor development
Facility-based interventions: Developmentally supportive family-centered intensive inpatient care for small and sick new born		
1. Establishment of Mother-Neonatal Intensive Care Unit (M-NICU), India 2. Family Participatory Care for Small & Sick Newborn in Neonatal Intensive Care Units India	Provision for Mothers' Stay at NICU with sick new born Adoption of developmentally supportive nurturing care practices in NICUs Enabling mothers in providing responsive care to their sick new born during the hospital stay and at home following discharge	Increased capacities of health providers in developmentally supportive inpatient care for sick newborn Enhanced skills & understanding of mothers in providing responsive care to sick new born Positive hospital care experience for parents Improved breastfeeding rates, at discharge Increased kangaroo mother care coverage in the facility and continuation at home No increase in any adverse event (nosocomial infection) Quality continuum of care at home post discharge and regular follow-up care visit Decline in mortality rate post-discharge

skills to provide universal support for child development and specialized support for infants/young children with additional needs.

(ii) Moreover investments should be made in building capacities of FLWs as well as facility-based providers to actively engage with both parents, especially fathers and other family members like grandparents to improve their responsive caregiving skills.

(iii) It is essential to adapt and scale up Infant and Family-Centred Developmental Care (IFCDC) or Family Participatory Care, as a key component of developmentally supportive inpatient care. This includes supportive policies and practices of zero separation including provision for mother to stay at NICU, optimal feeding with breastmilk, kangaroo mother care, a supportive sensory environment with acoustic adjustments, stress and pain reduction, the protection and promotion of sleep, the engagement of parents in caregiving processes, facilitation of a smooth transition to home care at discharge, appropriate follow-up care, and mental health and other support services for parents. Facility-based healthcare providers need to be appropriately trained and mentored in implementing such an approach.

(iv) The existing touchpoints in the health system for maternal, newborn and child health and HIV prevention and care services that already interface with HIV-affected children and their caregivers can be leveraged to integrate nurturing care to alleviate risks of poor development in HIV-exposed children. This will also support better mental health, improve adherence to ART as well as greater utilization of health services by mothers [39].

It is important that national pre-service and in-service training curriculum of health-care professionals including nursing professionals and community-based health and nutrition workers are updated to include competency based content on nurturing child development. This includes improved knowledge and skills on multi-dimensional nurturing care approach to optimal child development developmentally supportive management of at-risk young children, ability to engage and enable parents and other family members and addressing parental well-being and mental health during child health consultations.

Parents and other primary caregivers need to be supported through policies, information and services to have knowledge, skills, time and material resources for providing nurturing and responsive care to children. It is crucial to focus attention on enhancing capacities of parents and families with premature, low birthweight and sick newborns, in crisis and displacement conditions (armed conflict, natural disaster), mothers/parents living with HIV and with children exposed to/affected by HIV. Psychosocial and mental health of parents and caregivers should be prioritized in this context.

Intensifying social and behavior change communication (SBCC) in creating a dialogue around positive parenting for optimal early childhood development through multiple and diverse platforms including using innovative platforms including digital platforms to engage with parents to discuss the issues they face. It is suggested that social mobilization leveraging diverse platforms such as PRI groups, women's self-help groups, religious leaders for social mobilization and (iii) developing communication packages on responsive parenting.

Engaging men in nurturing care must be part of a broader goal of achieving gender equality. Services need to be strengthened and healthcare professionals oriented to engage men in their children's care, right from the start. This requires paradigm shift in traditional norms and policy frameworks for adopting supportive policies for men.

Comprehensive smoke-free policies are vital for young children healthy development. Child health and development linkages and relevant actionable areas should be clearly articulated in national tobacco control plans.

Improving coordinated and coherent actions through non-health sectors is crucial. These actions include expanding access of maternity benefits to informal sector women workers, paid parental leave, strengthening implementation of workplace facilities/creches, and accelerating provision of quality and affordable childcare services through both public and private sector.

There is an urgent need to integrate the Nurturing Care Framework into humanitarian policies, programs, and services with increased investment.

Regular early childhood development program evaluation should be made integral to health planning, to undertake continuous monitoring and evaluate progress in quality and coverage of the implementation and their outcomes. Comprehensive monitoring frameworks needs to be developed to ensure systematic progress tracking using child development nurturing care-relevant indicators through routine health data systems.

It is relevant that research gaps are addressed to inform policy, planning, and financing. There is need to generate local evidence of what works (and what does not) to improve equitable, quality early childhood development program implementation at scale, for identifying mechanisms for facilitating effective multi-sectoral approaches and the impact of integrating maternal mental health programs with child development programs.

Conclusion

Early childhood development requires a government-led, whole-of-society approach to establish a supportive and enabling health and community ecosystem, ensuring every child's right to survive and thrive. Leadership and commitment across sectors, including health, nutrition, education, child and social protection, and community leadership beyond the sectors is crucial to enable and empower families to provide responsive care and facilitate equitable access to strong nurturing environments for all children globally. The health sector is uniquely positioned to play a critical leadership role to strengthen and expand comprehensive nurturing health and child development interventions for all children, including those at risk and with special needs, embedded in comprehensive primary health care approach while ensuring safe continuum of care across all levels of health care. It can also mobilize action through all relevant sectors through multi-stakeholder engagement and forging strategic partnerships across both the public and private sectors. This requires adequate evidence-based investment in systems strengthening, with a focus on quality, equity and prioritizing capacity building and mentoring of the health workforce, both community and facility-based health work force and allied workforce along with family/community empowerment.

References

1. World Health Organization (WHO), United Nations Children's Fund (UNICEF), & World Bank Group. (2018). *Nurturing Care for Early Childhood Development: A Framework.*
2. WHO, UNICEF. (2023). *Nurturing Care Framework Progress Report.*
3. UNICEF & Countdown to 2030 Women's, Children's and Adolescents' Health. (2023). *Country Profiles for Early Childhood Development.* https://countdown2030.org
4. Ministry of Health and Family Welfare. (n.d.). Government of India. https://nhm.gov.in
5. Ministry of Women and Child Development. (n.d.). Government of India. https://wcd.gov.in
6. Ministry of Labour and Employment. (n.d.). Government of India. https://labour.gov.in
7. Ministry of Women and Child Development. (n.d.). Pradhan Mantri Matru Vandana Yojana. http://pmmvy.wcd.gov.in
8. Government of India. (n.d.). National Portal of India. https://www.india.gov.in
9. Black, M. M., Walker, P., Fernald, L. C. H., Andersen, C. T., DiGirolamo, A. M., Lu, C., & Lancet Early Childhood Development Series Steering Committee. (2017). Early Childhood Development Coming of Age: Science through the Life Course. *The Lancet, 389*(10064), 77–90. https://doi.org/10.1016/S0140-6736(16)31389-7
10. USAID FANTA II Project FHI 360, Maalouf-Manasseh, Z., et al. (2016). *Technical Brief: Giving Children the Best Start in Life.*
11. World Health Organization. (2024). *World Health Statistics 2024: Monitoring Health for the SDGs.*
12. UNICEF, World Health Organization (WHO), & World Bank Group. (2023). *Joint Child Malnutrition Estimates: Key Findings of the 2023 Edition.*
13. Shonkoff, J. P., Garner, A. S., & Committee on Psychosocial Aspects of Child and Family Health. (2012). The Lifelong Effects of Early Childhood Adversity and Toxic Stress. *Pediatrics, 129*(1), e232–e246. https://doi.org/10.1542/peds.2011-2663.
14. Chan, J. C., Nugent, B. M., & Bale, T. L. (2019). Parental Advisory: Maternal and Paternal Stress Can Impact Offspring Development.*Biological Psychiatry, 83*(10), 886–894.
15. Fleming, T. P., Watkins, A., Velazquez, M. A., Mathers, J. C., Prentice, A. M., Stephenson, J., et al. (2018). Origins of Lifetime Health Around the Time of Conception: Causes and Consequences. *The Lancet, 391*(10132), 1842–1852. https://doi.org/10.1016/S0140-6736(18)30312-X.
16. Li, J., Tsuprykov, O., Yang, X., & Hocher, B. (2016). Paternal Programming of Offspring Cardiometabolic Diseases in Later Life. *Journal of Hypertension, 34*(11), 2111–2126.
17. Stephenson, J., Heslehurst, N., Hall, J., Schoenaker, D., Hutchinson, J., Cade, J., Poston, L., et al. (2018). Before the Beginning: Nutrition and Lifestyle in the Preconception Period and Its Importance for Future Health. *The Lancet, 391*(10132), 1830–1841. https://doi.org/10.1016/S0140-6736(18)30311-8
18. Barker, M., Dombrowski, S., Colbourn, T., Fall, C., Kriznik, N., Lawrence, W., Norris, S., et al. (2018). Intervention Strategies to Improve Nutrition and Health Behaviours Before Conception. *The Lancet, 391*(10132), 1853–1864. https://doi.org/10.1016/S0140-6736(18)30313-1
19. Leonardi-Bee, J., Britton, J., & Venn, A. (2011). Secondhand Smoke and Adverse Foetal Outcomes in Non-Smoking Pregnant Women: A Meta-Analysis. *Pediatrics, 127*(4), 734–741. https://doi.org/10.1542/peds.2010-3041

20. Hackshaw, A., et al. (2014). Maternal Smoking during Pregnancy and Birth Defects in Children: A Systematic Review with Meta-Analysis. *Cadernos de Saúde Pública, 30*(12), 2491–2529. https://doi.org/10.1590/0102-311X00115813.
21. WHO, Nurturing Care. (2021). *Thematic Brief: Tobacco Control to Improve Child Health and Development.*
22. Tomlinson, M., Cooper, P., & Murray, L. (2005). The Mother-Infant Relationship and Infant Attachment in a South African Peri-Urban Settlement. *Child Development, 76*(5), 1044–1054.
23. WHO, UNICEF. (2022). *Thematic Brief: Nurturing Care and Men's Engagement.*
24. World Health Organization. (2020). *Monitoring Children's Development in Primary Care Services: Moving from a Focus on Child Deficits to Family Centred Participatory Approach.* Report of a Virtual Technical Meeting.
25. Aboud, F. E., & Yousafzai, A. K. (2016). Global Health and Development in Early Childhood. *Annual Review of Psychology, 67*(1), 115–137.
26. Britto, P. R., et al. (2017). Nurturing Care: Promoting Early Childhood Development. *The Lancet, 389*(10064), 91–102.
27. World Health Organization. (2019). *Operationalizing Nurturing Care for Early Childhood Development.*
28. Bouchane, K., Yoshikawa, H., Murphy, K. M., & Lombardi, J. (2018). *Early Childhood Programs for Refugees.* UNESCO.
29. UNICEF. (2023). The Early Childhood Development Index 2030: A New Measure for Early Childhood Development.
30. Grantham-McGregor, S. M., et al. (1991). Nutritional Supplementation, Psychosocial Stimulation, and Mental Development of Stunted Children: The Jamaican Study. *The Lancet, 338*, 1–5.
31. Walker, S. P., et al. (2006). Effects of Psychosocial Stimulation and Dietary Supplementation in Early Childhood on Psychosocial Functioning in Late Adolescence: Follow-Up of Randomized Controlled Trial. *BMJ, 333*, 472–476.
32. Vazir, S., Engle, P., Balakrishna, N., Griffiths, P., Johnson, S., Creed-Kanashiro, H., et al. (2013). Cluster-Randomized Trial on Complementary and Responsive Feeding Education to Caregivers Found Improved Dietary Intake, Growth, and Development Among Rural Indian Toddlers. *Maternal & Child Nutrition, 9*(1), 99–117. https://doi.org/10.1111/j.1740-8709.2012.00413.x
33. Frongillo, E. A., Nguyen, P., Saha, K., Tina Sanghvi, T., Kaosar Afsana, K., Haque, R., et al. (2016). Large-Scale Behavior-Change Initiative for Infant and Young Child Feeding Advanced Language and Motor Development in a Cluster-Randomized Program Evaluation in Bangladesh. *The Journal of Nutrition, 147*, 256–263. https://doi.org/10.3945/jn.116.240861.
34. Lozoff, B., et al. (2010). Home Intervention Improves Cognitive and Social-Emotional Scores in Iron-Deficient Anemic Infants. *Pediatrics, 126*, e884–e894.
35. Gope, R. K., et al. (2019). Effects of Participatory Learning and Action with Women's Groups, Counselling through Home Visits, and Crèches on Undernutrition among Children under Three Years in Eastern India: A Quasi-Experimental Study. *BMC Public Health, 19*(962). https://doi.org/10.1186/s12889-019-7274-3
36. Government of Meghalaya. (n.d.). Official Website of Meghalaya Government. https://meghalaya.gov.in
37. UNICEF, Nurturing Care, WHO, & PMNCH. (2020). *Thematic Brief: Nurturing Care for Children Affected by HIV.*
38. Gupta, P., Raut, A., Kothekar, P., Maliye C. H., Kalantri, A., Bahulekar, P., et al. (2021). Nurturing Care Interventions for Realizing the Development Potential of Every Child: From Pilot to Scale Up in Maharashtra. *Indian Pediatrics, 58*, Supplement 1, S46–S52.
39. Luoto, J. E., et al. (2020). Group-based Parenting Interventions to Promote Child Development in Rural Kenya: A Multi-Arm, Cluster-Randomized Community Effectiveness Trial. *The Lancet Global Health.* https://doi.org/10.1016/S2214-109X(20)30469-1
40. World Health Organization. (2018). *Survive and Thrive: Transforming Care for Small and Sick Newborns.*

41. Verma, A., et al. (2017). Family-Centered Care to Complement Care of Sick Newborns: A Randomized Controlled Trial. *Indian Pediatrics, 54*, 455–459.
42. USAID Maternal and Child Survival Program. (2019). *Nurturing Care for Small and Sick Newborns: Evidence Review and Country Case Studies.*
43. Nurturing Care for Every Newborn. (n.d.). *Nurturing Care Thematic Brief.* https://nurturing-care.org/thematic-briefs/

Chapter 12
Identifying and Addressing Health Disparities in Child Health and Nutrition

Neha Sanwalka

Introduction

India, one of the world's most populous countries, has around 30% of its population under 18 years. Despite rapid economic growth and expanding healthcare infrastructure, significant health disparities persist among Indian children. These disparities indicate variations in health outcomes and access to healthcare services among different population groups [1]. Health disparities stem from various factors including socioeconomic status (age, sex, education, and income), geographical location, ethnicity, culture (caste and religion), and environmental conditions [1]. Health disparities can stem from variations in health behaviors and access to nutritious food, which are influenced by education, income, and culture. Addressing these determinants is crucial for reducing disparities and promoting health equity. This chapter offers an in-depth overview of health and nutrition disparities in Indian children aged 0–24 months, the contributing factors, and actionable recommendations for healthcare workers, researchers, and policymakers to mitigate these disparities.

Definition

Health disparity, also known as health inequality, refers to the absence of equity in health outcomes.

Braveman P. (2006) defined health disparity/insecurity as "a particular type of difference in health or in the most important influences on health that could potentially be shaped by policies; it is a difference in which disadvantaged social groups (such as the poor, racial/ethnic minorities, women, or other groups that have persistently

N. Sanwalka (✉)
Hirabai Cowasji Jehangir Medical Research Institute, Jehangir Hospital, Pune, India
e-mail: neha.sanwalka@gmail.com

S. Suri (ed.), *Child Health and Nutrition from Conception to Age Two*,
https://doi.org/10.1007/978-981-95-7868-9_12

experienced social disadvantage or discrimination) systematically experience worse health or greater health risks than more advantaged groups" [1].

Braveman P (2006) also briefly summarized the definition as "health disparities/inequalities are potentially avoidable differences in health (or in health risks that policy can influence) between groups of people who are more and less advantaged socially; these differences systematically place socially disadvantaged groups at further disadvantage on health" [1].

Need to Assess Health Disparities in Indian Children

The first 1,000 days of life, from conception to a child's second birthday, are critical for laying a strong foundation for lifelong health and development. During this period, adequate nutrition plays a crucial role in supporting the growth of the fetus, development of the brain, and strengthening of the immune system [2, 3]. Nutritional deficiencies or excesses can affect metabolic health later in life [2]. Additionally, the formation of microbiome during the early stages of life plays a vital role in immune system development and may influence the risk of developing inflammatory and autoimmune conditions later in life [4, 5]. Beyond nutrition, external influences such as maternal substance use and limited access to healthcare can trigger epigenetic modifications. These changes affect a child's health and development without altering their genetic code [6, 7].

Despite India's growing economy, infant mortality, malnutrition, anaemia, and incomplete immunization persist [8]. These issues are unevenly distributed across regions and communities, driven by social, economic, environmental, and geographic disparities [9, 10].

As the first 1,000 days are crucial for laying the foundation for good health in later life, it is essential to understand the factors that cause health and nutritional disparities. An in-depth understanding of these factors will help policymakers, researchers, doctors, and nutritionists plan targeted interventions to reduce these disparities. The objectives of this chapter are as follows:

- To understand the disparities observed in health and nutrition in children aged 0–24 months
- To identify the multifactorial causes of disparities
- To discuss evidence-based strategies to reduce inequalities in child health and nutrition

Health and Nutrition Disparities in Indian Children

The primary health concerns for children under two years of age encompass a range of developmental and physical health issues, such as low birthweight, malnutrition, early initiation of breastfeeding, inadequate complementary feeding, mortality, and incomplete immunization. Inequality exists in the distribution of health concerns across the country. Factors such as poverty, limited access to education, inadequate healthcare infrastructure, geographical location, and maternal factors contribute to these disparities [10]. This section enumerates the major health and nutritional concerns of Indian children from birth to two years and the factors responsible for these disparities.

Low Birth Weight (LBW)

Low birth weight (LBW), defined by the World Health Organization (WHO) as birth weight less than 2,500 g [11], remains a pressing concern in India, with the National Family Health Survey 5 (NFHS-5) reporting that 18% of children in India are born with LBW [12]. LBW has several far-reaching health consequences as such hypothermia, hypoglycaemia, fluid-electrolyte imbalance, hyperbilirubinemia, respiratory lung syndrome, infections, necrotizing enterocolitis, intra-ventricular hemorrhage, hearing and sight issues, apnoea of prematurity, and anaemia [13]. These adverse outcomes underline the critical need to address the multitude of risk factors that contribute to LBW.

Maternal factors and antenatal care (ANC) play pivotal roles. Women with fewer than four ANC visits, maternal anaemia, poor dietary diversity, and tobacco use significantly increase the likelihood of LBW infants. Young maternal age below 20 years, limited education, and limited exposure to health information through media further compound LBW prevalence. This highlights the role of education and communication in maternal decision-making.

Geographically, the Northeast reports the lowest LBW prevalence (9.87%), while the Central (20.73%), Western (20.43%), and Northern (20.64%) regions show the highest prevalence [15]. Urban slums and tribal areas exhibit elevated LBW rates due to limited healthcare and economic constrains [14, 16, 17]. Environmental exposure to biomass fuel, industrial proximity, unclean water, pesticide use, and smoking impact intrauterine growth and increase LBW risk [18]. Socio-demographic factors like religion and income modulate risk. Children born in lower wealth quartiles or Hindu households, particularly in under-resourced districts, have a higher LBW prevalence [14, 16]. To reduce disparities in LBW, targeted interventions must focus on improving maternal nutrition, antenatal care access, and education among underserved populations.

Immunization

Immunization is important because it protects infants and children from various life-threatening diseases. Immunization helps build a child's immunity and increases their resistance to infection. It also plays a role in creating herd immunity and preventing the spread of the disease in the community of unvaccinated individuals [19]. Despite the Universal Immunization Program (launched in 1985) offering free vaccines against 12 preventable diseases in newborns and pregnant women, NFHS-5 data revealed that only 62.4% of children in India are fully immunized.

The reasons for low immunization coverage are multifactorial. Economic disparities are the most significant. Children from the poorest wealth quartiles have the lowest coverage (53.4%). Children from the wealthiest quartiles are also not universally protected [20]. Socio-demographic factors such as caste and religion also influence immunization rate with Schedule Castes, Scheduled Tribes, and Muslim communities showing the lowest coverage [20, 21]. Geographical location (Fig. 12.1) and area of residence also impact immunization coverage.

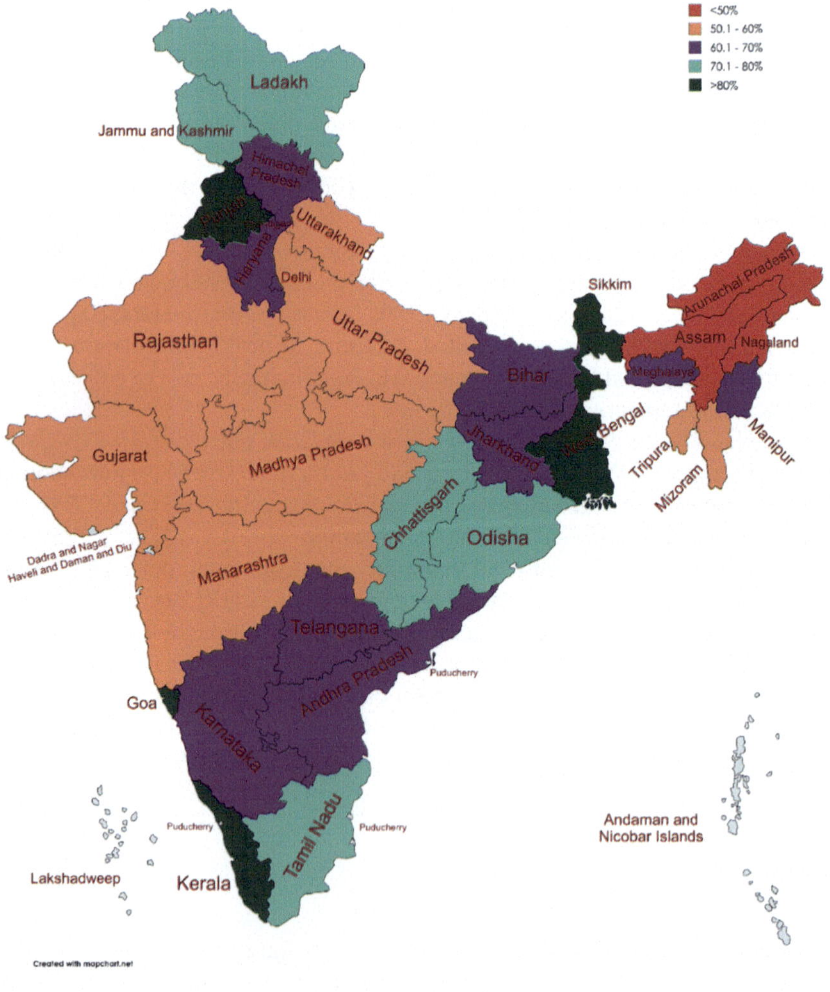

Fig. 12.1 State-wise immunization coverage in India in 2015–2016 [20]

Rural and tribal areas, especially those with poor infrastructure, limited cold chain facilities, and low awareness, are particularly vulnerable [21, 22]. Several factors contribute to the low immunization coverage in India's tribal regions, such as insufficient cold storage for vaccines, shortage of vaccines and syringes, low awareness of immunization schedules, distrust of government healthcare, and language and social barriers. Additionally, fear of post-vaccination illnesses, such as fever, and myths about vaccines causing impotence, pain, or other side effects, further reduces immunization rates in these areas. Birth order and sex of the child also play a role in immunization disparities. Girls, especially those with higher birth orders are less likely to be immunized [21]. Reducing immunization disparities requires strengthening last-mile delivery, addressing vaccine hesitancy, and ensuring equitable access in marginalized and remote communities.

Infant and Child Mortality

The neonatal mortality rate (NMR) is the number of deaths per 1,000 live births in the first 28 days of life, whereas the infant mortality rate (IMR) is the number of deaths per 1,000 live births from birth until 12 months of life. While positive reductions in NMR (30 vs. 25) and IMR (50 vs. 35) have been observed from NFHS-4 to NFHS-5, significant disparities persist across socioeconomic and geographic lines [12].

Children born in the lower wealth index face the highest risk, especially when combined with low paternal education and low exposure to health-related information [23, 24]. Birth order and spacing affect the mortality rate. Firstborns from lower income households and children born within 2 years of their siblings are especially vulnerable [23, 25]. Children born in Scheduled Castes and Scheduled Tribes show higher mortality due to restricted access to healthcare [23].

Maternal age patterns present a dual challenge. IMR is higher in younger mothers in the poorer income quartiles, whereas it is higher in older mothers in the richer income quartiles [25]. Geographically, Central India has the highest mortality rates followed by Northern and Eastern states while Southern states have the lowest mortality rates [23, 24]. Rural areas have higher mortality than urban areas [25]. Improving access to healthcare and enhancing quality antenatal and postnatal care, especially in high-burden regions can be key to reducing disparities in mortality.

Exclusive Breastfeeding

Breastmilk provides all nutrients in optimum quantities necessary for the growth and development of a child, enhances immunity, reduces the risk of infections and diseases, and promotes healthy weight gain and neurological development. UNICEF and WHO recommend exclusive breastfeeding (EBF) for the first six months, continuing up to two years, and starting within one hour of birth. Despite these guidelines, NFHS-5 data shows that only 41% of Indian mothers initiated breastfeeding within the first hour of birth while the average duration for EBF was approximately 3.9 months, well below the global standards [12]. Maternal factors had the most significant impact on EBF practices.

Maternal factors positively influencing breastfeeding practices

- **Education:**
  - Higher education associated with early initiation of breastfeeding and longer duration of EBF especially in rural areas [26, 27],
  - Less educated women sustain EBF longer in urban slums [28]
- **Work Status:** Non-working mothers are more likely to maintain EBF [26, 29]
- **Health Care:**
  - Four or more ANC visits,
  - Institutional delivery
  - Presence of trained healthcare professionals [26, 27]
- **Previous birth history:** Multiparous mothers are more likely to practice EBF as they have previous experience [26]

Geographical location and socioeconomic differences further compound this issue. Northeastern states lead early initiation and EBF practices whereas North and Central India lag behind [26, 27]. Women from poor economic quartiles (45.6%) tend to initiate breastfeeding earlier than women from rich economic quartiles (33.3%), often due to limited access to alternatives such as infant formulas. The middle economic quartiles women (21.1%) have the lowest EIB trends [26]. Women from the middle and wealthiest quartiles may cease EBF early due to time constrains, early return to work and lack of breastfeeding support at work [27].

Increasing maternal awareness regarding breastfeeding is the key to reducing disparities in breastfeeding practices.

Complementary Feeding

Complementary feeding is a critical transition phase in infant nutrition where food is introduced in the diet in addition to milk when breast milk or milk formula alone is no longer adequate to meet the infant's nutritional requirements and continues until 23 months [30] (Fig. 12.2).

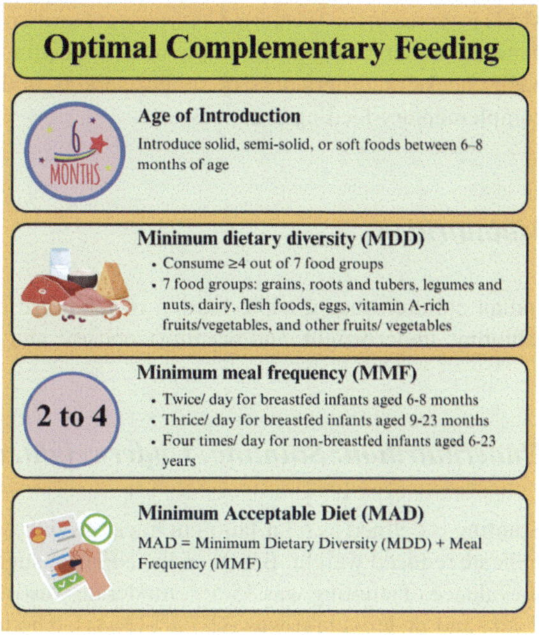

Fig. 12.2 Four features of optimal complementary feeding [31, 32]

According to NFHS-5 data, in India, only 24–32% of children meet MMF whereas 5–9% achieve MAD [31, 32]. A diet lacking in MDD fails to meet the micronutrient requirements of toddlers, whereas a diet lacking in MMF is deficient in macronutrients. Failure to achieve appropriate complementary feeding may lead to delay in growth and development; increased macro and micronutrient deficiencies and increase the risk of infections and diseases, thereby increase morbidity and mortality. Factors contributing to inadequate complementary feeding are multifaceted, spanning maternal, socioeconomic, and regional dimensions.

Maternal education is a key determinant of optimal complementary feeding practices. Mothers without formal education or those with less than secondary schooling are less likely to adopt optimal complementary feeding practices. Fewer ANC visits or postnatal check-ups are associated with poor complementary feeding practices. Maternal exposure to knowledge regarding complementary feeding via media (newspaper, radio, or television) improves complementary feeding practices in mothers [31].

Mothers from Scheduled Castes, Scheduled Tribes and other backwards classes follow suboptimal complementary feeding practices which may be due to lower exposure to knowledge regarding complementary feeding [32]. Mothers who follow Hinduism tend to delay the introduction of complementary feeding. All religions except Christianity are associated with higher odds of not meeting MMF [31]. Regional disparities in complementary feeding practices are also stark in India. The Central region on India has the worst MDD whereas the Northeastern and Southern regions have a better MDD. The lowest MMF was observed in the Western region.

MAD is worse in the Western, Central, and Northern regions of India [32]. Improving maternal understanding of complementary feeding via improved ANC visits, postnatal checks, and networks of social workers is the key to reducing disparities in complementary feeding practices.

Malnutrition

Indian children face a triple burden of malnutrition, encompassing undernutrition (stunting, underweight, and wasting), obesity, and micronutrient deficiencies.

Undernutrition: Stunting, Underweight, and Wasting

Stunting is defined as retardation in linear growth, whereas underweight and wasting indicate reduced weight. Based on the NFHS-5 survey, in children aged <5 years, the prevalence of stunting was 35.5%, moderate wasting was 19.3%, severe wasting was 7.7%, and underweight was 32.1% [33, 34]. The high prevalence of undernutrition is largely rooted in poverty and inequality, disproportionately affecting rural, tribal, and marginalized communities.

Identifying stunting, underweight, and wasting

When a child's measurements are less than two standard deviations from the WHO Child Growth Standards.

- Height/length for age—Stunted
- Weight for age—Underweight
- Weight for height/length—Wasted

Geographically, the Central, Eastern, and Western regions of India show the highest prevalence of undernutrition. Districts with higher economic development experience lower rates of childhood undernutrition than their less economically advanced counterparts [35]. Rural areas and urban slums, marked with poor sanitation, open defecation, and lack of access to clean water, further increase the burden of undernutrition [36]. Caste and religion further exuberate these disparities as children from Scheduled Tribes and Muslim-majority districts have a higher prevalence of undernutrition. This is largely attributed to reduced access to healthcare and long-standing sociocultural marginalization [35].

Low maternal height which serves as a proxy for chronic maternal undernutrition is strongly correlated with stunting. Maternal education has an equal impact on the prevalence of undernutrition. Mothers with no formal education are less likely to adopt optimal feeding practices which in turn increases the risk for undernutrition [35]. Birth order has an impact on the prevalence of undernutrition. Higher birth order is associated with a higher prevalence of stunting while lower birth order is associated with a higher prevalence of underweight [35] (Table 12.1).

Overnutrition: Overweight and Obesity

Paradoxically, India is now witnessing a rising trend in overnutrition among children. According to the NFHS-5 survey, 3.4% of children below the age of 5 years were overweight [37].

Identifying overweight and obesity:

In comparison to WHO Child Growth Standards, a child is defined as

- Overweight—weight for height ≥ 2 SD and < 3 SD
- Obese—weight for height ≥ 3 SD

Overnutrition is more prevalent in wealthier households. The prevalence of obesity rises with every increase in income quartiles from poorest to richest. A high prevalence is observed in children from Scheduled Tribes and from Hindu families. Maternal factors such as high education, overweight and obesity and working status are associated with an increase in prevalence. Mothers' lack of time to monitor their children's eating habits and physical activity levels are mediating factors associated with obesity in children. Boys and children with low birth ranks (1–3) are particularly vulnerable. High media exposure may contribute to sedentary lifestyle behaviors and consumption of unhealthy foods through marketing also plays a role in the increased prevalence of obesity [38] (Table 12.1).

Micronutrient Deficiencies

Several micronutrient deficiencies are prevalent in Indian infants and children, the most common deficiencies being anaemia (indicators of iron, vitamin B12, or folic acid deficiency) and Vitamin D deficiency. Anaemia affects 75.2% of 6–8 months old infants, 78.7% of 9–11 months old infants, 80% of children aged 12–17 months, and 78.2% of 18–23 months children [39]. Almost 40–90% of infants and children have vitamin D deficiencies [40]. Approximately 13.8% of children aged 1–4 years have vitamin B12 deficiency, and 22.8% have folate deficiency [41].

Low maternal education, maternal anaemia and high birth order are factors associated with disparities in the prevalence of anaemia [39, 41]. Lower income quartiles

Table 12.1 Factors increasing risk of malnutrition

Determinants	Undernutrition	Overnutrition	Micronutrient deficiencies
Geographical Region	Central, Eastern, Western India	–	Gujarat, Maharashtra, Bihar, Northeast
Economic Status	Low-income households; inverse correlation with district economy	High income households	Lower income groups (anaemia); Vitamin D deficiency not correlated
Caste	Scheduled Tribes	Scheduled Tribes	Scheduled Tribes
Religion	Muslim-majority district	Hindu families	–
Area of Residence	Rural areas and urban slums	–	Urban slums
Maternal Height	Low maternal height linked to stunting	–	–
Maternal Education	Low or no education	Higher education	Low education
Birth Order	Higher order = stunting; lower order = underweight	Birth rank 1–3	Higher birth order = higher anaemia
Maternal Work Status	–	Working mothers	–
Media Exposure	Lack of exposure	High media exposure	
Maternal Overweight/ Obesity	–	Strongly associated	–
Child's Sex	–	Boys	
Environmental Factors	Poor sanitation and lack of access to clean water	–	Low sunlight and pollution (vitamin D deficiency)

are associated with a higher prevalence of anaemia but no correlation with Vitamin D deficiency is observed [39, 40]. The prevalence of anaemia is significantly higher in children from Scheduled Tribes [39]. The prevalence of anaemia is higher in the districts of Gujarat, Maharashtra, Bihar, Himachal Pradesh, and Northeastern states [42]. B12 deficiency is more prevalent in Central India whereas folic acid deficiency is more prominent in Northeast [41]. Less or no exposure to sunlight, high levels of pollution, and living in crowded urban slums increase the risk for vitamin D deficiency [40] (Table 12.1).

Reducing malnutrition disparities requires integrated efforts to improve dietary diversity, maternal education, food security, and access to community-based nutrition services in vulnerable populations.

All health and nutrition inequalities are multifaceted, ranging from maternal factors to socio-demographic factors, economic factors, sex, birth order of the child, geographical location, environmental factors, and area of residence. The next section describes the underlying linkages between these characteristics and the disparities observed in children's health and nutrition.

Causes and Consequences of Health Disparities

Health disparities among Indian children are not incidental. They are a consequence of layered, systemic inequities embedded in geography, socioeconomic status, maternal wellbeing, and access to public health infrastructure. Understanding these disparities is crucial for developing targeted interventions and policies to promote health equity. The causes and consequences of health disparities are discussed in detail below.

Regional Disparities

India's vast geographical diversity has contributed to significant regional disparities. States with better healthcare infrastructure, literacy rates, and socioeconomic conditions tend to have more favorable health indicators, while others lag.

Geographical Location

India's vast geographic diversity creates stark contrasts in child health outcomes. States with higher literacy rates and health facilities like Kerala and Tamil Nadu have relatively better health outcomes. In contrast, less access to government health and nutrition programs, such as the Integrated Child Development Services (ICDS) in Central and Eastern states, increases inequalities in health outcomes such as malnutrition and mortality [23]. The geographical conditions and inaccessible mountainous terrain of Northeast India, language barriers and reduced infrastructure lead to limited healthcare accessibility and widen health disparities in Northeast India [43].

Urban Versus Rural

Urban areas generally have better access to healthcare services, nutrition, and sanitation than rural areas. Children in rural regions face higher risks of malnutrition and mortality owing to limited healthcare facilities and poor socioeconomic conditions.

Studies have also shown that women in rural areas tend to have a longer duration of EBF than women in urban areas, which may be due to the unavailability of alternatives to breast milk [28]. Even within urban areas, a socioeconomic divide is evident. Lower parental education, economic inability to avail the best medical treatment, lack of access to clean water, and sanitation are the causes of the high prevalence of infections, malnutrition, and mortality in urban slums.

Tribal Areas

Remote locations and lack of healthcare facilities are the primary reasons for the high disease burden observed in tribal areas. Lower parental education, poor income quartiles, lack of access to clean water and sanitation, and lower immunization rates in tribal areas increase the risk of disease and mortality.

Socio-Demographic Disparities

The socio-demographic impact on health disparities in India is multifaceted. Caste, religion, and economic status play important roles in determining the prevalence of diseases.

Caste and Religion

Marginalized castes such as Scheduled Castes and Scheduled Tribes often face systemic discrimination and have limited access to healthcare, education, and income opportunities. This leads to inappropriate breastfeeding practices, inadequate complementary feeding, and a higher prevalence of disease and mortality rates in marginalized castes. Deep-rooted religious beliefs have resulted in various health and nutritional disparities in India.

Economic Factors

Income remains one of the most significant factors affecting health disparities. Financial insecurity limits access to healthcare, nutritious food, and safe living conditions. Economic stability is crucial for ensuring children's wellbeing.

Maternal Factors

Various maternal factors are associated with disparities in health and nutrition including maternal health, education, exposure to the media, and work status.

Maternal Health and Nutrition

Maternal health, including mental health and nutrition, significantly affects child nutrition and development. Maternal depression is associated with negative health outcomes such as LBW, developmental delays, incomplete immunization schedules, and disrupted sleep patterns in infants and young children. Maternal depression also impairs childcare practices related to breastfeeding, healthcare, safety, and development, contributing to inadequate nutrition during pregnancy and infancy [44]. Adequate maternal nutrition during pregnancy and the peri-gestational period is essential for children's cognitive, motor, speech, and socio-emotional development [45]. A maternal diet low in dietary diversity leads to inadequate micronutrient intake and increases the risk of LBW and anaemia [16, 39]. Maternal mental health conditions such as postpartum anxiety, depression, and psychosis can lead to childhood delays in milestones, language development, and growth [46].

Maternal Education

As discussed earlier, lower maternal education is associated with a high prevalence of LBW [14], higher mortality rates [25], inadequate breastfeeding [27], inadequate complementary feeding practices [31], and high prevalence of undernutrition [35]. Low maternal education is associated with a lack of understanding of appropriate nutrition and dietary habits, which leads to disparities in health status. ANC visits are associated with a better understanding of child health, breastfeeding practices, and complementary feeding techniques. Hence, mothers with a higher number of ANC visits had children with a lower incidence of health and nutritional inadequacies. Similarly, exposure to media in the form of newspapers or radio is associated with improved knowledge in mothers, thereby reducing health and nutrition inequalities.

Maternal Work Status

The work status of women has varied impacts on health disparities in infants and children. On one hand, working mothers are financially independent and have better economic resources, enabling them to avail better health and nutrition facilities for their children. On the other hand, working women lack time to personally supervise their children's eating habits and physical activity levels, contributing to weight gain in their children [38]. Work status is inversely associated with EBF and complementary feeding. Working women initiate complementary feeding earlier as they need to return to work, and their workplaces are too far from home and do not have daycare facilities. In addition, a lack of knowledge regarding the importance of breast milk, and its expression and storage causes working women to initiate complementary feeding earlier than non-working women [29]. In addition, women working in unorganized sectors, such as hawkers in urban areas, need to return to work earlier to earn money, and many times the workplace is far from home, which induces early complementary feeding. Lack of family support is another reason for early cessation of breastfeeding in poor economic quartiles where women are working [28, 29].

Environmental Factors and Sanitation

Environmental factors such as exposure to biomass fuel, use of pesticides, and smoking have been associated with LBW in India [18]. High pollution levels can increase the risk of respiratory disorders in children. Lack of access to clean water also increases the risk of infections, thereby increasing the risk of malnutrition and mortality. Lack of access to clean drinking water accounts for 3% of the socioeconomic disparity in childhood stunting and approximately 4% of socioeconomic inequality in underweight cases in India [35]. Climate change, including constant floods and droughts in different parts of India, increasing temperatures, and carbon dioxide emissions also impact health equality in Indian children.

Understanding and addressing these root causes of health disparities is essential not only to improve immediate child health outcomes but also to break the intergenerational cycle of inequity and poor development.

Addressing Health Disparities

Multiple disparities in health and nutrition have been observed in India. To address these disparities, it is essential to provide not only resources but also improve the knowledge and understanding of the public. A multiparty approach involving the government, private healthcare centers, and the community is essential. This section focuses on various government initiatives, healthcare innovations in the private sector, and community-based approaches to bring about greater equity in Indian health and nutrition care for infants and children.

International Initiatives

The efforts of Global International organizations such as the WHO and UNICEF have significantly influenced India's strategies to reduce health and nutrition disparities. Several of the Sustainable Development Goals (SDGs) by the United Nations directly or indirectly focus on reducing inequalities in health and nutrition [47]. Programs like Every Woman Every Child Movement (2010), Committing to Child Survival: A Promise Renewed (2013), and Every Newborn—An Action Plan to End Preventable Deaths (2014) aim to improve health systems, improve women and newborn health, improve quality of life, and reduce mortality rates [47]. Government of India and UNICEF jointly fund the ICDS initiative in India [48]. Collaboration with agencies like UNICEF and WHO provides technical and financial support, as well as global accountability and scale models. As a result, India's key programs such as the National Health Mission and Poshan Abhiyan have integrated the best global practices to address systemic health inequalities.

Initiatives by the Government of India

Over the years, the Government of India has launched multiple policies to strengthen the health and wellbeing of Indian citizens, reduce malnutrition, provide immunization, and reduce inequalities in health outcomes. These policies are designed to address the needs of marginalized/ vulnerable groups. This subsection discusses various health and nutrition schemes that address disparities between infant and child health.

National Health Mission (NHM)

The National Health Mission (NHM) launched by the Government of India in 2013 encompasses two submissions: the National Rural Health Mission (launched in 2005) and the National Urban Health Mission. The NHM aims to achieve universal access to equitable, cost-effective, and high-quality healthcare services that are both accountable and responsive to the needs of the population. The major objectives of NHM are to improve reproductive health, reduce IMR and MMR, reduce communicable and non-communicable diseases, and boost health facilities at the district and sub-district levels [49, 50].

Table 12.2 Initiatives for infant and child health by the government of India

Initiative	Impact on reducing disparities
Accredited Social Health Activists (ASHAs)	ASHAs are trained community health volunteers who promote immunization, availability of iron and folic acid supplementation, breastfeeding and optimal complementary feeding practices, and optimal sanitation practices [49, 51]
Janani Suraksha Yojana	Promotes institutional delivery to reduce maternal and neonatal mortality [49]
Janani Shishu Suraksha Karyakram	Free medical service for pregnant women and infants for one year to reduce economic disparities [49]
Rashtriya Bal Swasthya Karyakram	Screen all children (birth to 18 years) for 32 health issues and offer free treatment to reduce disease burden and income disparities [52]
National Iron + Initiative	Provides free iron and folic acid supplementation to pregnant mothers and infants to reduce maternal and child anaemia [51]
Mission Indradhanush	Provide 12 vaccines free of cost to children under five years of age to [49]

Integrated Child Development Scheme (ICDS)

The Integrated Child Development Scheme (ICDS) provides food to children under six years of age and their mothers to combat malnutrition, poor health, and sex disparities. Under this initiative, Anganwadi Centers offers vaccinations, health screenings, nutritious meals, and informal educational activities. The ICDS also delivers nutrition and health education, immunizations, medical check-ups, referral services, non-formal preschool instruction, and contraceptive guidance to adolescents [48]. Table 12.2 illustrates the other infant and child health programs lead by government of India to promote health equity.

Pradhan Mantri Poshan Shakti Nirman–PM POSHAN

The Mid-day Meal Program (MDM) or Pradhan Mantri Poshan Shakti Nirman-PM POSHAN provides meals to disadvantaged children to reduce malnutrition. The program offers cooked MDM containing 300 cal and 8–12 g protein to school children. In India, MDM is one of the most successful nutrition supplementation programs [48, 53].

National Food Security Act (NFSA)

The National Food Security Act (NFSA) covers up to 75% of the rural population and 50% of the urban population. Under the NFSA, the poorest households receive free or subsidized food grains. The aim of NFSA is to bring food security and reduce nutritional inequalities [48, 54].

National Nutrition Mission/Poshan Abhiyan

Poshan Abhiyan or National Nutrition Mission (2018) was initiated to promote optimal nutrition for children from birth to six years of age, adolescent girls, and expectant and nursing mothers. The program objectives include decreasing stunting and wasting in children and reducing the occurrence of anaemia. Poshan Abhiyan uses information and communication technology applications, convergence, community engagement, large scale behavioral change initiatives, skill development, incentives and recognition, and innovative approaches to reduce nutritional inequalities in India [55].

Healthcare Initiatives

Improving healthcare access and quality is fundamental to reducing health disparities. This includes enhancing the healthcare infrastructure, increasing the healthcare workforce capacity, and ensuring the availability of essential medical supplies and services.

Strengthening Primary Healthcare

Primary healthcare centers (PHCs) are the backbone of rural healthcare in India. Strengthening PHCs by increasing budgetary allocations is essential for reducing health inequality. Training and empowering PHC professionals to prevent and treat maternal and child health conditions are imperative for reducing health disparities. PHC teams should be adequately supported through regular upskilling workshops and incentives [56].

Mobile Health Units

Mobile health units have emerged as an innovative solution to bridge the geographic barriers. These mobile van units provide basic healthcare services, immunization, and nutrition counseling to rural and underserved areas or areas where healthcare is not easily accessible, often in collaboration with district hospitals or non-government organizations (NGOs).

Telemedicine

Telemedicine is a promising strategy to close the access gaps, especially where speciality care is scarce. Telemedicine can be used for consultations, follow-up, and health education and to reduce urban–rural–tribal disparities in access to healthcare [57].

Referral Services and Community Intervention Programs

Urban healthcare facilities can organize various community intervention programs and health camps in rural and tribal areas. These camps provide free health check-ups, diagnoses, treatments, and follow-ups. Referral services can be offered via health camps to those who need specialized referrals.

Private–Public Partnerships

Private healthcare facilities can initiate public–private partnerships with government hospitals. Under such partnerships, private hospitals can improve the quality of care available in government facilities, thereby reducing health disparities.

Other Strategies to Bridge Health and Nutrition Inequalities

Several other approaches such as community initiatives, maternal education, and decentralization of healthcare via local governance, can be used to reduce health disparities.

Community Initiatives

Integrating health, hygiene, and nutrition education into the school curriculum and community workshops can build lifelong awareness. Community-based awareness programs can promote early breastfeeding initiation, EBF, appropriate complementary feeding and immunization while dispelling myths about immunization. The help of community leaders and social workers can be pivotal in promoting healthier choices and decreasing health inequalities. Nutrition and health science colleges can support these efforts through community awareness campaigns regarding optimal nutrition and a balanced diet.

Equitable Access to Healthcare

People are more inclined to use government health facilities when there is assured service availability, including medication and diagnostic services. Guaranteed access encourages utilization especially in underserved areas. An increase in government funding for medicine and diagnostics would ensure equitable access to healthcare in rural and tribal areas and help reduce healthcare disparities [50].

Maternal Education

Maternal education plays a critical role in shaping infant and child health and nutrition. Improving maternal education and knowledge via ASHAs, community intervention programs, ANC visits, and postnatal visits contributes to reducing health disparities. Media such as newspapers, radio, and social media can be leveraged to increase maternal education on various aspects of child health and nutrition.

Decentralization of Healthcare Initiatives

In India, healthcare falls under state jurisdiction. Along with major national initiatives, individual states should explore and implement strategies to address healthcare disparities. Empowering municipal and regional authorities enhances responsiveness, as they are best equipped to effectively identify and address community-specific healthcare disparities [50].

Regular Monitoring

India's health data system needs strengthening to provide timely and valuable information for action. It is crucial to gather and utilize up-to-date and reliable health data, broken down by factors such as sex, age, income, education, migration status, disability, geographic location, and other relevant characteristics specific to the national context. This level of detail is essential for identifying disparities among different population subgroups and implementing effective measures to address them [50].

Thus, an integrated approach involving government policies, PHCs, and community initiatives is needed to address various inequalities in health and nutrition in India.

Conclusion

This chapter provides a comprehensive overview of health and nutrition disparities among Indian children aged 0–24 months, addressing key issues such as low birth weight, immunization coverage, mortality rates, breastfeeding practices, complementary feeding, and malnutrition. The chapter also highlights significant disparities across regions, socioeconomic groups, and maternal factors. To mitigate these disparities, it is essential to enhance the implementation of existing programs, such as the ICDS, NHM, and Poshan Abhiyan and to improve monitoring and evaluation mechanisms for effective delivery. The equitable distribution of healthcare resources, focusing on rural and tribal areas, is important. Key strategies include strengthening PHCs and Anganwadi services and promoting maternal education at the grassroots level. Cross-sector collaboration, innovative healthcare delivery such as mobile health units and telemedicine, community engagement, and a data-driven approach can further promote health equity in India. Addressing health and nutrition disparities in Indian children requires a multifaceted approach that combines program enhancement, targeted interventions, grassroots investments, cross-sector collaboration, and community engagement to address significant health inequities and improve child health outcomes.

References

1. Braveman, P. (2006). Health Disparities and Health Equity: Concepts and Measurement. *Annual Review of Public Health, 27*, 167–194. Retrieved from https://doi.org/10.1146/ANNUREV.PUBLHEALTH.27.021405.102103.
2. Zhou, Y., & Xu, Y. (2023). Nutrition and Metabolism in the First 1000 Days of Life. *Nutrients, 15*(11), 2554. Retrieved from https://doi.org/10.3390/nu15112554.

3. Choong, Z., & Cheah, F. (2023). Early Life Nutrition During the First 1,000 Days from a Malaysian Perspective. *Medicine and Health, 18*(2), 279–299. Retrieved from https://doi.org/10.17576/MH.2023.1802.01.
4. Ratsika, A., Codagnone, M. C., O'mahony, S., Stanton, C., & Cryan, J. F. (2021). Priming for Life: Early Life Nutrition and the Microbiota-Gut-Brain Axis. *Nutrients, 13*(2), 423. Retrieved from https://doi.org/10.3390/NU13020423
5. Aires, J. (2021). First 1,000 days of life: Consequences of Antibiotics on Gut Microbiota. *Frontiers in Microbiology, 12*, 681427. Retrieved from https://doi.org/10.3389/FMICB.2021.681427.
6. Indrio, F., & Marchese, F. (2024). Microbiota in the First 1000 Days: Effect on Health and Diseases. *Global Pediatrics, 8*, 100162. Retrieved from https://doi.org/10.1016/J.GPEDS.2024.100162.
7. Vaiserman, A. M. (2013). Long-Term Health Consequences of Early-Life Exposure to Substance Abuse: An Epigenetic Perspective. *Journal of Developmental Origins of Health and Disease, 4*(4), 269–279. Retrieved from https://doi.org/10.1017/S2040174413000123
8. Pappachan, B., & Choonara, I. (2017). Inequalities in Child Health in India. *BMJ Paediatrics Open, 1*(1), e000054. Retrieved from https://doi.org/10.1136/BMJPO-2017-000054
9. Balarajan, Y., Selvaraj, S., & Subramanian, S. (2011). Health Care and Equity in India. *Lancet, 377*(9764), 505–515. Retrieved from https://doi.org/10.1016/S0140-6736(10)61894-6
10. Arokiasamy, P., Jain, K., Goli, S., & Pradhan, J. (2013). Health Inequalities Among Urban Children in India: A Comparative Assessment of Empowered Action Group (EAG) and South Indian states. *Journal of Biosocial Science, 45*(2), 167–185. Retrieved from https://doi.org/10.1017/S0021932012000211
11. World Health Organization. (2024). *Low Birth Weight*. Retrieved from https://www.who.int/data/nutrition/nlis/info/low-birth-weight.
12. Tripathi, S., Pathak, V. K., & Lahariya, C. (2023). Key Findings from NFHS-5 India Report: Observing Trends of Health Indicators Between NFHS-4 and NFHS-5. *Journal of Family Medicine and Primary Care, 12*(9), 1759–1763. Retrieved from https://doi.org/10.4103/JFMPC.JFMPC_377_23.
13. Sharma, M., & Mishra, S. (2003). Maternal Risk Factors and Consequences of Low Birth Weight in Infants. *IOSR Journal of Humanities and Social Science, 13*(4), 39–45. Retrieved from https://doi.org/10.9790/0837-1343945.
14. Banerjee, A., Singh, A. K., & Chaurasia, H. (2020). An Exploratory Spatial Analysis of Low Birth Weight and Its Determinants in India. *Clinical Epidemiology and Global Health, 8*(3), 702–711. Retrieved from https://doi.org/10.1016/j.cegh.2020.01.006.
15. Mallick, A. (2021). Prevalence of Low Birth Weight in India and Its Determinants: Insights from the National Family Health Survey (NFHS), 2015–2016. *Anthropologischer Anzeiger, 78*(3), 163–175. Retrieved from https://doi.org/10.1127/ANTHRANZ/2021/1317.
16. Girotra, S., Mohan, N., Malik, M., Roy, S., & Basu, S. (2023). Prevalence and Determinants of Low Birth Weight in India: Findings From a Nationally Representative Cross-Sectional Survey (2019–21). *Cureus, 15*(3), e36717. Retrieved from https://doi.org/10.7759/CUREUS.36717
17. Kumari, N., Algur, K., Chokhandre, P. K., & Salve, P. S. (2021). Low Birth Weight Among Tribal in India: Evidence from National Family Health Survey-4. *Clinical Epidemiology and Global Health, 9*, 360–366. Retrieved from https://doi.org/10.1016/J.CEGH.2020.10.010
18. Pinaki, P., Bijaya Kumar, P., & Leslie, E. (2013). Prevalence and Determinants of Low Birth Weight and Prematurity Among Rural, Urban, and Indigenous Tribal Communities in India. In *ISEE Conference Abstracts* (Vol. 1). Retrieved from https://doi.org/10.1289/ISEE.2013.P-1-33-04.
19. Wahyuni, S., et al. (2024). Education on the Importance of Immunization for Infants at Puskesmas Tamalanrea Jaya Makassar City. *Jurnal Pengabdian Masyarakat Edukasi Indonesia, 1*(1), 15–21. Retrieved from https://doi.org/10.61099/JPMEI.V1I1.33.
20. Wahl, B., et al. (2021). Change in Full Immunization Inequalities in Indian Children 12–23 Months: An Analysis of Household Survey Data. *BMC Public Health, 21*(1), 841. https://doi.org/10.1186/S12889-021-10849-Y

21. Mathew, J. L. (2012). Inequity in Childhood Immunization in India: A Systematic Review. *Indian Pediatrics, 49*(3), 203–223. Retrieved from https://doi.org/10.1007/S13312-012-0063-Z.
22. UNICEF. (2021). *Immunization Among Tribal Population in India: A Need Assessment Report*. Retrieved from https://www.unicef.org/india/media/6716/file/Immunization%20among%20Tribal%20Population%20in%20India.pdf.
23. Jain, N., Singh, A., & Pathak, P. (2013). Infant and Child Mortality in India: Trends in Inequalities Across Economic Groups. *Journal of Population Research, 30*(4), 347–365. Retrieved from https://doi.org/10.1007/S12546-013-9110-4.
24. Kumar, A., & Singh, A. (2014). Is Economic Inequality in Infant Mortality Higher in Urban Than in Rural India? *Maternal and Child Health Journal, 18*(9), 2061–2070. Retrieved from https://doi.org/10.1007/S10995-014-1452-9.
25. Bhatia, M., Ranjan, M., Dixit, P., & Dwivedi, L. K. (2018). Mind the Gap: Temporal Trends in Inequalities in Infant and Child Mortality in India (1992–2016). *SSM–Population Health, 5*, 201–209. Retrieved from https://doi.org/10.1016/J.SSMPH.2018.05.001.
26. Senanayake, P., O'Connor, E., & Ogbo, F. A. (2019). National and Rural-Urban Prevalence and Determinants of Early Initiation of Breastfeeding in India. *BMC Public Health, 19*(1), 896. Retrieved from https://doi.org/10.1186/S12889-019-7246-7.
27. Valappil, H. C., Jayalakshmi, R., & Sewor, C. (2023). Intersectional Inequalities in Exclusive Breastfeeding Practices in India: Analysis of National Family Health Survey-4. *International Breastfeeding Journal, 18*(1), 44. Retrieved from https://doi.org/10.1186/S13006-023-00577-X.
28. Nishimura, H., Krupp, K., Gowda, S., Srinivas, V., Arun, A., & Madhivanan, P. (2018). Determinants of Exclusive Breastfeeding in Rural South India. *International Breastfeeding Journal, 13*(40). Retrieved from https://doi.org/10.1186/S13006-018-0178-5.
29. Chowdhury, A. R., Surie, A., & Bhan, G. (2021). Breastfeeding Knowledge and Practices of Working Mothers in the Informal Economy in New Delhi: A Formative Study to Explore New Intervention Pathways Towards Improved Maternal and Child Health Outcomes. *Social Science & Medicine, 281*, 114070. Retrieved from https://doi.org/10.1016/J.SOCSCIMED.2021.114070.
30. World Health Organization. (2023). *WHO Guideline for Complementary Feeding of Infants and Young Children 6–23 Months of Age*. Retrieved from https://www.ncbi.nlm.nih.gov/books/NBK596427/.
31. Patel, A., Pusdekar, Y., Badhoniya, N., Borkar, J., Agho, K. E., & Dibley, M. J. (2012). Determinants of Inappropriate Complementary Feeding Practices in Young Children in India: Secondary Analysis of National Family Health Survey 2005–2006. *Maternal & Child Nutrition, 8*(1), 28–44. Retrieved from https://doi.org/10.1111/J.1740-8709.2011.00385.X.
32. Dhami, M. V., Ogbo, F. A., Osuagwu, U. L., & Agho, K. E. (2019). Prevalence and Factors Associated with Complementary Feeding Practices Among Children Aged 6–23 Months in India: A Regional Analysis. *BMC Public Health, 19*(1), 1034. Retrieved from https://doi.org/10.1186/S12889-019-7360-6.
33. Ministry of Health and Family Welfare Government of India. (2022). *National Family Healthy Survey 5 (2019–2021)—India Fact Sheet*. http://rchiips.org/nfhs/NFHS-5_FCTS/India.pdf. Accessed 5 March 2024
34. Ministry of Health and Family Welfare Government of India. (2013). *National Health Mission (NHM)—A Report*. Retrieved from https://nhm.gov.in/images/pdf/NHM/NHM_more_information.pdf.
35. Singh, S., Srivastava, S., & Upadhyay, A. K. (2019). Socio-Economic Inequality in Malnutrition Among Children in India: An Analysis of 640 Districts from National Family Health Survey (2015–16). *International Journal for Equity in Health, 18*(1), 203. Retrieved from https://doi.org/10.1186/S12939-019-1093-0.
36. Nguyen, P. H., et al. (2021). The Double Burden of Malnutrition in India: Trends and Inequalities (2006–2016). *PLoS ONE, 16*(2), e0247856. Retrieved from https://doi.org/10.1371/JOURNAL.PONE.0247856

37. Ministry of Health and Family Welfare Government of India. (2022). *National Family health Survey (NFHS-5), 2019–21, India Report*. Retrieved from https://dhsprogram.com/pubs/pdf/FR375/FR375.pdf.
38. Saha, J., et al. (2022). Overweight/Obesity Prevalence Among Under-Five Children and Risk Factors in India: A Cross-Sectional Study Using the National Family Health Survey (2015–2016). *Nutrients, 14*(17), 3621. Retrieved from https://doi.org/10.3390/NU14173621.
39. Singh, S. K., Lhungdim, H., Shekhar, C., Dwivedi, L. K., Pedgaonkar, S., & James, K. S. (2023). Key Drivers of Reversal of Trend in Childhood Anaemia in India: Evidence from Indian Demographic and Health Surveys, 2016–21. *BMC Public Health, 23*(1), 1574. Retrieved from https://doi.org/10.1186/s12889-023-16398-w.
40. Khadilkar, A., et al. (2022). Vitamin D Status and Determinants in Indian Children and Adolescents: A Multicentre Study. *Scientific Reports, 12*(1), 1–13. Retrieved from https://doi.org/10.1038/s41598-022-21279-0.
41. Shalini, T., et al. (2023). Prevalence of Vitamin B12 and Folate Deficiencies in Indian Children and Adolescents. *Nutrients, 15*(13), 3026. Retrieved from https://doi.org/10.3390/NU15133026.
42. Puranik, A., & N, S. (2022). Anemia Among Children Under 5 Years in India: A District-Level Spatial Analysis Using NFHS-5 Data. Asia-*Pacific Journal of Public Health, 34*(2–3), 206–212. Retrieved from https://doi.org/10.1177/10105395211058288.
43. Hossain, F. (2019). Levels of Health Care and Health Outcomes in Northeast India. *Indian Journal of Human Development, 13*(2), 221–232. Retrieved from https://doi.org/10.1177/0973703019870881
44. Madlala, S. S., & Kassier, S. M. (2018). Antenatal and Postpartum Depression: Effects on Infant and Young Child Health and Feeding Practices. *South African Journal of Clinical Nutrition, 31*(1), 1–7. Retrieved from https://doi.org/10.1080/16070658.2017.1333753.
45. de Reis, Á. E. M., et al. (2024). Maternal Nutrition and Its Effects on Fetal Neurodevelopment. *Nutrition, 125*, 112483. Retrieved from https://doi.org/10.1016/J.NUT.2024.112483.
46. Handa, A., Gaidhane, A., Quazi, Z., & Chaudhari, S. (2024). Association of Maternal Mental Health on Development and Growth of Children Under Two Years Old from Wardha: Protocol for a Cross-Sectional Study. *F1000Research, 13*, 23. Retrieved from https://doi.org/10.12688/f1000research.142774.1.
47. Brizuela, V., & Tunçalp, Ö. (2017). Global Initiatives in Maternal and Newborn Health. *Obstetric Medicine, 10*(1), 21–5. Retrieved from https://doi.org/10.1177/1753495X16684987.
48. Narayan, J., John, D., & Ramadas, N. (2019). Malnutrition in India: Status and Government Initiatives. *Journal of Public Health Policy, 40*(1), 126–141. Retrieved from https://doi.org/10.1057/S41271-018-0149-5.
49. Ministry of Health and Family Welfare Government of India. (2024). *National Health Mission (NHM)*. Retrieved from https://nhm.gov.in/.
50. World Health Organization. (2021). *Health Equity in India–A Technical Paper*. Retrieved from https://cdn.who.int/media/docs/default-source/wrindia/document/health-equity-in-india7cee19b6-1324-4de4-a9c7-13f24cee0976.pdf?sfvrsn=816d1189_4.
51. Ministry of Health and Family Welfare Government of India. (2013). *Guidelines for Control of Iron Deficiency Anaemia*. Retrieved from https://www.nhm.gov.in/images/pdf/programmes/wifs/guidelines/Guidelines_for_Control_of_Iron_Deficiency_Anaemia.pdf#:~:text=The%20National%20Iron%2B%20Initiative%20is%20an%20attempt%20to,to%20make%20both%20administration%20and%20compliance%20much%20simpler.
52. Ministry of Health and Family Welfare Government of India. (2024). *Rashtriya Bal Swasthya Karyakram*. Retrieved from https://rbsk.mohfw.gov.in/RBSK/.
53. Ministry of Education Government of India. (2024). *Pradhan Mantri Poshan Shakti Nirman–PM POSHAN*. Retrieved from http://www.pmposhan-ams.education.gov.in/About_mdm.aspx.
54. National Food Security Portal Department of Food & Public Distribution Government of India. (2024). *National Food Security Act, (NFSA)*. Retrieved from https://nfsa.gov.in/portal/NFSA-Act.

55. Ministry of Women and Child Development Government of India. (2021). *National Nutrition Mission*. Retrieved from https://www.pib.gov.in/PressReleaseIframePage.aspx?PRID=1777745.
56. Mohan, P., & Kumar, R. (2019). Strengthening Primary Care in Rural India: Lessons from Indian and Global Evidence and Experience. *Journal of Family Medicine and Primary Care, 8*(7), 2169–2172. Retrieved from https://doi.org/10.4103/JFMPC.JFMPC_426_19.
57. Price, J. C., & Simpson, D. C. (2022). Telemedicine and Health Disparities. *Clinical Liver Disease, 19*(4), 144. Retrieved from https://doi.org/10.1002/CLD.1171.

Chapter 13
Promoting Equity in Early Breastfeeding Practices: Examining Associated Factors for Policy Improvements in Early Initiation and Exclusive Breastfeeding in Urban Informal Settlements

Jennifer Spencer, Manjula Bahuguna, and Sushmita Das

Background

Breastfeeding stands out as a highly effective way to safeguard the health and longevity of children. It protects infants against various communicable and non-communicable diseases and promotes their overall development [1, 2]. Introducing breastfeeding from day one potentially saves 16% of neonatal fatalities, with this figure increasing to 22% if breastfeeding is initiated within the first hour after birth [3].

Early breastfeeding practices are measured by the World Health Organisation's (WHO) Infant and Young Child Feeding (IYCF) indicators. This includes 'Early initiation of breastfeeding (EIBF)' defined as the number of children who are given breast milk within the first hour of birth. In 2021, WHO added one new indicator 'Exclusively breastfed for the first two days after birth (EBF2D)' in its list of IYCF indicators [4]. It reiterated that not only initiating early breastfeeding but exclusive breastfeeding during the initial days is important for child health.

Globally, only 48% of newborns were breastfed within the first hour after birth between 2013 and 2018 [5]. In low- and middle-income countries (LMICs) despite numerous efforts, there is a notable gap between breastfeeding practices and recommendations outlined by the WHO. During 2010–2018, in 57 LMICs, the global weighted prevalence of EIBF was 52% [6]. In India, progress has been minimal with

J. Spencer (✉) · M. Bahuguna · S. Das
Society for Nutrition, Education and Health Action (SNEHA), Mumbai, India
e-mail: jennifer.spencer@snehamumbai.org

S. Das
e-mail: sushmita@snehamumbai.org

S. Suri (ed.), *Child Health and Nutrition from Conception to Age Two*,
https://doi.org/10.1007/978-981-95-7868-9_13

early breastfeeding rates remaining stagnant. The National Family Health Surveys (NFHS) conducted by the Government of India reported early breastfeeding initiation rates of 41.6% in NFHS-4 (2015–16) and 41.8% in NFHS-5 (2019–21) [7, 8]. Exclusive breastfeeding (EBF) for six months has shown improvement from 55% to 64% in the same period [7, 8]. This highlights the need for coordinated efforts to tackle the factors causing the lack of progress in early breastfeeding practices. There is also lack of available information about the newly added indicator of 'EBF2D', and factors that influence exclusive breastfeeding during initial days post birth. Particularly, breastfeeding practices need to be assessed in urban areas where a considerable proportion of the population lives in inadequate housing with unequal access to health services. NFHS data have shown minimal improvement in EIBF (42.8% in NFHS-4 to 44.7% in NFHS-5) in urban India while EBF rates in NFHS-5 were lower in urban (59.6%) than rural (65.1%) areas [7, 8].

This points to the need for specific interventions among underserved populations in urban areas of LMICs to improve equity in healthcare services.

Breastfeeding and Equitable Access to Healthcare

Equity in health involves eliminating systematic disparities in health outcomes between different social groups, ensuring that everyone has the right to achieve the highest possible standard of health, irrespective of their social advantages or disadvantages [9]. It depends on equitable access to healthcare, ensuring that everyone, regardless of their economic, social, or demographic background, has fair access to preventive, promotive, and curative information, resources, and care [10]. It is about distributive justice within the health system, ensuring that marginalized and most vulnerable members of the community are adequately cared for [11]. The equity lens can guide us in making ethical decisions about where to focus efforts to improve overall health outcomes, particularly for high-risk groups, underserved areas, and women and children.

In LMICs, significant progress has been observed in reproductive, maternal, newborn, and child health, however, much remains to be done in terms of reaching the marginalized and the most vulnerable [12]. In India, cities have witnessed rapid urbanization, resulting in a substantial population influx. However, the provision of basic services, including housing, water, sanitation, and healthcare, has not kept pace with this growth. As a result, a large proportion of the population resides in inadequate housing within urban informal settlements, commonly referred to as slums. These demographic experience significant disparities in the availability of and access to basic services and healthcare [13]. Despite numerous health programs and policies, the utilization of maternal healthcare services among disadvantaged population segments remains below the desired level [14]. Women in these vulnerable environments experience poor health due to inadequate nutritional intake, poor sanitation, congested living environments and limited access to quality obstetric care, which often leads to complications during pregnancy and delivery [15]. A majority of women in urban informal settlements access public healthcare services which are more affordable. However, public health services are heavily overburdened, often with limited and overworked staff. Patients also report encountering limitations of service availability, accessibility, and potential discrimination at public health facilities [13].

Among interventions for maternal and childcare, breastfeeding stands out as a highly effective way to safeguard the health and longevity of children [1]. Equitable access to breast milk for all infants is a key component of newborn care [16]. From an equity perspective, it is crucial to ensure that all women, regardless of their background or circumstances, have access to the necessary information and support to breastfeed successfully [17]. However, it is observed that women in vulnerable settings face various barriers that prevent them from breastfeeding adequately—a contributing factor to neonatal mortality, poor child growth, and inadequate nutrition, including an increased risk of child malnourishment [3, 18].

Various studies have highlighted how socio-demographic parameters like poor education among lower-income groups act as barriers toward effective breastfeeding [19, 20]. Cultural practices in communities also act as hindrances to follow early breastfeeding practices [21, 22]. Institutional barriers such as poor access, awareness, and lack of interventions toward aiding early breastfeeding practices are also considered one major hindrance toward equitable breastfeeding [21, 23]. It is therefore important to address barriers that might prevent women in vulnerable settings from receiving adequate breastfeeding education and assistance and promote equal opportunities for all mothers to provide optimal nutrition for their infants.

Equity in access to healthcare can be achieved through a multifaceted approach that addresses both the supply and demand sides of an intervention. Comprehensive and intersectoral interventions are considered essential to overcome barriers to adopting early breastfeeding practices [24]. This involves ensuring that healthcare services are readily available, accessible, and of high quality, while also empowering individuals and communities to seek and utilize these services effectively.

Some of the strategies targeted at healthcare workers include educational training, outreach, practice facilitation, audit, and feedback [25, 26]. Additionally, for specific types of problems, these strategies can include training healthcare workers to adopt a more patient-centered approach in clinical consultations [27]. Strategies also include promoting diversity within the health workforce and enhancing the cultural competence of healthcare workers [28, 29]. This can help ensure that healthcare providers better understand, respect, and meet the diverse needs of the populations they serve. Strategies targeted at healthcare recipients include mass media campaigns, educational programs, community outreach, and tailored interventions designed to raise awareness, improve health literacy, and encourage healthy behaviors. These approaches aim to empower individuals to take an active role in their health and make informed decisions about their care [30]. Vilar-Compte and colleagues [31] highlight four levels of interventions to ensure equity in breastfeeding-individual level such as improving mothers' awareness and education; community level such as support and counseling by community health workers; institutional or organizational level including adoption of Baby-Friendly Hospitals Initiative (BFHI) in healthcare facilities and workplace breastfeeding interventions; and structural level such as change in government policies regarding medical procedures, use of milk substitutes, etc.

Situating Equity and Breastfeeding in Mumbai's Urban Informal Settlements

Recognizing the need for equitable healthcare services to improve maternal and newborn health, there is a need to focus on breastfeeding practices among vulnerable populations such as those living in urban informal settlements. Indian cities have experienced rapid urbanization; the provision of basic services has however not kept pace with this growth, resulting in socio-economic vulnerability among a considerable proportion of the urban population. Disparities in access to basic services and healthcare facilities among this population, particularly for women, has heightened inequities related to maternal and child health outcomes, including early breastfeeding practices [13, 15]. Examining the extent of breastfeeding and factors influencing breastfeeding practices in this setting, can help frame possible solutions for more equitable access to maternal and newborn healthcare services.

The chapter analyses this using primary data from the Society for Nutrition, Education, and Health Action (SNEHA), a non-governmental organization based in Mumbai, India working to improve the health and nutritional status of mothers and children residing in urban informal settlements. The data was drawn from a quantitative survey conducted in four urban informal settlements in Mumbai with 1,049 mothers of under-two children. Urban informal settlements in Mumbai comprise 41% of the city's population [32] and are characterized by inadequate housing, congested living environment, inadequate sanitation and poor access to quality healthcare services.

Mothers of children under two years of age were primary respondents of the survey. One-third (33%) of the respondents were under 25 years of age. Majority had attended secondary school (50%) and nearly one-third (34%) of the respondents had three or more children. More than half (51%) of the respondents lived in nuclear families. Most respondents (85%) had made four or more ANC visits, primarily at public health facilities (69%). Additionally, 64% of the respondents delivered at public health facilities, and one-third (31%) underwent caesarean sections (C-sections). The proportion of girl children was (47%) and less than half (45%) of the children were aged 0–11 months.

The survey included information on feeding practices such as whether the baby was ever breastfed, time gap between birth and the initiation of breastfeeding, and whether the infant was given any liquids (details of the type) other than breast milk during the first two days after delivery. The computation of all breastfeeding related IYCF indicators adhered to WHO guidelines [4].

Extent of Early Breastfeeding Practices in Urban Informal Settlements of Mumbai

The study showed that among the 1,049 children born in the two years preceding the survey, majority (99%) were ever breastfed. However, only 33% were initiated into breastfeeding within the first hour after birth. Seen through an equity lens, the 33% presents a chasm- most mothers from urban informal settlements were unable to timely initiate breastfeeding. Further, compared to other studies, such as in slums of Dhaka, Bangladesh [33] where this rate was 64%, Mumbai's 33% is less than half, illuminating how site-specific constraints undermine equity even within LMIC slum contexts.

Compared to EIBF, EBF2D rates in the study were more promising- 65% infants were exclusively breastfed during the initial two days post birth. This prevalence is similar to other studies in urban informal settlements of Indian cities [19, 34] showing that exclusive breastfeeding for two days is being followed better than EIBF.

Apart from the indicators of EIBF and EBF2D, various studies in urban informal settlements of India indicate low rates of EBF for the first six months of birth. A study conducted in the urban slums of Patna, India revealed that only 28% of mothers practiced EBF for six months [20]. Another study in South India found that the prevalence of EBF decreased steadily from the first to the sixth month with only 11% of the mothers surveyed continuing EBF up to six months [35]. In comparison, this study documented a higher rate of EBF in the first six months (63%). Figure 13.1 shows information regarding various breastfeeding related IYCF indicators from the study.

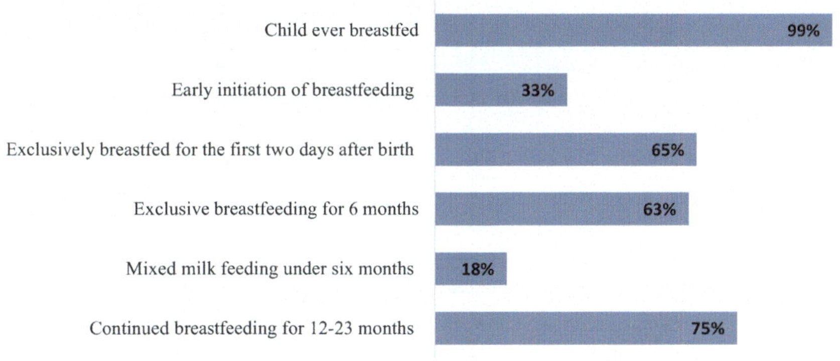

Fig. 13.1 Breastfeeding practices from four urban informal settlements of Mumbai. *Source* Authors

Factors Influencing EIBF and EBF2D in Urban Informal Settlements of Mumbai

To offer recommendations for enhancing early breastfeeding practices, it is essential to identify factors influencing these indicators in the context of urban informal settlements. A detailed analysis was conducted to understand respondents' demographic characteristics and health seeking behavior in relation to EIBF and EBF2D.

For the analysis, early breastfeeding practices of EIBF and EBF2D were employed as dependent variables where children whose mothers reported following these practices and those who did not report following them were separately categorized. Independent variables used for the analysis included child and maternal characteristics of the sample. Variables describing maternal characteristics were age in years (<25, 25–29, ≥30), education (no formal education, primary education, secondary education, higher education), number of children (1–2, ≥3), type of family (nuclear, joint), health facility used for antenatal care (ANC) visits (public, private), number of ANC visits (<4, ≥4), health facility used for delivery (public, private, home), and type of delivery (vaginal, caesarean). Variables related to the child characteristics were sex (male, female) and age (0–11 months, 12–23 months). Chi-squared tests, unadjusted and multivariate logistic models were used to explore the associations between independent variables and EIBF and EBF2D (Fig. 13.2).

The graph presents the Adjusted Odds Ratios (AOR) and Confidence Intervals (CI) for various factors influencing EIBF and EBF2D. Each point on the graph represents the OR for a specific factor, and the horizontal line extending from the

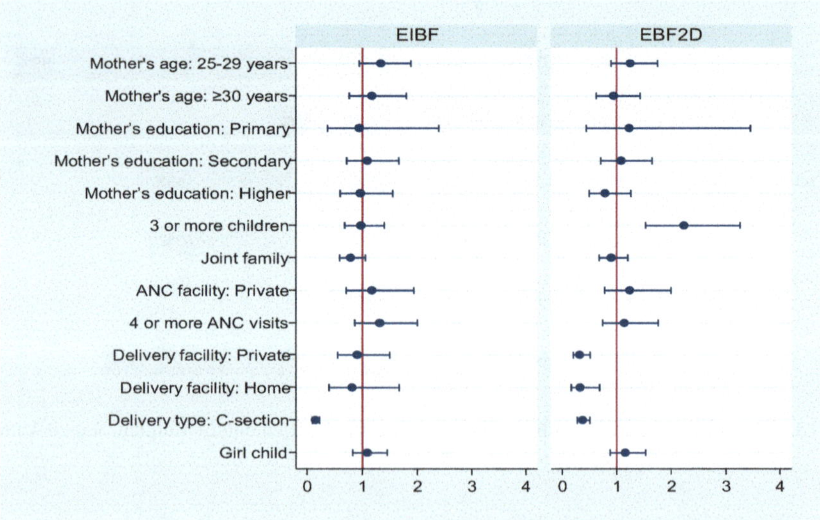

Fig. 13.2 Factors associated with early initiation of breastfeeding (EIBF) and exclusive breastfeeding for the first two days after birth (EBF2D) in four informal settlements of Mumbai, India. *Source* Authors

point illustrates the 95% Confidence Interval (CI) for that estimate. If the CI does not cross 1, the factor is considered to have a statistically significant effect on early breastfeeding practices.

The analysis showed that parents' education level and EBF2D had a significant association, with women having higher education being less likely to practice EBF2D compared to those with no education. However, this association lost statistical significance after adjusting for other factors. Another study conducted in South India revealed a negative correlation between education level and adherence to exclusive breastfeeding [35]. Higher education is linked to increased exposure to information about, and a greater preference for, the use of milk substitutes or formula milk, acting as one reason for such a negative association [36]. While several other studies report a positive association between education of the mother and EBF practices there is a need to focus on the level of awareness regarding accurate EBF practices which need not be a function of education [19, 20]. This is particularly relevant for improving equity in breastfeeding practices among those living in urban informal settlements with lesser formal education. ANC visits are considered one way of receiving such information and improving awareness of parents toward breastfeeding. However, as seen in this study, the number of ANC visits had no significant association with breastfeeding practices, indicating that more than frequency of visits it is the quality of ANC counseling which can matter in improving early breastfeeding practices. This is corroborated by evidence from other studies in India where women who received prenatal and antenatal counseling regarding early breastfeeding practices were more likely to follow EIBF and EBF compared to those who did not receive such advice [26, 37].

Another factor linked to the level of education and awareness of early breastfeeding is the influence of cultural practices. Such practices extend beyond parents' education or awareness and are often imposed by in-laws or elders in the family and neighborhood, which have to be followed without much choice [21, 22]. Such beliefs include not feeding the 'first milk' or initiation of breastfeeding only after 48 hours, since such milk is considered to be impure and not good for infants, a key reason for low EIBF rates [38, 39]. Such practices also surround not feeding colostrum, which is otherwise considered to be important in building the immunity of the infant [21]. Other cultural practices include feeding pre-lacteals such as jaggery, honey, or water [33, 34], hindering the adherence of EBF2D. In this study, such practices were evident, with 41% of infants being fed pre-lacteals. Conversely, research has emphasized that supportive family attitudes and norms play a crucial role in encouraging mothers to practice exclusive breastfeeding effectively [40]. A combination of cultural practices, level of education and awareness are thus key determinants of individual and community-level perspectives influencing early breastfeeding practices.

At the institutional and systemic levels, the analysis showed that the place of delivery and type of facility (public/private) for delivery significantly influenced EIBF and EBF2D. Poor EBF practices have been associated with deliveries in facilities where the child is taken away from the mother for a longer period, as compared to home deliveries. A study in Bangladesh found that a higher proportion of women who delivered at home, initiated breastfeeding within one hour as compared to those who delivered in facilities [37]. Nevertheless, given the essentiality of institutional delivery for ensuring positive maternal and child outcomes, understanding and addressing factors hindering early breastfeeding in healthcare institutions needs to be done. Among the type of delivery facility, the study indicates that the proportion of women practicing EIBF and EBF2D was higher among those who delivered in public facilities. However, this difference was not significant for EIBF in the adjusted regression model. Women delivering in a private health facility had lower odds [AOR 0.31, 95% CI 0.19–0.51] of EBF2D compared to women delivering in a public health facility.

Various studies in South Asia including India have shown that breastfeeding practices have been followed more diligently in public hospitals. One study showed how government schemes adopting the BFHI implemented in public health facilities ensures better EIBF and EBF2D rates [20]. Studies have also shown that patients who received counseling and assistance from health professionals were more likely to initiate early breastfeeding practices [26, 37]. Given that a majority of residents in urban informal settlements access public healthcare, this bodes well for enhancing healthcare equity. However, evidence also shows that in the public sector health professionals are overburdened with a high inflow of patients, giving them lesser time to explain and assist mothers for initiating breastfeeding [21]. In the case of health facilities in the private sector, promotion of formula feed supplementation has been reported, which impedes the practice of exclusive breastfeeding during the initial days after birth. Extensive marketing of formula feeds, especially by health professionals can diminish mothers' confidence in their breastfeeding capabilities [41].

Another factor related to delivery in health facilities is the method of childbirth, particularly C-sections, which have been increasing in urban India, especially in private facilities [23]. The study found that the odds of EIBF [AOR 0.15, 95% CI 0.10–0.22] and EBF2D [AOR 0.37, 95% CI 0.27–0.50] were significantly lower following a C-section compared to vaginal delivery. This finding aligns with results from several other studies, reinforcing the importance of the method of delivery in influencing early breastfeeding practices [42, 43]. Studies on EIBF in Ethiopia and Nepal showed high association of C-section with delays in initiating breastfeeding [44, 45], while studies from Bangladesh and Ghana show how C-section is associated with a lower chance of practicing exclusive breastfeeding [46, 47]. This is a matter of concern since C-sections are among the most frequently performed surgical procedures in many LMICs [48] and their prevalence is also rising among vulnerable populations. A rise in C-section deliveries is often attributed to an overburdened health system where doctors prefer to plan deliveries via C-section in order to save time and resources [49, 50]. In the private sector, conducting C-sections is also considered to be much more profitable for hospitals than vaginal deliveries [51]. C-sections are also associated with lifestyle-related factors such as poor nutrition, which is prevalent among women in urban informal settlements [52].

For timely initiation of breastfeeding, it is suggested that after birth every effort should be made to keep the mother–baby dyad together to alter the mother's behavior, strengthen the bonding process, and initiate breastfeeding [53–55]. However, in most cases of C-sections, it is observed that infants are separated from their mothers and kept waiting for their first feed until the mother has been transferred to the postnatal ward. Some of the reasons like delayed mother-to-infant skin-to-skin contact, physical complications, and effects of anesthesia, among mothers who undergo C-sections lead to late initiation of breastfeeding [42, 43]. In some cases, where emergency C-sections have been carried out, or the baby is preterm, infants are kept separately in neonatal intensive care units, increasing the possibility of delayed initiation of breastfeeding [56]. Similarly, in cases of vaginal delivery, factors such as exhaustion from labor, delay in mother-to-infant skin-to-skin contact facilitated by healthcare staff, may inhibit EIBF [57, 58]. The increasing use of labor pain medications is also being associated with delayed onset of milk production among mothers [59]. This is reflected in the study, where a majority of mothers who underwent vaginal delivery were also unable to initiate breastfeeding within one hour of birth. Such delay in initiating breastfeeding also increases the chances of introducing pre-lacteal foods, breast milk substitutes, or formula feed.

Policy Suggestions for Improving Early Breastfeeding Practices

Based on the extent and factors associated with EIBF and EBF2D rates found in the study, we attempt to provide possible suggestions for improvement in these practices. We employ a four-fold framework [31] of interventions—at the individual, community, institutional, and structural level—to ensure equity in breastfeeding. Our policy suggestions can be applied in the context of urban informal settlements in India but are also valuable for wider policy change related to early breastfeeding practices in other LMICs.

First, at the individual and community level, awareness regarding the importance of EIBF and EBF2D is essential among parents, family, and in the community to ensure that these practices are followed. Community health centers providing ANC services need to ensure that adequate information regarding the importance and need for EIBF and EBF are provided to registered women and their spouses. In the context of urban informal settlements, community-based awareness interventions should extend beyond health centers to include the broader community, particularly elders in families and neighbourhoods, whose cultural norms often influence the practice of EIBF and EBF [21, 22]. Such community-based interventions also help reach out to pregnant women who are unable to register for ANC services or regularly visit health centers for ANC check-ups [60]. Such awareness programs can be especially beneficial for primigravida women who are known to have lesser knowledge and experience of birthing and breastfeeding [21, 61]. To enable this, community health workers such as Accredited Social Health Activists (ASHAs) and Anganwadi Workers (AWWs) can play an essential role. ASHAs and AWWs can ensure individual and community-level counseling of pregnant women and their families to inculcate the importance of early breastfeeding practices and dispel cultural misconceptions associated with discarding colostrum or giving pre-lacteal feeds. Post-delivery, ASHAs and AWWs need to monitor the practice of exclusive breastfeeding, providing continued awareness and support for addressing common challenges such as perceived insufficient milk supply, nipple soreness, and the use of artificial feeders.

Awareness and interventions at the community level also need to include strategies for holistic health support, because the living environment of pregnant women and their overall health before and during pregnancy have lasting impacts on the extent of breastfeeding practices. For instance, poor nutritional intake before and during pregnancy can lead to complications in delivery (at times leading to C-section) and difficulty in breastfeeding (such as not producing milk), both of which adversely impact EIBF and EBF. Strengthening nutritional support for pregnant women through maternal and child health policies as well as improving the staff strength and services provided at primary health centers can go a long way in ensuring continued health support to women and infants during and after pregnancy.

At the institutional level, changes and initiatives are primarily required to improve EIBF and EBF rates given that women are encouraged to deliver in health facilities. The BFHI recommended by the WHO, addresses all aspects valuable to protect, promote, and support breastfeeding and the well-being of young children [62]. It includes ten comprehensive steps for maternity facilities to ensure optimal breastfeeding practices. First, it mandates that institutions have a written breastfeeding policy and follow national policies related to marketing and use of breastmilk substitutes. Secondly, it requires that healthcare staff have adequate knowledge and skills to support breastfeeding. This relates to the next two steps of healthcare staff being equipped to provide ANC education, advising pregnant women and their families, and ensuring immediate and uninterrupted skin-to-skin contact between the mother and baby after birth. Another guideline includes 'rooming-in' or ensuring that the mothers and infants remain together in close proximity. In cases of emergency or C-section deliveries, where mothers are separated from their newborn, BFHI guidelines also provide for mothers to be given information on how to maintain lactation. Next, BFHI steps mandate for exclusive breastfeeding—healthcare staff of hospitals need to ensure that any food or fluids other than breastmilk are not given to babies unless medically indicated. While relatively a common practice, BFHI guidelines also include providing information to mothers on the risks associated with feeding bottles, teats, and pacifiers. Finally, the guidelines call for a smooth institution to home transition for mothers by stressing on continued breastfeeding and support.

In India, BFHI was launched in the year 1993 but still not all health facilities in the country follow the ten steps of BFHI or are certified as baby-friendly [63]. The implementation of this initiative needs to be ensured through clearly stated policies on breastfeeding by the health facility and developing required resources for the same [64]. During labor/delivery/post-delivery women are largely dependent on the health system staff to guide and support them, highlighting their importance in ensuring the adherence of accurate breastfeeding practices. The training of the healthcare professionals and support staff involved in obstetric care needs to be conducted to ensure that requisite information is provided to mothers and their family, and that EIBF and EBF2D are practiced [25, 27, 28]. A crucial aspect here is training staff in providing support to mothers by ensuring skin-to-skin contact and assisting the mothers to initiate breastfeeding within one hour of birth [26]. Such training must include hands-on skills to assist new mothers for latching, positioning, and addressing common breastfeeding difficulties, while having a considerate and caring attitude toward patients.

Specific quality improvement interventions implemented at the facility level shown to have improved early breastfeeding initiation especially among mothers who underwent C-section delivery can also be adopted to improve outcomes [65, 66]. In one case, EIBF rates in a tertiary hospital were increased from 0% to 82% in the case of C-section deliveries using a series of plan-do-study-act cycles in collaboration with a team of obstetricians, pediatricians, and nurses. Adopting mother-baby contact and putting the baby to the mother's breast in the transition room after the surgery with the help of labor room nurses and female attendants, as compared to previous practice of initiating mother-baby bonding after being shifted to the ward, helped improve EIBF rates [65].

A majority of women in urban informal settlements access public healthcare for deliveries and other health issues. Public health systems in urban areas, especially in megacities like Mumbai are heavily overburdened due to vacancy in staff positions, high inflow of patients and challenges related to facility infrastructure [21, 49, 50]. At the structural level, it is therefore essential to strengthen public health services by allocating adequate finances to the sector, ensuring filling of vacant posts and additional openings to reduce the burden on existing staff, expanding hospital infrastructure including setting up of new public health facilities/strengthening existing facilities in nearby cities and towns to reduce the patient inflows on few tertiary-level facilities [67]. This will not only enable better support for women during and after pregnancy, ensuring the early initiation of breastfeeding but also reduce the probability of avoidable C-sections that are carried out more due to convenience than medical need [50]. Private health facilities also regularly need to evaluate their patient load vis à vis staff adequacy to ensure adequate support and attention to new mothers and infants. Significant policy focus and financing needs to be directed toward implementing the BFHI in healthcare facilities. Similarly, community-level policies such as the Integrated Child Development Services scheme needs to be strengthened by increasing training regarding early breastfeeding practices among AWW enabling their role as community breastfeeding counsellors. Particularly, AWW can act as a crucial link to enable continued support for new mothers post discharge to ensure exclusive breastfeeding practices.

Regulatory policies governing breastfeeding practices and delivery procedures need to be reinforced both at the healthcare facility level and within government policy frameworks. A qualitative study from Delhi, India, found that the absence of monitoring the ratio of C-sections to total deliveries for each health professional, coupled with the financial incentives that increase hospital profitability, encourages doctors to perform C-sections [51]. If the proportion of C-sections to total deliveries is better monitored as a part of facility-wise reporting to the government, it can go a long way in reducing the number of C-sections conducted based on convenience rather than medical need. Similarly, facility-wise rules and monitoring of breastfeeding practices such as EIBF can help improve the rates. For instance, regulations on the marketing and sale of formula feeds should be strictly enforced, and its unnecessary prescriptions by health practitioners should be curtailed, particularly when breastfeeding is a possible alternative. This does not imply neglecting medical conditions like premature infants facing an increased risk of complications needing such substitutes for survival. Decisions based on individual cases, considering the woman and family's informed choice, should be encouraged at the health facility level.

While we have outlined the most essential suggestions related to four-fold interventions for equity in breastfeeding, breastfeeding practices and their initiation need to be seen comprehensively. A combination of various strategies needs to be adopted to improve early breastfeeding outcomes which include awareness, counseling and support during and post pregnancy through a combination of community-level, facility-level and government policy-related interventions [31, 68, 69]. Sri Lanka has been one such example in the South Asian region, achieving EIBF rates of 90% and EBF rates of 82% [70]. This was made possible by robust implementation of BFHI in healthcare institutions prioritizing immediate skin-to-skin contact, rooming-in and providing skilled lactation support for mothers. Primarily, the establishment of 'Lactation Management Centres' (LMC) in public hospitals enabled comprehensive support for breastfeeding [70]. The LMC staffed with trained lactation consultants and nurses provided breastfeeding counseling and support, guidance on latching, positioning, expressing breastmilk, and addressing difficulties in feeding. Some LMCs also included human milk banks providing breastfeeding support in emergency cases. Most importantly, LMCs provided for follow-up visits establishing referrals with community health workers and community support groups to ensure continuity of care. We can learn from such successful initiatives in order to improve early breastfeeding practices among socio-economically vulnerable populations in India's cities.

The study has a few limitations. The cross-sectional nature of the study design limited the possibility of causal inference. Additionally, as the survey was part of a broader maternal and child health assessment, limited information was available on health status of the child post birth that may have influenced breastfeeding practices. Self-reported breastfeeding practices may be subject to positive bias; however, this bias is likely consistent among all mothers in the surveillance data. Another possible limitation is the presence of recall bias, as respondents were asked to retrospectively report on early breastfeeding practices, which they may have forgotten or misreported.

Concluding Reflections: Toward a More Equitable Health System

Mumbai's informal settlements exemplify both the promise and the pitfalls of urban health equity. While nearly all mothers breastfeed, only a fraction achieve the timeliness and exclusivity that science shows can save lives. The study highlights the need for improvements in exclusive breastfeeding rates especially the need for specific focus on EIBF. The study indicates that among other factors, the type of delivery facility and the mode of delivery significantly impact early breastfeeding practices. The factors identified provide crucial insights on the kind of interventions required at the level of the community and in health systems to ensure adequate breastfeeding practices are followed. Through multi-level interventions—from community-level awareness initiatives to state-level policy advocacy—the chapter illuminates a pathway for strengthening health systems so that breastmilk becomes a right, not a privilege. But the work is far from over: training healthcare staff in counseling and postnatal support, monitoring delivery and breastfeeding outcomes, and ensuring that BFHI is implemented will require sustained commitment. Only then will every newborn, regardless of circumstance, have an equal start.

References

1. Brahm, P., & Valdés, V. (2017). Benefits of Breastfeeding and Risks Associated with Not Breastfeeding. *Revista Chilena de pediatría, 88*(1), 15–21. Retrieved from https://doi.org/10.4067/S0370-41062017000100001.
2. Marandi, S., & Ezzeddin-Zanjani, N. (2012). On the Occasion of the World Breastfeeding Week: The Promotion of Breastfeeding in the I. R. Iran. *International Journal of Preventive Medicine, 3*(8), 520–21.
3. Edmond, K., Zandoh, C., Quigley, M., Amenga-Etego, S., Owusu-Agyei, S., & Kirkwood, B. (2006). Delayed Breastfeeding Initiation Increases Risk of Neonatal Mortality. *Pediatrics, 117*(3), 380–86. Retrieved from https://doi.org/10.1542/peds.2005-1496.
4. World Health Organization. (2021). *Indicators for Assessing Infant and Young Child Feeding Practices: Definitions and Measurement Methods.* World Health Organisation. Retrieved from https://www.who.int/publications/i/item/9789240018389.
5. World Health Organization. (2021). *Global Breastfeeding Scorecard 2021: Protecting Breastfeeding Through Bold National Actions During the COVID-19 Pandemic and Beyond.* World Health Organisation. Retrieved from https://www.who.int/publications/i/item/WHO-HEP-NFS-21.45.
6. Zong, X., Wu, H., Zhao, M., Magnussen, C., & Xi, B. (2021). Global Prevalence of WHO Infant Feeding Practices in 57 LMICs in 2010–2018 and Time Trends Since 2000 for 44 LMICs. *Lancet, 37*, 1–9. Retrieved from https://doi.org/10.1016/j.eclinm.2021.100971.
7. Ministry of Health and Family Welfare. (2022). *National Family Health Survey-5 India Factsheet.* Ministry of Health and Family Welfare. Retrieved from https://main.mohfw.gov.in/sites/default/files/NFHS-5_Phase-II_0.pdf.
8. Ministry of Health and Family Welfare. (2017). *National Family Health Survey-4 India Factsheet.* Ministry of Health and Family Welfare. Retrieved from https://www.iipsindia.ac.in/content/nfhs-project.

9. Braveman, P., & Gruskin, S. (2003). Defining Equity in Health. *Journal of Epidemiology and Community Health, 57*(4), 254–58. Retrieved from https://doi.org/10.1136/jech.57.4.254.
10. Banerjee A. (2020). Equity and Quality of Health-Care Access: Where Do We Stand and the Way Forward? *Indian Journal of Community Medicine, 45*(1), 4–7. Retrieved from https://doi.org/10.4103/ijcm.IJCM_183_19.
11. Galiatsatosa, P., et al. (2020). Health Equity and Distributive Justice Considerations in Critical Care Resource Allocation. *The Lancet Respiratory Medicine, 8*(8), 758–760.
12. Hasan, M., *et al.* (2020). Meeting the Global Target in Reproductive, Maternal, Newborn, and Child Health Care Services in Low- and Middle-Income Countries. *Global Health Science and Practice, 8*(4), 654–65. Retrieved from https://doi.org/10.9745/GHSP-D-20-00097.
13. Tata Institute of Social Sciences. (2015). *Social Economic Conditions and Vulnerabilities: A Report of the Baseline Survey of M(East) Ward, Mumbai.* Tata Institute of Social Sciences. Retrieved from https://urk.tiss.edu/wp-content/uploads/2020/08/M-Ward-Report.pdf.
14. Agarwal, P., Singh, M., & Garg, S. (2007). Maternal Health-Care Utilization Among Women in an Urban Slum in Delhi. *Indian Journal of Community Medicine, 32*(3), 203–205.
15. Kabir, R. (2013). Utilization of Antenatal Care Among Pregnant Women of Urban Slums of Dhaka City, Bangladesh. *IOSR Journal of Nursing and Health Science, 2*(2), 15–19.
16. Chawla, P. (2020). Global Nutrition Report 2020-An Action on Equity to End Malnutrition. *Jus Corpus Law Journal, 1*(2), 86–92.
17. Rollins, N., et al. (2016). Why Invest, and What It Will Take to Improve Breastfeeding Practices? *Lancet, 387*(10017), 491–504. Retrieved from https://doi.org/10.1016/S0140-6736(15)01044-2
18. Robinson, K., Fial, A., & Hanson, L. (2019). Racism, Bias, and Discrimination as Modifiable Barriers to Breastfeeding for African American Women: A Scoping Review of the Literature. *Journal of Midwifery & Womens Health, 64*(6), 734–742. Retrieved from https://doi.org/10.1111/jmwh.13058.
19. Dave, V., Shah, V., Sonaliya, K., & Solanki, A. (2014). Assessment of Breastfeeding Practices: Findings from Urban Slum Area at Ahmedabad City, India. *GCSMC Journal of Medical Sciences, 3*(2), 9–15.
20. Kazmi, S., Akparibo, R., Ahmed, D., & Faizi, N. (2021). Prevalence and Predictors of Exclusive Breastfeeding in Urban Slums, Bihar. *Journal of Family Medicine and Primary Care, 10*(3), 1301–1307. Retrieved from https://doi.org/10.4103/jfmpc.jfmpc_2000_20.
21. Gala, Z., Shetye, S., Sadawarte, D., & Autade, M. (2023). Barriers in Exclusive Breastfeeding Encountered by Mothers in Urban Slum Area of a Metropolitan City. *Journal of Family Medicine and Primary Care, 12*(11), 2690–2695. Retrieved from https://doi.org/10.4103/jfmpc.jfmpc_990_23.
22. Choudhry, U. (1997). Traditional Practices of Women from India: Pregnancy, Childbirth, and Newborn Care. *Journal of Obstetric, Gynecologic, & Neonatal Nursing, 26*(5), 533–539. Retrieved from https://doi.org/10.1111/j.1552-6909.1997.tb02156.x.
23. Pandey, A., Raushan, M., Gautam, D., & Neogi, S. (2023). Alarming Trends of Cesarean Section-Time to Rethink: Evidence From a Large-Scale Cross-sectional Sample Survey in India. *Journal of Medical Internet Research, 25*, 1–16. Retrieved from https://doi.org/10.2196/41892.
24. Zamora, G., Lutter, C., & Pena-Rosas, J. (2015). Using an Equity Lens in the Implementation of Interventions to Protect, Promote, and Support Optimal Breastfeeding Practices. *Journal of Human Lactation, 31*(1), 21–25. Retrieved from https://doi.org/10.1177/0890334414561477.
25. Balyakina, E., Fulda, K., Franks, S., Cardarelli, K., & Hinkle, K. (2016). Association Between Healthcare Provider Type and Intent to Breastfeed Among Expectant Mothers. *Maternal and Child Health Journal, 20*(5), 993–1000. Retrieved from https://doi.org/10.1007/s10995-015-1884-x.
26. Namasivayam, V., *et al.* (2021). Association of Prenatal Counselling and Immediate Postnatal Support with Early Initiation of Breastfeeding in Uttar Pradesh, India. *International Breastfeeding Journal, 16*(26), 1–11. Retrieved from https://doi.org/10.1186/s13006-021-00372-6.

27. Edgman-Levitan, S., & Schoenbaum, S. (2021). Patient-centered Care: Achieving Higher Quality by Designing Care Through the Patient's Eyes. *Israel Journal of Health Policy Research, 10*(21), 1–5. Retrieved from https://doi.org/10.1186/s13584-021-00459-9.
28. Rosenkranz, K., et al. (2021). Diversity, Equity and Inclusion in Medicine: Why It Matters and How do We Achieve It? *Journal of Surgical Education, 78*(4), 1058–1065. Retrieved from https://doi.org/10.1016/j.jsurg.2020.11.013.
29. Williams, J., Walker, R., & Egede, L. (2016). Achieving Equity in an Evolving Healthcare System: Opportunities and Challenges. *The American Journal of the Medical Sciences, 351*(1), 33–43. Retrieved from https://doi.org/10.1016/j.amjms.2015.10.012.
30. Pantoja, T. et al. (2017). Implementation Strategies for Health Systems in Low-income Countries: An Overview of Systematic Reviews. *Cochrane Database of Systematic Review, 9*(9), 1–19. Retrieved from https://doi.org/10.1002/14651858.
31. Vilar-Compte, M., Pérez-Escamilla, R., & Ruano, A. (2022). Interventions and Policy Approaches to Promote Equity in Breastfeeding. *International Journal for Equity in Health, 21*(63), 1–7. Retrieved from https://doi.org/10.1186/s12939-022-01670-z.
32. Ministry of Home Affairs. (2011). *Census of India, 2011*. Ministry of Home Affairs. Retrieved from https://censusindia.gov.in/census.website/.
33. Khatun, H., Comins, C., Shah, R., Munirul Islam, M., Choudhury, N., & Ahmed, T. (2018). Uncovering the Barriers to Exclusive Breastfeeding for Mothers Living in Dhaka's Slums: A Mixed Method Study. *International Breastfeeding Journal, 13*(44), 1–11. Retrieved from https://doi.org/10.1186/s13006-018-0186-5.
34. Roy, S., Dasgupta, A., & Pal, B. (2009). Feeding Practices of Children in an Urban Slum of Kolkata. *Indian Journal of Community Medicine, 34*(4), 362–363. Retrieved from https://doi.org/10.4103/0970-0218.58402.
35. Velusamy, V., Premkumar, P., & Kang, G. (2017). Exclusive Breastfeeding Practices Among Mothers in Urban Slum Settlements: Pooled Analysis from Three Prospective Birth Cohort Studies in South India. *International Breastfeeding Journal, 12*(35), 1–7. Retrieved from https://doi.org/10.1186/s13006-017-0127-8.
36. Barennes, H., et al. (2012). Breast-Milk Substitutes: A New Old-Threat for Breastfeeding Policy in Developing Countries: A Case Study in a Traditionally High Breastfeeding Country. *PLoS ONE, 7*(2), 1–9. https://doi.org/10.1371/journal.pone.0030634
37. Senanayake, P., O'Connor, E., & Ogbo, F. (2019). National and Rural-urban Prevalence and Determinants of Early Initiation of Breastfeeding in India. *BMC Public Health, 19*(896), 1–13. Retrieved from https://doi.org/10.1186/s12889-019-7246-7.
38. Bandyopadhyay, M. (2009). Impact of Ritual Pollution on Lactation and Breastfeeding Practices in Rural West Bengal, India. *International Breastfeeding Journal, 4*(2), 1–8. Retrieved from https://doi.org/10.1186/1746-4358-4-2.
39. Raval, D., Jankar, D., & Singh, M. (2011). A Study of Breast Feeding Practices Among Infants Living in Slums of Bhavnagar City, Gujarat, India. *Healthline, 2*(2), 73–83.
40. Ramani, S., Shaikh, N., Das, S., Pantvaidya, S., Fernandez, A., & Jayaraman A. (2019). "Everybody Breastfeeds if They Have Milk": Factors That Shape Exclusive Breastfeeding Practices in Informal Settlements of Mumbai, India. *International Breastfeeding Journal, 14*(10), 1–10. Retrieved from https://doi.org/10.1186/s13006-019-0204-2
41. Parry, K., Taylor, E., Hall-Dardess, P., Walker, M., & Labbok, M. (2013). Understanding Women's Interpretations of Infant Formula Advertising. *Birth, 40*(2), 115–124. Retrieved from https://doi.org/10.1111/birt.12044.
42. Hobbs, A., Mannion, C., McDonald, S., Brockway, M., & Tough, S. (2016). The Impact of Caesarean Section on Breastfeeding Initiation, Duration and Difficulties in the First Four Months Postpartum. *BMC Pregnancy Childbirth, 16*(90), 1–9. Retrieved from https://doi.org/10.1186/s12884-016-0876-1.
43. Kitsantas, P., & Palla, H. (2017). Mode of Delivery and Breastfeeding Practices. *International Journal of Pregnancy and Child Birth, 2*(6), 167–172. Retrieved from https://doi.org/10.15406/ipcb.2017.02.00042.

44. Khanal, V., Scott, J., Lee, A., Karkee, R., & Binns, C. (2015). Factors Associated with Early Initiation of Breastfeeding in Western Nepal. *International Journal of Environmental Research and Public Health, 12*(8), 9562–9574. Retrieved from https://doi.org/10.3390/ijerph120809562.
45. Tilahun, G., Degu, G., Azale, T., & Tigabu, A. (2016). Prevalence and Associated Factors of Timely Initiation of Breastfeeding Among Mothers at Debre Berhan Town, Ethiopia: A Cross-Sectional Study. *International Breastfeeding Journal, 11*(27), 1–9. Retrieved from https://doi.org/10.1186/s13006-016-0086-5.
46. Yeboah, J., Forkuor, D., & Agyemang-Duah, W. (2019). Exclusive Breastfeeding Practices and Associated Factors Among Lactating Mothers of Infants Aged 6–24 Months in the Kumasi Metropolis, Ghana. *BMC Research Notes, 12*(689), 1–6. Retrieved from https://doi.org/10.1186/s13104-019-4723-0.
47. Ali, N. et al. (2020). Are Childbirth Location and Mode of Delivery Associated with Favorable Early Breastfeeding Practices in Hard to Reach Areas of Bangladesh? *PLoS One, 15*(11), 1–16. Retrieved from https://doi.org/10.1371/journal.pone.0242135
48. Boatin, A., Ngonzi, J., Ganyaglo, G., Mbaye, M., Wylie, B., & Diouf. K. (2021). Cesarean Delivery in Low- and Middle-income Countries: A Review of Quality of Care Metrics and Targets for Improvement. *Seminars in Fetal and Neonatal Medicine, 26*(1), 1–8. Retrieved from https://doi.org/10.1016/j.siny.2021.101199.
49. Nantume, S., Baluku, E., Kwesiga, D., & Waiswa, P. (2023). Factors Associated with High Rates of Caesarean Deliveries: A Cross-Sectional Study Classifying Deliveries According to Robson in Mengo Hospital Kampala. *Risk Management and Healthcare Policy, 16*, 2339–56. Retrieved from https://doi.org/10.2147/RMHP.S422705.
50. Panda, S., Begley, C., & Daly, D. (2018). Clinicians' Views of Factors Influencing Decision-Making for Caesarean Section: A Systematic Review and Meta Synthesis of Qualitative, Quantitative and Mixed Methods Studies. *PLoS ONE, 13*(7), 1–27. Retrieved from https://doi.org/10.1371/journal.pone.0200941.
51. Peel, A., Bhartia, A., Spicer, N., & Gautham, M. (2018). "If I Do 10–15 Normal Deliveries in a Month I Hardly Ever Sleep at Home." A Qualitative Study of Health Providers' Reasons for High Rates of Caesarean Deliveries in Private Sector Maternity Care in Delhi, India. *BMC Pregnancy Childbirth, 18*(470), 1–11. Retrieved from https://doi.org/10.1186/s12884-018-2095-4.
52. Wells, J., Wibaek, R., & Poullas, M. (2018). The Dual Burden of Malnutrition Increases the Risk of Cesarean Delivery: Evidence From India. *Frontiers in Public Health, 6*:292. https://doi.org/10.3389/fpubh.2018.00292.
53. Awi, D., & Alikor, E. (2006). Barriers to Timely Initiation of Breastfeeding Among Mothers of Healthy Full-term Babies Who Deliver at the University of Port Harcourt Teaching Hospital. *Nigerian Journal of Clinical Practice, 9*(1), 57–64.
54. Smith, L. J. (2007). Impact of Birthing Practices on the Breastfeeding Dyad. *Journal of Midwifery and Women's Health, 52*(6), 621–630. Retrieved from https://doi.org/10.1016/j.jmwh.2007.07.019.
55. Widstrom, A. et al. (1990). Short-term Effects of Early Suckling and Touch of the Nipple on Maternal Behaviour. *Early Human Development, 21*(3), 153–163. Retrieved from https://doi.org/10.1016/0378-3782(90)90114-x.
56. Sharma, M., Anand, A., Goswami, I. & Pradhan, M. (2023). Factors Associated with Delayed Initiation and Non-exclusive Breastfeeding among Children in India: Evidence from National Family Health Survey 2019–21. *International Breastfeeding Journal, 18*(28), 1–13. Retrieved from https://doi.org/10.1186/s13006-023-00566-0.
57. Raihana, S., Alam, A., Huda, T., & Dibley, M. (2021). Factors Associated with Delayed Initiation of Breastfeeding in Health Facilities: Secondary Analysis of Bangladesh Demographic and Health Survey 2014. *International Breastfeeding Journal, 16*(14), 1–13. Retrieved from https://doi.org/10.1186/s13006-021-00360-w
58. Ahluwalia, I., Li, R., & Morrow, B. (2012). Breastfeeding Practices: Does Method of Delivery Matter? *Maternal and Child Health Journal, 16*(2), 231–237. Retrieved from https://doi.org/10.1007/s10995-012-1093-9.

59. Lind, J., Perrine, C., & Li, R. (2014). Relationship Between Use of Labor Pain Medications and Delayed Onset of Lactation. *Journal of Human Lactation, 30*(2), 167–173. Retrieved from https://doi.org/10.1177/0890334413520189.
60. Gamberini, C., Angeli, F. & Ambrosino, E. (2022). Exploring Solutions to Improve Antenatal Care in Resource-limited Settings: An Expert Consultation. *BMC Pregnancy Childbirth, 22*(449), 1–11. Retrieved from https://doi.org/10.1186/s12884-022-04778-w.
61. Nkoka, O., Ntenda, P., Kanje, V., Milanzi, E., & Arora, A. (2019). Determinants of Timely Initiation of Breast Milk and Exclusive Breastfeeding in Malawi: A Population-Based Cross-sectional Study. *International Breastfeeding Journal, 14*(37), 1–9. Retrieved from https://doi.org/10.1186/s13006-019-0232-y.
62. World Health Organization. (2020). *Promoting Baby-friendly Hospitals.* World Health Organisation. Retrieved from https://www.who.int/activities/promoting-baby-friendly-hospitals.
63. Ministry of Health and Family Welfare. (2020). *Baby Friendly Hospital Initiative (BFHI).* Ministry of Health and Family Welfare. Retrieved from https://www.bfhi-india.in.
64. Hirani, S., & Ahmadi, R. (2022). Barriers and Strategies for Successful Implementation of Baby-Friendly Hospital Initiative: A Scoping Review. *Clinical Lactation, 13*(3), 139–155. Retrieved from https://doi.org/10.1891/CL-2022-0003.
65. Kalita, P., Dey, P., & Begum, S. (2023). A Quality Improvement Study on Breast Feeding Within First Hour of Caesarean Delivery in a Tertiary Care Centre. *The New Indian Journal of OBGYN, 10*(1), 142–148. Retrieved from https://doi.org/10.21276/obgyn.2023.10.1.25.
66. Maria, A., Shukla, A., Wadhwa, R., Kaur, B., Sarkar, B., & Kaur, M. (2018). Achieving Early Mother-Baby Skin-to-Skin Contact in Caesarean Section: A Quality Improvement Initiative. *Indian Paediatrics, 55*(9), 765–767.
67. Narain, J. (2016). Public Health Challenges in India: Seizing the Opportunities. *Indian Journal of Community Medicine, 41*(2), 85–88. Retrieved from https://doi.org/10.4103/0970-0218.177507.
68. Patyal, N., et al. (2021). A Quality Improvement Initiative: Improving First-Hour Breastfeeding Initiation Rate Among Healthy Newborns. *Paediatric Quality and Safety, 6*(4), 1–6. Retrieved from https://doi.org/10.1097/pq9.0000000000000433.
69. Sinha, B., et al. (2015). Interventions to Improve Breastfeeding Outcomes: A Systematic Review and Meta-analysis. *Acta Paediatrica, 104*(467), 114–134. Retrieved from https://doi.org/10.1111/apa.13127.
70. World Health Organisation. (2023). *WHO Joins Hands to Sustain Breastfeeding Promotion Efforts in Sri Lanka.* World Health Organisation. Retrieved from https://www.who.int/srilanka/news/detail/02-08-2023-who-joins-hands-to-sustain-breastfeeding-promotion-efforts-in-sri-lanka.

Part V
Stregthening Health System

Chapter 14
Strengthening Health Systems for Child Health: Policy Challenges and Future Priorities

Sanjay Zodpey and Habib Hasan Farooqui

Introduction

Investments in the health sector in terms of financial allocation and supportive policy ecosystem led to significant improvement in population-level health indicators and outcomes over the last few decades, particularly maternal and child health outcomes. For example, the maternal mortality ratio (MMR) has significantly decreased from 398/100,000 live births (95% CI 378–417) in 1997–98 to 99/100,000 (90–108) in 2020 [1]. Similarly, between 1990 and 2021, the country witnessed significant reductions in neonatal mortality rate (NMR), infant mortality rate (IMR), and under-5 mortality rate (U5MR) [2]. However, wide inter-state and intra-state disparities persist across socioeconomic strata at the population level. It may be argued that to improve population-level health outcomes, not only are investments in health needed, but also in social determinants of health, such as safe drinking water and sanitation, nutritional interventions, health awareness, and education, are essential. As an example, a study analysing data from 15 South Asian Association for Regional Cooperation (SAARC) and Association for South East Asian Nations (ASEAN) countries demonstrated that improved sanitation facilities were associated with increased life expectancy and reduced infant mortality rate [3]. Recent evidence suggests that investments in the health sector, such as strengthening health services delivery and improved access and coverage of essential health services such as emergency obstetric care, immunisation, and other maternal and child healthcare services, are critical to ensuring improvements in maternal and child outcomes and in achieving population health impact [2]. It may be noted that continuous monitoring of health outcomes and health indicators is essential to assess the performance and effectiveness of health interventions as well as the responsiveness of the health systems.

S. Zodpey (✉) · H. H. Farooqui
Public Health Foundation of India, New Delhi, India
e-mail: sanjay.zodpey@phfi.org

S. Suri (ed.), *Child Health and Nutrition from Conception to Age Two*,
https://doi.org/10.1007/978-981-95-7868-9_14

What Is a Health System?

A health system consists of all the organisations, institutions, resources, and people whose primary purpose is to improve health [4]. The health system is designed to deliver promotive, preventive, curative, and rehabilitative care to the population. This population-level care is delivered through a network of healthcare facilities. To provide health care services at health centres, the health system requires several inputs such as financial resources, human resources (e.g., doctors, nurses, pharmacists, laboratory technicians, paramedical staff, and other health workers), health infrastructure, information systems, health commodities (e.g., medicines, laboratory material, surgical supplies, etc.), health technology (e.g., machines and equipment), and a governance structure and regulatory framework. Hence, the health system can also be thought of as a system that converts inputs (such as financial resources, human resources, and health commodities) into health outputs such as population health services, maternal and child health services, immunisation services, surgeries, and consultations, which ultimately impact population health outcomes (Fig. 14.1).

Building Blocks of the Health System

The WHO framework defines the health system using the concept of 'building blocks' (Fig. 14.2). The six building blocks that are critical to the proper functioning and performance of the health system are health financing, health workforce, health information systems, access to essential medicines, service delivery, and leadership/governance [5]. It is worth noting that building blocks related to leadership/governance and health information systems are overarching, cross-cutting, and facilitate seamless information sharing, decision-making, transparency, and accountability in the system. They are essential for regulating other building blocks, such as medical products and technology that are essential for healthcare services delivery, using inputs such as financial and human resources. The governance and regulatory framework are critical to managing interactions and interdependencies among building blocks to ensure that the health system achieves its objectives and goals. These goals include (a) optimal health for all, i.e., reducing premature mortality and

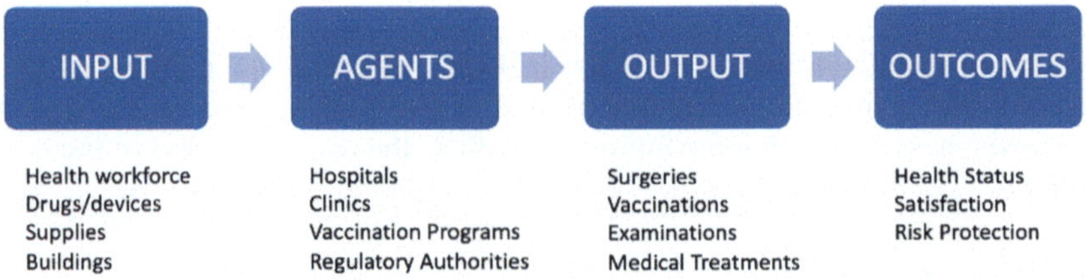

Fig. 14.1 Health system as converter

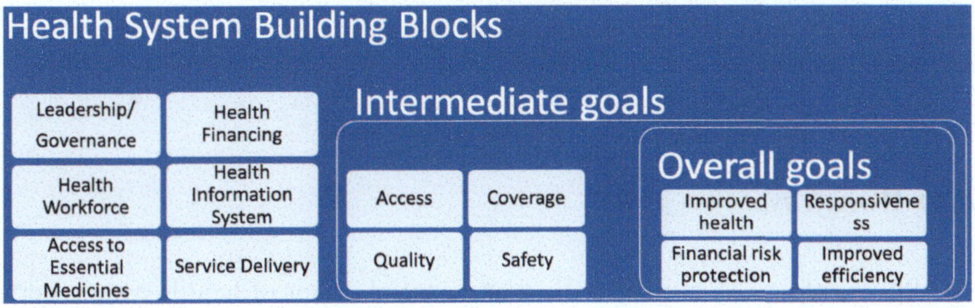

Fig. 14.2 WHO's health system framework

improving non-fatal health outcomes, (b) fairness in financing, i.e., ensuring financial risk protection; and (c) equity and responsiveness in meeting legitimate non-health needs, such as ensuring dignity and confidentiality. It has been empirically demonstrated that investments in the health system pay rich dividends in terms of a healthy population and economic growth. Robust health systems with universal coverage not only ensure improved population health and financial risk protection but also contribute to economic growth through improved labour productivity.

Health Financing

The performance of the building blocks largely drives the health system's performance and, hence, population-level outcomes. Financing is one of the most critical factors driving the performance and outcomes of a health system. In a tax-based financing approach, national health systems are funded through general revenue tax, health services provision is through public providers, and health coverage is comprehensive, whereas in a compulsory social health insurance-based system, health systems are funded through earmarked health insurance premiums that are levied on employers and employees, health services provision is through both public and private providers, and basic 'basket' of services are covered. However, in a free market system, health services provision is predominantly through private providers, and healthcare is treated as a commodity, and the ability to pay determines the level of coverage. As a result, health services are purchased through out-of-pocket (OOP) payments at the point of care or through pre-payment for private health insurance. Hence, the choice of the health financing mechanism at the country level determines not only the performance of the health system but also the burden of the OOP payments on the households and thus equity in the utilisation of health services and their benefits. An analysis of panel data from the South Asian Association for Regional Cooperation (SAARC) and Association for Southeast Asian Nations (ASEAN) countries for 20 years (1995–2014) demonstrated that total health expenditure had a significant effect in reducing the infant mortality rate. Furthermore, the study also demonstrated that both private and public health expenditures are essential for improving the population's health. However, the extent of the effect of private health expenditure was found to be higher than that of public health expenditure [3].

Health Workforce

The health workforce is another critical and central driver of health system performance. Their knowledge, skills, and motivation play a crucial role in delivering health services to those in need. The quality, quantity, and skill mix of the health workforce determine the quality of health services, patient-level clinical outcomes, and population-level health outcomes. The Global Burden of Disease (GBD) 2019 Human Resources for Health Collaborators estimated minimum workforce density thresholds required to meet a specified target of 80 out of 100 on the Universal Health Coverage (UHC) effective coverage index, and shortages with respect to those thresholds. The study estimated that to reach 80 out of 100 on the UHC effective coverage index, at least 20×7 physicians, 70×6 nurses and midwives, 8×2 dentistry personnel, and 9×4 pharmaceutical personnel would be needed per 10,000 population [6]. Furthermore, the study also highlighted that national health workforces fell short of minimum thresholds in all categories of health workforce. Another study has also reported that the density of skilled human resources directly impacts the health system's performance and population-level health outcomes [7]. Hence, managing human resources for health through training, recruitment, and retention is an important governance issue within the health system.

Access to Essential Medicines

Essential medicines are a subset of the total range of pharmaceuticals that satisfy the priority healthcare needs of the population. They are selected with due regard to public health relevance, evidence on efficacy and safety, and cost-effectiveness. Hence, it is important to ensure that essential medicines are readily available at all times in the health system to satisfy patient needs. Furthermore, their availability in appropriate dosage forms for the intended uses and patients, quality, and affordability for individuals and the health system are critical to ensure seamless health services delivery. Research has demonstrated that access to essential medicines has substantial impacts not only on population health outcomes and related economic indicators but also causes economic burden and impoverishment of households because the cost of medicines is a major contributor to the treatment cost [8, 9]. Hence, ensuring access to quality-assured, safe, and effective medicines and other health commodities such as vaccines and medical devices is critical to the proper functioning of a health system.

Health Information System

The health information systems comprise infrastructure that facilitates the monitoring of health policies, health service delivery, and population health outcomes. Health information systems, hence, encompass the people, institutions, interinstitutional relationships, legislation, values, technologies, and standards that contribute to data sharing and processing for decision-making [10]. Health information systems play a key role in information exchange across all building blocks of the health system, which not only ensures transparency and accountability in the system but also keeps the system responsive to population health needs and population-level outcomes.

Governance/ Leadership

WHO defines health systems governance as the processes, structures, and institutions that are in place to oversee and manage a country's healthcare system [11]. An effective health system governance mechanism ensures that healthcare systems are responsive to the needs of all members of society, regardless of their socioeconomic status, ethnicity, gender, or other factors. Investments in health system governance are required to ensure that the proper functioning of the health system and health service delivery are of high-quality, accessible, affordable, efficient, and equitable.

Indian Healthcare System

India currently has a mixed healthcare delivery system. Historically, based on the Sir Joseph Bhore committee's policy recommendations in the 1940s, a government-funded, three-tiered public health system was established to deliver preventive and curative healthcare services. However, by the 1980s, the private sector's role in health began to gain prominence. In mixed healthcare systems, such as India, health services are delivered not only through public healthcare facilities but also at private healthcare facilities and non-governmental healthcare facilities. In general, across the country, health services are free at the point of care in the public health system. However, this may not be universally applicable, and at some public sector facilities, individuals may be required to make payment for some services or may be required to purchase those services from the private sector, such as medicines and laboratory and radiology services. The health services delivered through the public and private sectors may be both supplementary and complementary. From the population access perspective, such an arrangement allows for a choice of providers and access to services at competitive prices; though from the economic perspective, there may be equity and efficiency concerns.

Latest estimates suggest that the public health sector covers around 30% of all outpatients and 42% of inpatient services and is a major provider of preventive and promotive health services and medical education. Whereas around 70% of all outpatient visits, about 58% of all inpatient episodes, and approximately 90% of medicines dispensed and diagnostic facilities are provided by either for-profit or not-for-profit providers in the private sector [12]. In the private sector, individuals are required to make OOP payments to access care and services. Furthermore, the magnitude of service delivery in the private sector indicates that the proportions of the health workforce employed in the private sector are commensurate. For example, around 65% of doctors, 89% of dentists, 93% of AYUSH professionals, and around 67% of other health workers are employed in the private sector. India's private healthcare sector is quite heterogeneous. It has over one million private healthcare enterprises, of which 75% are micro-enterprises and the rest are medium to large medical establishments [13]. However, only 66% of the medical facilities are registered under any act or society. It is important to note that the cost, quality, and effectiveness of health services vary across healthcare providers.

Current Challenges

Though the Performance of the Indian Health system Has Improved Significantly over the Past Few Decades, Several Areas of Improvement Remain. Some of them Are Discussed below for each Building Block

Health Financing

One of the fundamental goals of the health system is to ensure financial risk protection. Out-of-pocket payments at the point of care to access health services can lead to catastrophic expenditure and impoverishment of poor households, undermining the goal of the health system. One of the core challenges that the Indian health system is grappling with is its inability to ensure financial risk protection because of OOP payments at the point of care, especially in the private sector. Several health surveys have indicated that the population's preference for access to care between the public and private sectors varies by type of care, such as maternal and childcare, outpatient care, and hospitalisation. Recent research from India has indicated that around 24.6% of households spent more than 20% of household consumption expenditure (HCE) on hospitalisation. A total of 20.4% of households faced catastrophic health expenditure (CHE) for hospitalisation based on the average per capita consumption expenditure. The study also reported that households that sought treatment in private health facilities had a higher burden of CHE and impoverishment. The disease conditions that more commonly led to economic burden were cancers, cardiovascular diseases, psychiatric conditions, injuries, and others [14].

Universal Health Coverage and Health Insurance are two major policy instruments that are used by governments to ensure that households do not have to incur OOP expenditures at the point of care to access treatment and care. Evidence suggests that the implementation of universal health care not only ensures financial risk protection but also improves population health outcomes. Theoretically, the public health system is best placed to provide universal health coverage; however, it is conditional on the magnitude of public health expenditure as a percentage of the gross domestic product. Poor financial allocation to the health sector results in poor health system performance because of the shortage of human resources, frequent stock-outs of essential medicines, and low utilisation rates. A cross-country panel analysis reported that transitions from OOP-dominant systems to government-financed systems improved most health outcomes. The study reported that transitions to government financing not only reduced catastrophic health expenditure incidence (−3.3%, $p < 0.05$) but also increased life expectancy (+1.3 years, $p < 0.05$) and reduced under-5 mortality (−8.7%, $p < 0.05$) [15]. This study indicated that one of the best mechanisms to improve child health outcomes is to strengthen the public health system by increasing financial allocation to the health sector.

In the absence of Universal Health Coverage, another policy instrument that is used to prevent catastrophic health expenditure and ensure financial risk protection is health insurance, especially in the event of hospitalisation. Health insurance provides both choice for access to care as well as financial risk protection to households. Social health insurance schemes such as the Central Government Health Scheme and Employee State Insurance Scheme are conditional on employment status and are available to certain employment sections, whereas private insurance coverage can be purchased by individuals and households to cover healthcare expenses by making pre-payment. Several State governments also provide public health insurance to a section of vulnerable and socioeconomically disadvantaged populations. Recently, the national government has introduced Ayushman Bharat (Pradhan Mantri Jan Arogya Yojana–PMJAY): a public health insurance scheme that is limited to poor and vulnerable populations with predefined eligibility criteria and a ceiling of INR 500,000 per household per year to improve access to hospital care and provide financial risk protection to vulnerable households. Theoretically, access to insurance and its usage for healthcare payment should ideally reduce OOP expenditure for households. However, an impact evaluation of the Rashtriya Swasthya Bima Yojana (RSBY) health insurance scheme reported no impact of the RSBY scheme on the level of outpatient OOP expenditure and the probability of incurring outpatient OOP expenditure; in contrast, the likelihood of incurring any OOPE increased by 30% due to RSBY [16]. Similarly, a systematic review of health insurance schemes in India reported no impact of health insurance on the reduction of OOP expenditures [17]. This could be due to the insurance provider's limited coverage of diagnosis-related conditions, high healthcare costs, limited financial coverage, and significant unmet needs at the household level, which become apparent only during hospitalisation. More recently, the national government has increased investments not only for infrastructure development to strengthen primary healthcare but also to strengthen financial risk protection mechanisms under the PMJAY scheme. The potential impact of these measures on improvement in maternal and child health outcomes is yet to be investigated.

Health Workforce

Another major challenge the Indian health system is trying to address is the shortage of the healthcare workforce. Health workforce shortages, both absolute and relative, adversely affect health services delivery and consequently population-level health outcomes. Furthermore, at the country level, the density of human resources for health is associated with heterogeneities in terms of population-level outcomes. Anand et al. reported that maternal and child health outcomes such as maternal mortality, infant mortality, and under-5 mortality are associated with doctor density (with elasticities ranging from −0.474 to −0.212, $p < 0.003$), whereas nurse density was associated with maternal mortality rates [7]. Another study reported that countries with a higher density of skilled health workers have a lower maternal mortality ratio, a lower under-5 mortality rate, a lower infant mortality rate, and a lower neonatal mortality rate compared with countries that had a lower density of skilled health workers [18].

Latest estimates suggest that the health workers' stock-to-population ratio in India is around 24.4 skilled health workers per 10,000 population. However, the health workforce density drops to only 11 skilled health workers per 10,000 population if the active health workforce is considered [19]. Furthermore, there are heterogeneities in the distribution of the health workforce across public and private sectors, rural and urban areas, and across Indian states. Estimates suggest that rural India and states in eastern India have a health workforce density lower than the WHO minimum threshold (22.8 per 10,000 population). The private sector remains a major employer of doctors and nurses in the country, with more than 80% of doctors and 70% of nurses and midwives employed, whereas around 20% of adequately qualified doctors were not in the current workforce. The study also reported that around 25% of the currently working health professionals lack the required qualifications as laid down by professional councils [20]. Some of the reasons for the shortage identified in the scoping review were inadequate health workforce production, job dissatisfaction, brain drain, regulatory issues, and lack of training, monitoring, and evaluation [21]. Hence, it is important to increase investment in human resources for health to improve the availability of the health workforce, [22] particularly the female health workforce, as such investments are critical not only in improving maternal and child health outcomes but also play a key role in enhancing female labour force participation.

Access to Essential Medicine

In India, access to essential medicines remains a critical building block as it influences both child health outcomes as well as financial risk protection. World Health Survey reported that poorer households in low and middle-income countries (LMICs) spent up to 9.5% of their total expenditure on medicines compared to 3.5% from their high-income countries (HICs) counterparts [9]. Recent studies from India have also indicated that medicines are the most significant component of households' OOP expenditure on healthcare. In terms of share of total consumption expenditure of the households, the total OOP payments and medicines OOP payments were estimated to be 6.77% (95%CI: 6.70–6.84%) and 4.49% (95%CI: 4.45–4.54%), respectively, in the year 2011–12 [8]. Furthermore, given the budget constraints and limited ability to pay at the household level, it was estimated that medicines OOP payments pushed around 38 million persons into poverty in the year 2011–12. Some of the common health conditions with high OOP payments were cancers, injuries, cardiovascular diseases, genitourinary conditions, and mental disorders.

High prices of medicines are another challenge concerning access to essential medicines, which makes them unaffordable to poor households and public and private payers, irrespective of the country's income level [23, 24]. For example, access to oncology medicines is particularly concerning because of the lack of universal health coverage, frequent drug shortages, inconsistent drug pricing, variations in cost between the private and public sectors, limited quality monitoring of generic medicines after regulatory approval, and delays in approval of new medicines [25]. Recent research in India has indicated that the mean availability of childhood anti-cancer medicines was 43% in public hospitals and 71% in private hospitals. Furthermore, the estimated treatment cost for leukaemia was INR 27,850, which translates to 88 days' wages for the lowest-paid government employee [26]. It may be noted that access to essential medicines and vaccines for the prevention and treatment of childhood illnesses has the highest potential to impact and improve child health outcomes at the country level.

Furthermore, ensuring the quality and safety of essential medicines is critical to maintaining public confidence in the health system. Given the fact that India is the pharmacy of the world and is a major exporter of generic medicines, quality assurance of medicines is critical. One of the major policy challenges is ensuring a balance between manufacturing high-quality assured generics and medicine prices at the country level. Another challenge pertains to establishing a balance between pharmaceutical policy goals and health policy goals. To ensure equitable access to medicines for universal health coverage, WHO recommends that national medicines policies and other legislation and policies on trade, innovation, commerce, and intellectual property work are aligned with national health policies and should support access to medicines. In addition to sustainable financing for the procurement of essential medicines, vaccines and medical products, strengthening national capacities to improve access to essential medicines is needed [27].

Health Information System

One of the important cross-cutting building blocks which play a key role in evidence-informed decision-making is the health information system. In India, though there is a deep penetration of technology, access to sophisticated hardware and software, and broadband networks across the country, the use of health information systems varies across the public and private sectors. For example, an electronic health records-based system is not as widely implemented in the public health system in comparison to the private sector super-speciality corporate hospitals. However, the use of information technology for population-level health and disease monitoring is at a much wider scale in the public sector. For example, digital technologies play a key role in the procurement and supply chain management of health commodities such as medicine and vaccines, surveillance of infectious diseases, monitoring of non-communicable diseases, and implementation and management of national health programmes. These systems have played a major role in the success of the universal immunisation programme, which has had a major impact on the prevention and control of common childhood diseases and has resulted in significant improvement in child health outcomes over the last few decades.

Another area for improvement in the health system is the implementation of tele-health and leveraging digital technologies to improve patient-level and population health outcomes. Health systems are increasingly focusing on the use of digital health and telehealth to improve population-level health, particularly in rural and remote locations. It may be argued that a wider range of smart devices and interconnected equipment, with due consideration to privacy and confidentiality, should be utilised to enhance individual-level clinical decision-making as well as policy-level decisions on health policies and programmes for population health. The potential of telemedicine, electronic health records, artificial intelligence, big data, blockchain, and other such technologies can be harnessed to achieve health system goals. Recent research on the application and challenges of telehealth during the COVID-19 pandemic in India indicated that, though there was effective utilisation of telehealth, insufficient technological infrastructure and other barriers to virtual consultations constrained the full implementation of telehealth in India. [28] The study also noted that telehealth is a cost-effective solution to bridge the rural-urban healthcare divide.

Recent research has highlighted that effective implementation and use of health information systems and digital technologies are conditional on broadly four interdependent factors [29]; (a) technical factors such as cost, system performance, integration and interoperability, stability and reliability, accessibility and adaptability of hardware; (b) organisational factors such as readiness for change, leadership and management, expectations, user ownership, teamwork and communication, learning and evaluation; (c) social factors which include attitudes and concerns, resistance and workarounds, user expectations, user input in design, training and support, integration with existing work practices; and (d) wider socio-political factors such as healthcare organisations, policy dimensions, professional groups, the wider economic environment, and international developments. However, there has been a limited application and implementation of telehealth solutions for maternal and child health programmes and related areas that have a direct impact on child health outcomes, though the use of technology in digital education, training, and capacity building is documented.

Health System Governance

Another important cross-cutting health system building block that determines the performance of a health system is governance and leadership. Health systems governance plays a crucial role in promoting equity and social justice in healthcare. In India, not only are there inter-state heterogeneities in terms of health system performance and consequent population-level health outcomes, but also intra-state variabilities. The differences in the health system governance approach and leadership can explain most of these heterogeneities. Furthermore, it may be argued that individual-level and population-level health outcomes are driven by access to quality health services. Recent research has indicated that to improve the quality of health care at the health system level, a focus on governance issues such as improving public sector management, building institutional capacity, and promoting a culture of data-driven policies is required [30]. It is important to note that these measures should not only include efficient and equitable allocation of healthcare resources, regulations guiding healthcare delivery, and mechanisms for monitoring and evaluating the healthcare system's performance, but also investments in developing leadership capacity at all levels through system-wide reform. For example, leadership practices influence staff motivation and teamwork, which have implications for health system performance. Hence, understanding the interdependencies among various stakeholders (such as patients and their families, healthcare providers, public, private, and non-governmental sectors) and their effective management through strategic health policies, sustainable financing, appropriate regulations, attention to system design, oversight, and accountability is critical. It is important to note that the realisation of universal health coverage requires not only massive investments in the health system but also a conducive policy environment and governance framework. Recent research has indicated that countries with resilient pandemic responses had capable and effective leaders who engaged with scientists and made evidence-informed decisions [31].

Case Studies on the Impact of Health System Strengthening Initiatives on Maternal and Child Health Services

In order to ensure financial risk protection for households and improve access and responsiveness of the health services, several initiatives have been implemented over the past few decades. The National Rural Health Mission was one of the flagship health system initiatives directed to improve access and responsiveness of the health system. Janani Suraksha Yojana was another initiative to improve institutional deliveries. More recently, Ayushman Bharat was implemented to achieve the vision of Universal Health Coverage (UHC). It adopts a continuum of care approach, by creating Health and Wellness Centres and Pradhan Mantri Jan Arogya Yojana (PMJAY), which is a publicly financed health insurance scheme for the poor and vulnerable populations to provide financial risk protection against out-of-pocket expenditures. The impact of the National Health Mission and Mission Indradhanush on maternal and child health outcomes is discussed below.

National Health Mission

In the past decades, several health system-strengthening initiatives were implemented with reasonable success in the country. One of the flagship initiatives was the National Health Mission, which encompassed the National Rural Health Mission (NRHM) for rural areas and the National Urban Health Mission (NUHM) for urban areas. The NHM aimed to develop an integrated network of all primary, secondary, and a substantial part of tertiary care, providing a continuum from the community level to the district hospital, with robust referral linkages to tertiary care. Furthermore, the primary focus was on strengthening the healthcare system at the primary level, including outreach services in rural areas and urban slums. The mission has resulted in significant improvement in maternal and child health outcomes. Using a logical evaluation framework of time series data of input, output, and impact indicators for NRHM, Kumar et al. reported that NRHM resulted in an increase in the fund allocation by nearly five times, and the number of auxiliary nurse midwives and nurses has doubled and tripled, respectively. As a result of increased fund allocation and health workforce, institutional deliveries increased by 40.2%, during 2005–15 and full immunisation coverage increased by 19%. Furthermore, infant mortality rate declined from 58 to 33 per 1000 live births, and the maternal mortality ratio declined from 254 to 122 per 100,000 live births during the implementation years [32].

Another major impact of the NRHM has been on reduction in inequity at the population level. A recent benefit incidence analysis suggests that the difference in utilisation rates between the poorest 20% and the richest 20% of households had significantly declined during the NRHM period in comparison to the pre-NRHM period. Similarly, the Concentration Index (CI) (which measures the magnitude and direction of inequity) for subsidies on prenatal services and post-natal services declined significantly, implying that the subsidy on prenatal and post-natal services was overwhelmingly received by the poor [33]. This could be explained by the improvement in infrastructure and service provisioning through the NRHM route in the public facilities, which predominantly benefited the poor. However, inequality continues to persist across all healthcare services in the private health sector. Another study reported that NRHM resulted in increased uptake of maternal healthcare and a decline in socioeconomic inequity. Particularly, greater effects were observed among the lowest and middle wealth tertiles compared to the highest tertile. Furthermore, larger equity impacts were observed in the late post-NRHM period, 2011–12, than in the early post-NRHM period, 2007–08 [34]. It may be noted that the reduction in inequity in utilisation of health services in the public sector predominantly improves maternal and child health outcomes.

Mission Indradhanush

Mission Indradhanush (MI) was another important initiative that was initiated to address socioeconomic inequalities in access to immunisation and to improve immunisation coverage to 90% in districts with poor coverage rates. Based on the concept of periodic intensification of routine immunisation (PIRI) approach, Intensified Mission Indradhanush (IMI) was implemented in India across 24 states between October 2017 and January 2018. Under-immunised children were identified by conducting door-to-door surveys, and appropriate locations for immunisation sites with particular emphasis on urban slums and nomadic populations were identified through district-level micro-plans. Recent research has indicated the success of Mission Indradhanush and IMI programmes in increasing overall immunisation coverage at the district level and coverage rates for specific vaccines. For example, IMI implementation resulted in an 18.5% increase in full immunisation coverage from pre-IMI levels [35]. Another quasi-experimental evaluation reported that IMI resulted in increased delivery of traditional UIP vaccines with a median effect of 10.6% (95% CI 5.1–16.5%) during the implementation period [36]. More recent evidence on the cost-effectiveness of IMI suggests that IMI was cost-effective when using a threshold of 1 × per capita GDP per disability-adjusted life year (DALY) averted. The study reported that periodic intensification of routine immunisation could be a cost-effective way to improve vaccination coverage and reach zero-dose children, as the estimated cost per incremental dose delivered was only $6.21, and the estimated cost per zero-dose child reached was $82.99 [37]. Though Mission Indradhanush adopted a targeted service delivery approach contrary to the health system strengthening approach of NRHM, it has benefited immensely from the system strengthening that was achieved under NRHM. It is important to note that both systems strengthening as well as targeted approaches are complementary and critical to achieving intended population health objectives. Both approaches have led to significant improvements in child health outcomes over the last few decades, particularly significant reductions in infant and under-five mortality rates.

Future Directions

A high-quality, robust health system is critical to ensure equitable and efficient health service delivery as it impacts both individual-level clinical outcomes as well as population-level health outcomes. A health system framework-based approach helps in the identification of bottlenecks and ensures appropriate and timely intervention to address those bottlenecks. Strengthening the health system through strengthening individual components has the potential to make the Indian health system more resilient and responsive to emerging healthcare needs and service delivery challenges.

One of the core areas of strengthening the health system and health services is developing pathways of care. The integration of primary, secondary, and tertiary care through a referral system across the public and private sector health facilities and at the same time ensuring financial risk protection through a universal access card or health insurance-based approach, is critical to improve maternal and child health outcomes. Ensuring the continuity of care is particularly important to improve maternal and child health outcomes. The continuum of care from the prenatal to post-natal period and early childhood period for both mother and child plays a critical role in improving survival rates as well as educational outcomes and consequently labour and economic outcomes.

Similarly, the referral system and integration of primary to tertiary and emergency care play a key role in managing mothers with high-risk pregnancies and individuals with chronic conditions such as diabetes and hypertension. The integration of care pathways to ensure the continuum of care can also be accomplished using innovative technological approaches such as telemedicine. The role and impact of telemedicine are now well-established. Telemedicine as a technological solution to several health system constraints can be rapidly adopted and scaled up to create alternative pathways of care for individuals residing in remote locations for disease conditions which require constant contact with healthcare providers, to situations where specialist care with more advanced diagnostic and therapeutic workups. Formal integration of telemedicine into the health system through policy directions and standardised protocols should be implemented to ensure holistic patient care and efficient utilisation of resources, particularly advanced medical care service provision.

Furthermore, enhancing the health workforce both quantitatively and qualitatively is essential to ensure high-quality service delivery and trust in the public system. The latest estimates published by the WHO suggest that to meet the density threshold of 34.5 skilled health workers per 10,000 population, around 0.16 million doctors and 0.65 nurses/midwives are further needed in the total health workforce by the year 2030. The estimated investment required to achieve the 34.5 health workers per 10,000 population threshold requirements ranges from INR 2127 to 2724 billion, considering 50% of health professionals are not working (or out of labour) [19]. In addition to increasing the quantity and quality of the health workforce through new recruitment, retention of a skilled and appropriately trained health workforce is critical to ensure the care delivered is of high-quality and has the potential to significantly improve maternal and child health outcomes.

There is also a need to consider redesigning the care pathways. For example, a team-based approach can be developed to provide holistic care to pregnant women with high-risk pregnancies, such as those with gestational diabetes or pregnancy-induced hypertension, without too much reliance on medical specialists and pharmacotherapy by using an appropriately skilled team comprising nutritionists, health educators, and other health professionals. Another pathway to achieve the intended objective of equitable access to health services and population-level health outcomes is by ensuring universal access to health commodities such as essential medicines, diagnostics, and vaccines, through increased financial allocations to the national health budget. Previously, a high-level expert group on universal health coverage has estimated that allocation of around half a per cent of gross domestic product (GDP) could provide universal access to essential medicines to the entire country. An increased budgetary allocation to the tune of 2.5% of GDP has been recommended to further strengthen the public health system to improve health service delivery [38]. Recent research on the comparison of differences in structural features, types of health care spending, and performance between the United States and 10 high-income countries suggests that utilisation rates in the United States were largely like those in other nations, though the United States spent approximately twice as much as other high-income countries on medical care. The major drivers of the difference in overall cost were prices of labour and goods, including pharmaceuticals, and administrative costs [39, 40]. It is important for India and other LMI countries to not only increase public health spending on health but also to ensure that health spending is efficient and equitable. Health technology assessment should be used for priority setting and decision-making for efficient utilisation of existing resources and new investments across levels of care, particularly for maternal and child health conditions.

Finally, it is important to ensure high levels of transparency and accountability in the health system, as it reflects the health system's governance. The defining characteristic between good and poorly performing health systems is the quality of governance. There is a need to ensure transparency in financial decision-making, particularly in the procurement of medical commodities and the recruitment of the health workforce. One of the important mechanisms to ensure a high level of accountability is through regular reviews and audits and the implementation of quality assurance systems. Ensuring public access to audit reports, quality assurance reports, and other key policy documents improves transparency in the system and ensures a high level of public trust.

Recommendations

To safeguard children's health, a well-funded public health system must prioritise recruiting and training skilled professionals, adopting cutting-edge health technologies, and ensuring access to critical medicines, vaccines, and diagnostics. A well-regulated private healthcare sector should work in tandem, supported by policies that align with national goals to enhance child health outcomes. The provision of promotive, preventive, curative, and rehabilitative services through the health system drives child health outcomes. Hence, it is critical to ensure equity in the distribution and utilisation of health services across population groups, with particular focus on poor and vulnerable populations.

Understanding how health system components interact and affect service delivery is crucial for optimising performance. One of the key areas of research and policy intervention is the development of systems thinking and health system design. Innovative policies, such as system diagnosis and priority-setting exercises, health technology assessment, strategic purchasing, innovative benefit packages for health insurance, and provider payment mechanisms, can ensure efficient use of resources. At its core, a future-ready health system must focus on improving access, quality, and responsiveness to deliver better health outcomes for every child.

References

1. Meh C, Sharma A, Ram U, Fadel S, Correa N, Snelgrove JW, et al. Trends in maternal mortality in India over two decades in nationally representative surveys. BJOG. 2022; 129(4):550–561. Epub 20210915. doi:https://doi.org/10.1111/1471-0528.16888. PubMed PMID: 34455679; PubMed Central PMCID: PMCPMC9292773.
2. Wahl, B., Nama, N., Pandey, R. R., Garg, T., Mishra, A. M., Srivastava, S., et al. (2023). Neonatal, infant, and child mortality in India: Progress and future directions. *Indian Journal of Pediatrics, 90*(Suppl 1), 1–9. Epub 20230911. https://doi.org/10.1007/s12098-023-04834-z
3. Rahman MM, Khanam R, Rahman M. Health care expenditure and health outcome nexus: New evidence from the SAARC-ASEAN region. Globalization and Health 2018;14(1):113. Epub 20181122. doi:https://doi.org/10.1186/s12992-018-0430-1. PubMed PMID: 30466452; PubMed Central PMCID: PMCPMC6249744.
4. WHO Monitoring the building blocks of health systems: a handbook of indicators and their measurement strategies. World Health Organization., 2010.
5. WHO. (2007). *Everybody's business — Strengthening health systems to improve health outcomes. WHO'S framework for action.* World Health Organization.
6. Collaborators GBDHRfH. Measuring the availability of human resources for health and its relationship to universal health coverage for 204 countries and territories from 1990 to 2019: A systematic analysis for the global burden of disease study 2019. Lancet. 2022; 399(10341):2129–2154. Epub 20220523. doi:10.1016/S0140-6736(22)00532-3. PubMed PMID: 35617980; PubMed Central PMCID: PMCPMC9168805.
7. Anand, S., & Barnighausen, T. (2004). Human resources and health outcomes: Cross-country econometric study. *Lancet, 364*(9445), 1603–1609. https://doi.org/10.1016/S0140-6736(04)17313-3
8. Selvaraj S, Farooqui HH, Karan A. Quantifying the financial burden of households' out-of-pocket payments on medicines in India: A repeated cross-sectional analysis of National Sample Survey data, 1994-2014. BMJ Open 2018; 8(5):e018020. Epub 20180531. doi:https://doi.org/10.1136/bmjopen-2017-018020. PubMed PMID: 29858403; PubMed Central PMCID: PMCPMC5988077.
9. Wagner AK, Graves AJ, Reiss SK, Lecates R, Zhang F, Ross-Degnan D. Access to care and medicines, burden of health care expenditures, and risk protection: Results from the world health survey. Health Policy. 2011; 100(2–3):151–158. Epub 20100909. doi:10.1016/j.healthpol.2010.08.004.

10. WHO. (2024). *Support tool to strengthen health information systems: Guidance for health information system assessment and strategy development*. World Health Organization. Regional Office for Europe.
11. WHO. Health system governance 2024. Available from: https://www.who.int/health-topics/health-systems-governance#tab=tab_1.
12. Selvaraj, S. K. S., Srivastava, S., Bhan, N., & Mukhopadhyay, I. (2022). *India health system review*. World Health Organization, Regional Office for South-East Asia.
13. Mackintosh M, Channon A, Karan A, Selvaraj S, Cavagnero E, Zhao H. What is the private sector? Understanding private provision in the health systems of low-income and middle-income countries. Lancet. 2016; 388(10044):596–605. Epub 20160626. doi:https://doi.org/10.1016/S0140-6736(16)00342-1.
14. Yadav J, Menon GR, John D. Disease-specific out-of-pocket payments, catastrophic health expenditure and impoverishment effects in India: An analysis of National Health Survey Data. Applied Health Economics and Health Policy. 2021;19(5):769–782. Epub 20210222. doi:https://doi.org/10.1007/s40258-021-00641-9.
15. Gabani J, Mazumdar S, Suhrcke M. The effect of health financing systems on health system outcomes: A cross-country panel analysis. Health Economics. 2023;32(3):574–619. Epub 20221208. doi:https://doi.org/10.1002/hec.4635. PubMed PMID: 36480236; PubMed Central PMCID: PMCPMC10107855.
16. Karan A, Yip W, Mahal A. Extending health insurance to the poor in India: An impact evaluation of Rashtriya Swasthya Bima Yojana on out of pocket spending for healthcare. Social Science & Medicine. 2017;181:83–92. Epub 20170327. doi:https://doi.org/10.1016/j.socscimed.2017.03.053. PubMed PMID: 28376358; PubMed Central PMCID: PMCPMC5408909.
17. Prinja S, Chauhan AS, Karan A, Kaur G, Kumar R. Impact of publicly financed health insurance schemes on healthcare utilization and financial risk protection in India: A systematic review. PLoS One 2017;12(2):e0170996. Epub 20170202. doi:https://doi.org/10.1371/journal.pone.0170996. PubMed PMID: 28151946; PubMed Central PMCID: PMCPMC5289511.
18. Liu J, Eggleston K. The association between health workforce and health outcomes: A cross-country econometric study. Social Indicators Research. 2022; 163(2):609–632. Epub 20220314. doi:https://doi.org/10.1007/s11205-022-02910-z. PubMed PMID: 35310535; PubMed Central PMCID: PMCPMC8919693.
19. WHO. (2022). Health workforce in India: Where to invest, how much and why? *World Health Organization.*
20. Karan A, Negandhi H, Nair R, Sharma A, Tiwari R, Zodpey S. Size, composition and distribution of human resource for health in India: New estimates using National Sample Survey and registry data. BMJ Open 2019;9(4):e025979. Epub 20190527. doi:https://doi.org/10.1136/bmjopen-2018-025979. PubMed PMID: 31133622; PubMed Central PMCID: PMCPMC6549895.
21. Mehta V, Ajmera P, Kalra S, Miraj M, Gallani R, Shaik RA, et al. Human resource shortage in India's health sector: A scoping review of the current landscape. BMC Public Health 2024;24(1):1368. Epub 20240521. doi:https://doi.org/10.1186/s12889-024-18850-x. PubMed PMID: 38773422; PubMed Central PMCID: PMCPMC11110446.
22. WHO. (2020). Decade for health workforce strengthening in SEAR 2015–2024, mid-term review of progress. *World Health Organization.*
23. Attaei MW, Khatib R, McKee M, Lear S, Dagenais G, Igumbor EU, et al. Availability and affordability of blood pressure-lowering medicines and the effect on blood pressure control in high-income, middle-income, and low-income countries: An analysis of the PURE study data. The Lancet Public Health. 2017;2(9):e411-e4e9. Epub 20170905. doi:https://doi.org/10.1016/S2468-2667(17)30141-X. PubMed PMID: 29253412.
24. Khatib R, McKee M, Shannon H, Chow C, Rangarajan S, Teo K, et al. Availability and affordability of cardiovascular disease medicines and their effect on use in high-income, middle-income, and low-income countries: An analysis of the PURE study data. Lancet. 2016;387(10013):61–69. Epub 20151020. doi:https://doi.org/10.1016/S0140-6736(15)00469-9.

25. Barrios C, de Lima Lopes G, Yusof MM, Rubagumya F, Rutkowski P, Sengar M. Barriers in access to oncology drugs-a global crisis. Nature Reviews. Clinical Oncology. 2023;20(1):7–15. Epub 20221115. doi:https://doi.org/10.1038/s41571-022-00700-7. PubMed PMID: 36380066; PubMed Central PMCID: PMCPMC9665041.
26. Faruqui N, Martiniuk A, Sharma A, Sharma C, Rathore B, Arora RS, et al. Evaluating access to essential medicines for treating childhood cancers: A medicines availability, price and affordability study in New Delhi, India. BMJ Global Health 2019;4(2):e001379. Epub 20190423. doi:https://doi.org/10.1136/bmjgh-2018-001379. PubMed PMID: 31139456; PubMed Central PMCID: PMCPMC6509613.
27. WHO. (2017). *Equitable access to medicines for universal health coverage by 2030*. World Health Organization. Regional Office for South-East Asia.
28. Rajkumar E, Gopi A, Joshi A, Thomas AE, Arunima NM, Ramya GS, et al. Applications, benefits and challenges of telehealth in India during COVID-19 pandemic and beyond: A systematic review. BMC Health Services Research 2023;23(1):7. Epub 20230104. doi:https://doi.org/10.1186/s12913-022-08970-8. PubMed PMID: 36597088; PubMed Central PMCID: PMCPMC9810518.
29. Cresswell KM, Bates DW, Sheikh A. Ten key considerations for the successful implementation and adoption of large-scale health information technology. Journal of the American Medical Informatics Association. 2013;20(e1):e9-e13. Epub 20130418. doi:https://doi.org/10.1136/amiajnl-2013-001684. PubMed PMID: 23599226; PubMed Central PMCID: PMCPMC3715363.
30. Mohanan M, Hay K, Mor N. Quality of health care in India: Challenges, priorities, And The Road Ahead. Health Aff (Millwood). 2016;35(10):1753–1758. doi:https://doi.org/10.1377/hlthaff.2016.0676. PubMed PMID: 27702945.
31. Phillips G, Kendino M, Brolan CE, Mitchell R, Herron LM, Kõrver S, et al. Lessons from the frontline: Leadership and governance experiences in the COVID-19 pandemic response across the Pacific region. Lancet Reg Health West Pac. 2022;25:100518. Epub 20220707. doi:https://doi.org/10.1016/j.lanwpc.2022.100518. PubMed PMID: 35818573; PubMed Central PMCID: PMCPMC9259208.
32. Kumar, R. (2021). Impact of National Health Mission of India on infant and maternal mortality: A logical framework analysis. *Journal of Health Management., 23*(1), 155–165. https://doi.org/10.1177/0972063421994988
33. Selvaraj S, Karan AK, Mao W, Hasan H, Bharali I, Kumar P, et al. Did the poor gain from India's health policy interventions? Evidence from benefit-incidence analysis, 2004-2018. International Journal for Equity in Health 2021;20(1):159. Epub 20210710. doi:https://doi.org/10.1186/s12939-021-01489-0. PubMed PMID: 34246269; PubMed Central PMCID: PMCPMC8272306.
34. Vellakkal S, Gupta A, Khan Z, Stuckler D, Reeves A, Ebrahim S, et al. Has India's national rural health mission reduced inequities in maternal health services? A pre-post repeated cross-sectional study. Health Policy and Planning. 2017;32(1):79–90. Epub 20160810. doi:https://doi.org/10.1093/heapol/czw100. PubMed PMID: 27515405; PubMed Central PMCID: PMCPMC5886191.
35. Gurnani V, Haldar P, Aggarwal MK, Das MK, Chauhan A, Murray J, et al. Improving vaccination coverage in India: Lessons from intensified Mission Indradhanush, a cross-sectoral systems strengthening strategy. BMJ. 2018;363:k4782. Epub 20181207. doi:https://doi.org/10.1136/bmj.k4782. PubMed PMID: 30530467; PubMed Central PMCID: PMCPMC6282735.
36. Clarke-Deelder, E., Suharlim, C., Chatterjee, S., Brenzel, L., Ray, A., Cohen, J. L., et al. (2021). Impact of campaign-style delivery of routine vaccines: A quasi-experimental evaluation using routine health services data in India. *Health Policy and Planning, 36*(4), 454–463. https://doi.org/10.1093/heapol/czab026
37. Clarke-Deelder, E., Suharlim, C., Chatterjee, S., Portnoy, A., Brenzel, L., Ray, A., et al. (2024). Health impact and cost-effectiveness of expanding routine immunization coverage in India through intensified Mission Indradhanush. *Health Policy and Planning, 39*(6), 583–592. https://doi.org/10.1093/heapol/czae024

38. Thakur J. Key recommendations of high-level expert group report on universal health coverage for India. Indian J Community Med. 2011;36(Suppl 1):S84–S85. PubMed PMID: 22628920; PubMed Central PMCID: PMCPMC3354908.
39. Bauchner, H., & Fontanarosa, P. B. (2018). Health care spending in the United States compared with 10 other high-income countries: What Uwe Reinhardt might have said. *Journal of the American Medical Association, 319*(10), 990–992. https://doi.org/10.1001/jama.2018.1879
40. Papanicolas, I., Woskie, L. R., & Jha, A. K. (2018). Health care spending in the United States and other high-income countries. *Journal of the American Medical Association, 319*(10), 1024–1039. https://doi.org/10.1001/jama.2018.1150

Index

S. Suri (ed.), *Child Health and Nutrition from Conception to Age Two*,
https://doi.org/10.1007/978-981-95-7868-9

The manufacturer's authorised representative in the EU is Springer Nature Customer Service Centre GmbH, Europaplatz 3, 69115 Heidelberg, Germany. If you have any concerns regarding our products, please contact ProductSafety@springernature.com

Printed and bound by CPI Group (UK) Ltd, Croydon, CR0 4YY
07/10/2026
02229349-0012